To Peter, Happy Reading,

Laz Bannock, PhD., is a member of the Institute of Biology (UK) as a Chartered Biologist, [illegible] of the Royal Society of Health, and a Member of the Royal Institute of Public Health and Hygiene. Academic qualifications include a BSc(Hons) in Human Physiology, an MPhil in Human Nutrition and PhD in Nutritional Physiology. He has lectured all over the world on Human Nutrition and is a senior lecturer in Nutrition for the European Academy of Biomedical Sciences as well as a tutor and lecturer in Nutrition and Health for the Royal Society of Health. Dr Bannock is the Creator and Editor of HumanNutrition.com – a critically acclaimed web-site for nutrition information with subscribers from all over the world. He frequently appears in the UK and international media and was the creator and 'expert' presenter on the recent UK Ch4 Daily Television Show 'Why Weight'. Personal Clients include many well-known celebrities from the Music, Film and Sporting Industries.

First printing 2001. Revised 2002.

Published by HumanNutrition.com

ISBN 0-9542017-0-1

GENERAL DISCLAIMER

The nutritional suggestions and research reported in this book are not offered to treat, mitigate or cure disease, and should not be used as a substitute for sound medical advice. This book is designed to be used in conjunction with the services provided by a trained, licensed healthcare practitioner.

CAUTION

Caution should be used in all conditions, especially concerning pregnancy and children, when taking herbal supplements or high potency nutrients. A physician knowledgeable in natural and preventative medicine should be consulted.

INFORMATION ON THE INTERNET

For more information on nutrition and health or purchasing information for this book, please refer to the following internet web addresses:

http://www.humannutrition.com

CONTENTS

PART I: THE PHYSIOLOGY AND SUBCLINICAL/PATHOLOGICAL CONDITIONS OF THE BODY SYSTEMS

PART II: NUTRIENT APPLICATIONS AND RESEARCH

PART III: INTERACTIONS

PART IV: BIBLIOGRAPHY AND INDEX

THE PHYSIOLOGY OF THE DIGESTIVE SYSTEM

Food - We need it to survive. However, to be able to use food for nourishment and energy, it must be broken down by an intricate process of **digestion**, preparing it for ultimate **absorption** into the bloodstream and utilization by tissues. The presence of food signals the brain to release hormones and enzymes to act on the food. This ultimate **absorption** provides for the delivery of **essential nutrients,** including: **water,** the **macronutrients (protein, carbohydrate and fat),** and the **micronutrients (vitamins and minerals).** The process begins with **starch/protein digestion (mouth- stomach)**. Moving on to the **small intestine**, the process continues with the digestion of fats and absorption of nutrients.

The small intestine is a key player in providing the energy we derive from food, as it is here that the **macronutrients (protein, carbohydrate and fat)** are broken completely down to their single elements, preparing them for ultimate **absorption** into the bloodstream and **utilization** by tissues. Essential **water** and **micronutrients (vitamins and minerals)** are also absorbed in the small intestine.

Finally, the large intestine, or **colon**, is the site for the **reabsorption** of most of our **water** and many **minerals. Beneficial bacteria** are produced and **flourish in the colon**, contributing to the **immune defense system.** The digestive system is an intricately organized system that changes the composition of food, and gets the nutrients to their final destination - the cells of the body that depend on them for their life-sustaining force.

DIGESTION PHYSIOLOGY

MOUTH to ESOPHAGUS

In the mouth, **starch digestion** is initiated by **amylase**. **Amylase** is an enzyme in saliva which breaks down starch into smaller chains of starch, known as **dextrins**. The action of swallowing moves food down the **esophagus** and closes the **epiglottis.** (This prevents food from entering the **trachea**, or windpipe).

The Lower Esophageal Sphincter (LES) is a band of muscle tissue located at the end of the esophagus. It contracts after food enters the stomach, preventing an efflux of acid contents from the stomach. Malfunctioning of the **LES** causes backup of acid into the esophagus, a condition commonly referred to as, "**heartburn**".

STOMACH

Once food reaches the stomach, it moves through by means of **peristaltic waves. Protein digestion** occurs in the stomach due to **hydrochloric acid production (HCL)**, and pepsin activation. **HCL**, secreted from the parietal cells in the stomach; provides the necessary pH for **protein digestion** (parietal cells also secrete **intrinsic factor**, which attaches to **B-12,** and is necessary for absorption of **B-12** into the small intestine). **HCL** secretion is an integral factor in proper protein digestion. Lack of optimal **HCL** secretion, which is a common problem, is known to create gastric disturbances. In addition to uncoiling protein, **HCL** cleaves **pepsinogen** (secreted by the chief cells in the stomach) to make the active hormone **pepsin. Pepsin** breaks the protein into smaller chains of amino acids known as **peptides**. **Intestinal mucosa glands** secrete **water, mucous and bicarbonate**, which protect the stomach lining from acidity. The stomach produces about 1-2 liters of this **gastric juice** (containing HCL, pepsin, mucous, bicarbonate and other gastric hormones) per day.

SMALL INTESTINE (Duodenum, jejunum, ileum)

Macronutrient digestion: **Pancreatic enzymes** travel through a duct to the small intestine to **break down fat** (pancreatic lipase) and to continue both **carbohydrate** breakdown (pancreatic amylase) and **protein** breakdown (proteases). Once the protein, carbohydrate and fat have been broken down into smaller molecules by pancreatic enzymes, **further breakdown** is accomplished by the **enzymes** present on the **surface of these microvilli.**

The Enzymes: **Peptidases** are enzymes on the surface of the **microvilli** which further break down peptides (formed by the action of **pepsin** on protein in the stomach) to **single amino acids**; **saccharidases** are enzymes which break starch dextrins to **single sugar molecules.** (The fat has been reduced in size by the pancreatic lipase).

The Absorption: **Villi** are folds in the intestinal lining that increase surface area for digestion and absorption. Approximately 20 ft. of small intestine provides an area about ¼ of a football field. **Microvilli** are tiny fingerlike projections on the **villi.** The minute particles then readily pass through the **microvilli** into the **blood**, and **circulate to the tissues**.

***Micronutrient absorption*:** **Vitamins, minerals and water** are mostly absorbed in the small intestine. Easily digested nutrients are absorbed at the top of the tract, so, for instance, the top portion of the **duodenum** is specialized for absorption of calcium and several B vitamins (ie thiamine and riboflavin), while vitamin B-12 is absorbed at the end of the **ileum.** Vitamin D aids in calcium absorption.

LIVER

The routing of the blood makes sure that all the nutrients absorbed into circulation from the digestive tract go to the liver first. The liver is a multi-faceted organ that screens, stores, manufactures, and detoxifies, among other things Vessels collect nutrients and water from all over the digestive tract, and then merge into the portal vein, which carries absorbed materials to the liver. In essence, the liver gets first crack at absorbed nutrients. Some long-chain fatty acids pass into the lymphatic system , bypassing the liver and entering main circulation by the heart.

Bile is manufactured in the liver and stored in **gall bladder.** It travels from the gall bladder through the **bile duct** into the small intestine when fat is present. **Bile** suspends fat in water and reduces it to an ultrafine emulsion, which **exposes** a greatly increased **surface** of fat molecules to the action of the **pancreatic lipase**. **Bile** also emulsifies **fat-soluble vitamins** and **aids** in their **absorption** with other fats.

PANCREAS

***Pancreatic secretions*:** The pancreas produces **hormones, enzymes, and fluids** that travel in ducts to the **duodenum** of the small intestine, aid in the digestive process, and allow for the **breakdown of carbohydrate, protein and fat** in the small intestine.

Pancreatic enzymes: **Amylase** is an enzyme continuing starch digestion. **Lipase** is an enzyme that breaks fat into monoglycerides, glycerol, and fatty acids. (Fat exists as fatty acids attached to a glycerol backbone. When one fatty acid is attached, it is a monoglyceride, two attached fatty acids make a diglyceride, and three attached fatty acids make a triglyceride, the most common form of fat). **Proteases** continue working on protein, breaking large peptides into smaller peptides and amino acids, and include **trypsin and chymotrypsin. Trypsin** attacks specific linkages next to amino acids arginine or lysine.

COLON

The **diameter of the colon** is much **larger** than the **small intestine**; three longitudinal bands make up the external muscular layer. The fact that the bands are shorter than the rest of the colon makes for "**outpouchings**" on the wall of the colon. The colonic mucosa has no villi, however it does have glands, short inward projections that secrete mucus.

When food leaves the stomach, the cecum relaxes, and the chyme passes through the ileocecal valve. This is thought to be a **vagal reflex**, and **sympathetic stimulation increases** the tonic **contraction** of the valve. Contractions and peristaltic waves move the contents through for eventual elimination.

The colon has an immense absorptive capacity, mainly for water, sodium and minerals. "Some enteric microorganisms synthesize vitamin K and a number of B complex vitamins, and the folic acid produced by bacteria can be shown to be absorbed in significant amounts" (Review of Medical Physiology, 1987, Appleton & Lange, San Mateo, Ca. p.425).

These microorganisms are the “healthy” bacteria, and they usually keep the “unhealthy” bacteria in check, partly by creating lactic acid from carbohydrate. However, an upset in the immune system, such as that caused by antibiotic administration, kills off the beneficial bacteria and ultimately allows the harmful bacteria to flourish.

Several vitamins are **synthesized** by some of these bacteria, and then **absorbed in the colon.** The colon is a necessary pathway for elimination of undigested matter, including some fat and cholesterol. In the **absence of good nutrition**, diseases such as **colon cancer and diverticulitis can arise**.

SUBCLINICAL AND PATHOLOGICAL CONDITIONS OF THE GASTRO-INTESTINAL SYSTEM

ESOPHAGEAL PROBLEMS

HEARTBURN

A burning sensation in the chest and stomach which may radiate into the neck; caused when hydrochloric acid (HCl) regurgitates back into the esophagus. The lower esophageal sphincter (LES) prevents acidic stomach contents from moving back up into the esophagus, but if the sphincter muscle isn't working correctly, it can be one of the major causes of heartburn.

Signs and Symptoms of Heartburn:

- burning sensation in the stomach
- acidic reflux into mouth
- pain in chest (may feel like heart attack)

Possible Causes:

1) Overconsumption of spicy, fried or fatty foods, coffee, alcohol, tomato-based foods, chocolate, citrus foods or carbonated beverages (soft drinks)
2) Hiatal hernia
3) Digestive enzyme deficiency
4) Food allergies
5) Gallbladder problems
6) Ulcers
7) Stress/Anxiety
8) Ileocecal valve problems
9) High or low HCl levels
10) Obesity
11) Cigarette smoking
12) Heavy metal/chemical toxicity
13) Infectious agents - Helicobacter pylori, candida/parasites, Epstein-Barr Virus (EBV)

Nutrient Applications:

1) Digestive Enzymes - taken with meals to aid digestion
2) Aloe vera - for soothing, healing properties
3) DGL (deglycyrrhizinated licorice) - to increase amount of mucus-secreting cells in the digestive tract
4) Cabbage - aids in cleansing mucous membranes of the stomach and the intestinal tract
5) Slippery Elm - soothes mucous membranes
6) Okra - rich source of vegetable fiber; beneficial effect on blood sugar, cholesterol and irritable bowel syndrome; it protects the internal membranes and relieves irritation of the linings of the digestive tract. (Editors of Prevention Magazine, The Complete Book of Natural and Medicinal Cures, Rodale Press, PA, pp. 76-78).
7) Glandular support - stimulate tissue specific organ or gland
8) HCl support if necessary - do stomach acid self-test
9) Calcium and Magnesium - potent antacids; great for symptomatic relief, but should not be used for prolonged periods of time

10) Vitamin D - essential for absorption and utilization of calcium from GI tract
11) Vitamin A - protects and regenerates the mucosa
12) Bismuth - inhibits Helicobacter Pylori

Dietary and Lifestyle Applications:

1) Eat small, frequent meals and drink liquids apart from meals to avoid distending the stomach - chew food well.
2) Avoid tight-fitting clothes, lying down, or bending over after meals, in order to decrease stomach pressure.
3) Sleep with head elevated.
4) Limit decaffeinated coffee, caffeine and red peppers, to avoid stimulation of HCl secretion.
5) Limit intake of fat, caffeine, alcohol, smoking, peppermint and spearmint oil, all of which decrease pressure on the LES and inhibits function.
6) Avoid acidic juices such as orange, tomato and grapefruit juices to decrease irritation to the esophagus.
7) Lose weight if necessary to decrease pressure in abdomen.
8) Avoid stress and/or repressed emotions.
9) Exercise moderately.
10) Drink plenty of water to soothe the irritated esophageal lining.

Considerations:

1) Do stomach acid self-test

When you are experiencing heartburn, take one tablespoon of **apple cider vinegar or lemon juice**. If your heartburn goes away, you are probably deficient in HCl. If heartburn gets worse, you have excess HCl. If the symptoms improve when taking the vinegar or lemon juice, sip pure apple cider vinegar and water with meals. (Balch, J., MD. and Balch, P., CNC, Prescription for Nutritional Healing, Avery Publishing Group, Inc. NY,NY, p. 304).

2) Antacids

Overuse of antacids can mask the underlying problem. **Calcium carbonate antacids** can produce a rebound effect by causing secretion of more acid to overcompensate for the neutralization by the antacids. The calcium carbonate antacids are strongly alkaline, and may also cause a potential **problem for kidney stone formers**. The **sodium bicarbonate antacids** are simply baking soda in effervescent form. They may **induce systemic alkalosis** (excessive pH throughout the body), which may lead to headaches, nausea, vomiting, mental confusion and kidney stone formation. Antacids containing **aluminum and sodium** should also be avoided. Absorption of aluminum is greatly enhanced in patients with **Alzheimer's disease or impaired kidney function, or if citric acid is ingested frequently** (citrus fruits, soda pop, orange juice).

Long-term use of antacids can create a problem. Antacids raise the pH of the stomach from 1.5-2.5 to above 3.5. This alkaline pH of the stomach inhibits the action of pepsin and interferes with HCl production. Regular use of antacids **can lead to malabsorption of nutrients, kidney stones, bowel problems and mineral imbalances**.

Note: Many people take antacids as a calcium supplement. In order for calcium to be absorbed, it must be solubilized and ionized by stomach acids. This is why people with low HCl (especially in older individuals) need to have their calcium needs addressed. Calcium lactate, gluconate or citrate are calcium forms that are in a soluble and ionized state and are much more readily absorbed than calcium carbonate.

HIATAL HERNIA

The hiatus is an opening in the diaphragm where the esophagus passes through to the stomach. When the tissue around the hiatus weakens, the stomach protrudes through the opening into the chest cavity. Hiatal hernias are not uncommon.

Signs and Symptoms of a Hiatal Hernia:

- belching
- heartburn
- discomfort behind the breastbone

Possible Causes:

1) Heavy lifting or bending
2) Trauma
3) Obesity
4) Tissue weakening due to vitamin/mineral deficiency
5) Ileocecal valve problems - tends to be a consistent pattern with hiatal hernias
6) Digestive problems - enzyme deficiency or biliary dysfunction

Nutrient Applications:

1) Proteolytic enzymes (avoid HCl unless it aids symptoms) - between meals to reduce inflammation
2) Manganese, calcium and magnesium - ligament nutrient support
3) Aloe vera - for soothing and healing properties
4) DGL (deglycyrrhizinated licorice) - to aid in healing
5) Slippery Elm - to soothe intestinal lining

Dietary and Lifestyle Applications:

1) Avoid heavy lifting or bending.
2) Do not lie down after eating.
3) Eat small, frequent meals.
4) Avoid allergenic foods, spicy or fried foods, caffeine, alcohol or smoking. Smoking encourages the production of stomach acid.
5) Avoid constipation or straining during bowel movements.
6) Lose weight if necessary.

STOMACH PROBLEMS

INDIGESTION (DYSPEPSIA)

It is a vague term used to describe any pain or discomfort in the upper abdomen after eating. The timing of the symptoms may offer a clue as to where the problem originates. Discomfort during eating may indicate esophagitis or gastritis. Discomfort several hours after eating may indicate an ulcer. The most common cause of indigestion is a lack of hydrochloric acid secretion.

Signs and Symptoms of Indigestion:

- discomfort in upper abdomen
- heartburn
- nausea
- bloated feeling, relieved by belching

Possible Causes:

1) Food allergies
2) Hypochlorhydria or achlorhydria
3) Swallowing excess air while eating
4) Stress

5) Lack of digestive enzymes or biliary problems

Nutrient Applications:

1) Highly active pancreatin - with meals as a digestive aid
2) Acidophilus - helpful to promote healthy intestinal flora
3) Gallbladder/liver support may be necessary
4) HCl support if necessary

Dietary and Lifestyle Applications:

1) For excess gas - lemon juice or bifidus enemas are helpful to balance pH.
2) Avoid refined foods, fatty or spicy foods, red meat, dairy products, caffeine and carbonated beverages.
3) The juice of a lemon or apple cider vinegar in water are excellent digestive aids.
4) Avoid food allergens.
5) Increase fiber-rich foods.

HYPOACIDITY (HYPOCHLORHYDRIA)

Many clinical conditions develop due to decreased gastric acid secretion

Hypochlorhydria - deficient gastric acid secretion
Achlorhydria - complete absence of gastric secretion

Signs and Symptoms of Low Gastric Acidity:

- bloating, belching or burning after eating
- excessive abdominal gas after eating
- multiple food allergies
- frequent indigestion, constipation and/or diarrhea
- vomiting of undigested food
- unsuccessful treatment for anemia
- B-12, folic acid or iron deficiency
- chronic intestinal infections - i.e. parasites, yeast, bacteria
- acne problems
- undigested food in stool
- weak, peeling or cracked fingernails

Low HCl production has been associated with:

1) **Iron-deficiency anemia** - due to poor iron absorption; also vitamin B-12 (which needs the intrinsic factor, secreted along with HCl, to be absorbed) and folic acid deficiency.
2) **Osteoporosis** - due to decreased calcium absorption.
3) **Multiple food allergies** - low HCl causes poor food absorption and assimilation, which can lead to "leaky gut syndrome". This, in turn, causes large proteins to enter the bloodstream and cause antigen/antibody reactions.
4) **Gallstones** - many people with gallstones exhibit decreased HCl secretion compared to gallstone-free patients.
5) **Diabetes Mellitus patients** - have shown decreased HCl secretion.
6) Eczema, psoriasis, dermatitis, vitiligo (skin condition characterized by lack of melanin production) - possibly due to association of low HCl with food allergies.
7) Tooth and periodontal disease
8) **Increased intestinal infection** including yeasts, parasites and bacteria.
9) **Low pancreatic enzyme secretion** since HCl is stimulus for pancreatic secretions.
10) **Asthma**.

11) **Chronic stress** could cause HCl production to decrease over time.
12) **Age** causes gastric acid secretion to decrease.
13) **Heavy metal toxicity** - the heavy metal lead binds HCl in the gut and makes HCl unavailable for digestion.

Nutrient Applications:

1) HCl - with meals for digestive support
2) Digestive enzymes - with meals for digestive support
3) B vitamins - to assist in production of HCl
4) Magnesium and Pyridoxal-5-Phosphate (form of B-6) - to stimulate production of HCl
5) Glandular support - to stimulate tissue specific organ or gland

Dietary and Lifestyle Applications:

1) The juice of half a lemon squeezed in water or a teaspoon of apple cider vinegar in warm water 15 minutes before meals has been shown to be helpful in stimulating gastric juices.
2) Ginger tea may be helpful.

Considerations:

1) **Heidelberg Gastric Analysis Test** - method for diagnosing HCl deficiency or excess.
   - An electronic capsule attached to string is swallowed and remains in stomach to measure pH of the stomach. A bicarbonate challenge is given to test the stomach's ability to secrete acid and the results are recorded by radio messages.

2) **Stomach Acid Self-Test** - see Heartburn section.

ULCERS

The term peptic ulcer usually refers to both gastric and duodenal ulcers. If the ulcer forms in the stomach it is known as a gastric ulcer. If it forms in the first portion of the small intestine it is called a duodenal ulcer. Ulcers are a result of the loss of integrity of the lining of the intestinal tract. Recent scientific evidence within the last ten years supports the theory that a bacterial infection of Helicobacter Pylori (HbP), rather than acid hypersecretion, is involved in the etiology of ulcers, and is probably the leading cause of ulcers. The bacterial infection causes an eroding of the mucosal lining. When the protective mucosal lining has disintegrated, stomach acid will cause pain. Non-steroidal, anti-inflammatory drugs (NSAIDs), such as ibuprofen, also erode the lining. When the protective mucosal lining has disintegrated, stomach acid will cause pain.

Signs and Symptoms of Ulcers:

- abdominal pain 45-60 minutes after eating or during the night
- gnawing, burning, aching pain or heartburn
- eating usually relieves symptoms

Possible Causes:

1) Food allergies.
2) Medications - excessive use of antacids (rebound effect), aspirin or other anti-inflammatory drugs, including steroids. Non-steroidal, anti-inflammatory drugs inhibit mucus producing prostaglandins.
3) Stress - can increase HCl secretion, especially in high-achieving people or intense worriers.
4) Excess alcohol, caffeine or smoking. Smoking has been associated with peptic ulcers based on three theories:
   1) decreases the pancreatic bicarbonate secretion, which neutralizes gastric acid.

2) increases reflux of bile salts into the stomach, which are highly irritating to the stomach lining.
3) increases gastric emptying.

5) Nutrient deficiency.
6) Helicobacter pylori (HbP) bacteria - found in 70-75% of gastric ulcer patients and 90-100% of duodenal ulcer patients. HbP secretes an enzyme that destroys the mucus which protects the intestinal lining. Eradication of HbP eliminates ulcer recurrence in a high percentage of people.

Nutrient Applications:

1) Digestive enzymes - to aid digestion
2) Aloe vera - known for its positive healing properties in ulcers
3) Slippery Elm - specific herb for ulcers to soothe mucus membranes
4) DGL (deglycyrrhizinated licorice) - known as a "remarkable anti-ulcer agent"
5) Cabbage - very beneficial in soothing ulcers; contains vitamin U, the anti-ulcer vitamin
6) Vitamins A, C, E and zinc - all have shown positive results in treatment of ulcers
7) Glutamine - aids in tissue healing
8) Bioflavonoids - inhibit histamine release

Dietary and Lifestyle Applications:

1) Increase fiber - aids in mucus production.
2) Avoid alcohol, smoking and stress.
3) Avoid milk (rebound effect - the calcium and protein in milk stimulate production of more acid).
4) Avoid hot, spicy foods, coffee, sugar, refined carbohydrates and chocolate.
5) Fresh cabbage juice may be very helpful in the treatment of ulcers.

Considerations:

1) **Antacids** - although they provide immediate relief of symptoms, they have side effects when used long term. Refer to Heartburn section. Antacids do not treat the underlying problem of a dysfunctional lining.
2) **Medications** - H-2 receptor antagonists - these block the action of H-2 histamine receptors, which normally stimulate secretion of HCl. These include cimetidine (Tagamet), ranitidine (Zantac), famotidine (Pepcid) and nizatidine (Axid). These drugs not only have side effects, they compound the problem by further deteriorating the lining.
   Note: 70-90% of people taking H2-receptor antagonists have a relapse within a year after discontinuing the drug.
3) **Helicobacter pylori (HbP) detection test** - measures the presence of antibodies in serum specific to HbP. Useful in identifying cause in ulcers and gastritis. HbP is the only known bacteria to live in the very acidic environment of the stomach. Low HCl has been indicated in association with HbP infection. HbP digests the mucus layer of the stomach lining, making it thin and runny. This allows HCl and pepsin to come into direct contact with the unprotected epithelial cells.

GASTRITIS

Inflammation of the mucus membrane that lines the stomach

Signs and Symptoms of Gastritis:

- upper abdominal discomfort
- nausea and possible vomiting
- diarrhea
- belching

Possible Causes:

1) Viral infection - "stomach flu".
2) Bacteria - helicobacter pylori.
3) Induced chemically by medications such as aspirin, ibuprofen, Motrin, steroids; people who take more than 2-3 aspirin daily may experience microscopic GI bleeding.
4) Heavy drinking, smoking or eating too much.
5) Food allergies.
6) Autoimmune reaction, which destroys the lining of the digestive tract. Resulting interference of vitamin B-12 absorption can lead to pernicious anemia.
7) Stress.
8) Sometimes seen in people who do not produce sufficient HCl, especially in the elderly. This condition may correlate with vitamin B-12 deficiency.

Nutrient Applications:

1) Refer to Ulcer section.
2) Immune stimulants if due to viral infection:
   Vitamin C - just below bowel tolerance
   Vitamin A, beta-carotene and zinc to help repair and regenerate the GI lining
3) Multi-vitamin/mineral support.
4) Use bismuth and acidophilus. Sometimes antibiotics may be necessary against helicobacter pylori bacteria.
5) Vitamin B-12 and HCl may be necessary for the elderly or in people with decreased HCl production.

Dietary and Lifestyle Applications:

1) Eliminate foods that cause allergies.
2) Eat a well-balanced diet. Avoid food irritants such as spicy or fatty foods, alcohol, etc.
3) No smoking.

Considerations:

1) Helicobacter pylori detection test - see Ulcer section.
2) Medications - see Ulcer section.
3) Antacids - see Heartburn section.

GALLBLADDER PROBLEMS

GALLSTONES - crystalline structures comprised mainly of cholesterol (80%) or calcium salts of bile pigment (20%). Usually no symptoms are present, but if the stone blocks the bile passageway (cystic duct), severe abdominal pain, nausea and vomiting may occur.

GALLBLADDER INFLAMMATION - causes severe pain in the upper right part of the abdomen, nausea, vomiting and fever; can lead to cholecystitis, which is life-threatening.

BILIARY COLIC - symptom of gallbladder disease, which is usually triggered by eating a fatty meal.

Signs and Symptoms of Gallbladder Problems:

- from no symptoms to severe abdominal pain, nausea and vomiting
- flatulence (gas)
- bloating
- pain after a heavy, fatty meal
- fever

- loss of appetite
- constipation

Possible Causes:

1) Cholesterol becoming saturated (insoluble) with bile in the gallbladder
2) Dietary factors - high fat, low fiber diets
3) Age - older men seem to have an increased risk of developing gallstones
4) Sex - women have a 4X higher incidence of gallstones compared to men
5) Cystic fibrosis and Crohn's disease
6) Digestive problems - especially low HCl
7) Food allergies
8) Parasites
9) Stress
10) Dental amalgams or chemical/heavy metal toxicity

Nutrient Applications:

1) Lipotropic factors - fat-metabolizing substances including choline, inositol, lecithin, betaine, vitamin B-12, folic acid and methionine
2) Lecithin - shown to increase cholesterol solubility
3) Fiber
4) Enzymes with bile acids
5) Vitamin C

Dietary and Lifestyle Applications:

1) Prevention is best.
2) Eliminate food allergies and food sensitivities, especially dairy products and eggs. Food allergies may cause the bile ducts to swell, creating bile flow problems.
3) Increase fiber, decrease meat and fat to increase cholesterol solubility. Fiber binds and decreases the formation of deoxycholic acid, which is a culprit in decreased cholesterol solubility, causing cholesterol to become saturated with bile.
4) Do not remove fat entirely from the diet. Studies have suggested that people who diet and eat less than three grams of fat per day have a tendency to develop gallstones. (Burton Goldberg Group, Alternative Medicine: The Definitive Guide, Future Medicine Publishing, Inc. WA, p. 924).
5) Eat regularly and do not overeat.
6) Carrot, beet and cucumber juice with a little garlic may be helpful.

Considerations:

1) Over ½ million people per year have gallbladder surgery to remove their gallbladders.

LIVER PROBLEMS

HEPATITIS

Inflammation of the liver associated with damage or death of liver cells.

Three types of viral hepatitis:

1. **Acute Hepatitis A** - highly infectious; transmitted by contaminated water or food and fecal contamination. Incubation period: 2-6 weeks.

2. **Acute Hepatitis B** - more serious; transmitted by contaminated blood, saliva and sexual secretions. Most common in intravenous drug users and homosexuals. Incubation period: 6 weeks - 6 months.

3. **Non-A, Non-B Hepatitis** - usually acquired through blood transfusions because it is hard to screen in the blood. Incubation period: 2 - 20 weeks.

Signs and Symptoms of Hepatitis:

- jaundice (yellowing of skin and eyes due to increased bilirubin levels in the blood) develops 1-2 weeks after infection
- fever
- nausea/vomiting
- loss of appetite
- elevated liver enzymes
- muscle aches and pains
- dark urine
- abdominal discomfort
- flu-like symptoms
- extreme fatigue
- headaches
- joint pain
- liver tenderness

Possible Causes:

1) Virus contamination from Type A, B or non-A, non-B
2) Drug abuse or reaction to prescription drugs
3) Chemical exposure
4) Excess alcohol consumption
5) Blood transfusions
6) Epstein-Barr Virus (EBV) or Cytomegalovirus (CMV)

Nutrient Applications:

1) Vitamin C (high doses to bowel tolerance) - have been shown to improve viral hepatitis (Murray, M. and Pizzorno, J., Encyclopedia of Natural Medicine, Prima Publishing, CA,. p. 352). (contraindicated in iron overload disease and or kidney stones).
2) Vitamin B-12 and folic Acid - may decrease recovery time
3) B-Complex - high amounts to support the system
4) Lipotropic factors - choline, inositol, methionine
5) Beta-Carotene
6) Methionine, L-Cysteine and Glutathione - detoxify harmful liver toxins
7) Carnitine
8) Free form amino acids - easily assimilated protein support takes digestive stress off the liver. Also, a low protein diet is recommended to decrease stress on the liver.
9) HCl - low HCl has been associated with chronic hepatitis
10) Dandelion (Taraxacum officinale) - one of the best herbs for the liver - clears liver heat and congestion
11) Milk Thistle (Silybum marianum) - protects and regenerates the liver
12) Artichoke (Cynara Scolymus) - contains silymarin - regenerates the liver
13) Licorice (Glycyrrhiza glabra) - antiviral activity and may inhibit EBV, CMV and hepatitis B virus
14) Glandular extracts (liver) - promote liver regeneration

Dietary and Lifestyle Applications:

1) No alcohol or caffeine.
2) Avoid medications, recreational drug use and strenuous exercise.
3) Eat a healthy diet, low in refined carbohydrates and fats and high in fiber, natural fruits and vegetables. High fiber diets help remove toxic substances from the body.
4) Bed rest is important in the acute stages.

5) Due to contagious aspect of the disease, close contact should be avoided during the contagious phase (approximately two weeks before symptoms appear to 1-2 weeks after jaundice appears). **NOTE:** The virus is in the feces, thus strict hygiene should be followed.
6) Drink plenty of filtered water.
7) Fresh lemon juice in water in the morning and evening is excellent for liver function. Follow this with fresh vegetable juice, especially carrot juice, beet juice and green drinks.

Considerations:

1) Indications of hepatitis include:
   a) positive antibody test for the virus.
   b) abnormal liver tests for a period of six weeks or longer.
   c) positive liver biopsy.

PANCREAS PROBLEMS

PANCREATITIS

Inflammation of the pancreas (acute or chronic), which is caused when the pancreatic duct is obstructed by stones, scarring, or cancer.

Signs and Symptoms of Pancreatitis:

Acute:

- severe pain in the abdomen that may radiate into the chest and back
- nausea/vomiting
- clammy skin or sweating
- abdominal bloating or tenderness
- fever
- pain often worse when lying down
- increased heartrate

Chronic:

- abdominal bloating
- upper abdominal pain
- flatulence (gas)
- muscle pain
- fever
- malabsorption problems (steatorrhea - fat in stools)
- nausea/vomiting
- weight loss
- onset of diabetes

Possible Causes:

1) Gallbladder inflammation or gallstones
2) Dietary habits - refined foods, fatty foods, alcohol, caffeine
3) Alcohol abuse - most common cause in adults
4) Drugs
5) Obesity
6) Infections (viral or bacterial)
7) Increased triglycerides or calcium level in the blood
8) Liver problems

9) Cystic fibrosis is most common cause in children. Cystic fibrosis is a hereditary disease that affects both the respiratory and digestive systems. Cystic fibrosis affects the mucus and sweat glands of the body.
10) Stress
11) Food allergies
12) Intestinal infections (dysbiosis)

Nutrient Applications:

1) Acidophilus
2) Glandular support (pancreas)
3) Pancreatic enzymes
4) Chromium
5) Lipotropic factors (inositol/choline)
6) B vitamins with extra pantothenic acid and niacin
7) Vitamin C (contraindicated in iron overload disease, gout and/or kidney stones)

Dietary and Lifestyle Applications:

1) Diet is very important. In acute stage, a liquid diet may be necessary and I.V.'s may be needed. A diabetic diet should be followed once appetite returns (see Diabetes section).
2) Avoid all refined foods, fatty foods, alcohol and caffeine.
3) Surgery may be necessary if pancreatic duct is blocked or gallstones are creating obstruction.
4) Address food allergies.

Considerations:

1) Chronic pancreatitis often causes digestive problems and diabetes, because the pancreas does not make enough enzymes or insulin.

SMALL AND LARGE INTESTINE PROBLEMS

MALABSORPTION PROBLEMS

Characterized by abnormal fecal excretion of fat (steatorrhea) and malabsorption of various nutrients.

Signs and Symptoms of Malabsorption Problems:

- weight loss
- gas and/or bloating
- diarrhea and/or constipation
- foul-smelling stool
- abdominal cramps
- gray or pale stool (from steatorrhea)
- flatulence
- floating stools
- amenorrhea
- dermatitis, acne, eczema
- anemia
- easily bruised
- chronic GI infections
- fatigue
- decreased immunity
- Irritable Bowel Syndrome
- nutrient deficiencies
- impotence
- food intolerances
- osteoporosis
- premature aging
- hair loss
- dry skin
- muscle weakness

Possible Causes:

1) Poor diet

2) Defective nutrient breakdown and assimilation (i.e. pancreatic insufficiency)
3) Inadequate bile salts
4) Rapid transit time
5) Infection
6) Celiac sprue (gluten intolerance)
7) Whipple's disease - unusual bacterial infection which causes diarrhea, chronic fatigue, abdominal pain, weight loss and general malabsorption
8) Crohn's disease
9) Lactose intolerance
10) Intestinal infections - parasites, yeast, bacteria
11) Food allergies or intolerances
12) Alcoholism - due to intestinal tissue damage from alcohol
13) Non-Steroidal Anti-Inflammatory Drugs (NSAIDs) - disrupt intestinal barrier function and increase permeability (key in people with arthritis)
14) Chemotherapy or other chemical ingestion
15) Excess use of laxatives or antacids
16) Diarrhea and/or constipation which may damage the intestinal mucosa
17) Chronic pancreatitis

Nutrient Applications:

1) Enzymes - to aid in digestion and counter inflammation
2) L-Glutamine - principle fuel for the upper intestinal tract
3) Acidophilus - supports intestinal flora
4) Chlorophyll - soothes the bowel
5) Bile - to aid digestion
6) HCl - as a digestive aid
7) Zinc and other antioxidants - to aid tissue healing and quench free radicals formed during detoxification
8) B-12 lozenges - if needed to prevent anemia
9) B vitamins and overall vitamin/mineral supplementation

Dietary and Lifestyle Applications:

1) Remove any offending agents (allergy foods, drugs, chemicals, etc.).
2) Eat bland, non-offending foods (millet, brown rice, mild fruits (no citrus fruits), steamed vegetables, fish
3) Avoid wheat, fried foods, excess fat (coats intestinal tract and further inhibits absorption), dairy products, processed foods and red meat.
4) Drink 6-8 glasses of filtered water daily.

Considerations:

1) Malabsorption increases with age.
2) Problems with fat malabsorption include:
    a) loss of highest energy source.
    b) essential fatty acid deficiency.
    c) vitamin deficiency of fat soluble vitamins A, D, E, K, B-12 and folic acid because of loss in stool.
3) **Malabsorption test**: Dual sugar technique (lactulose and mannitol), which measures the ability of two non-metabolized sugars to be absorbed. Mannitol (a monosaccharide) and lactulose (a disaccharide) are water-soluble and not metabolized by the body.
    Mannitol - easily absorbed - marker for transcellular uptake.
    Lactulose - slightly absorbed - marker for mucosal integrity to denote increased intestinal permeability.

The test requires that a patient drink a liquid containing lactulose and mannitol; measures amounts recovered in a six-hour urine sample.

Low levels of mannitol - indicate malabsorption
Elevated levels of lactulose - indicate increased permeability
i.e. Crohn's disease and Ulcerative Colitis - show increased lactulose and decreased mannitol
Celiac disease - shows increased ratio of lactulose to mannitol

4) Low blood levels of vitamin B-12 and folic acid strongly suggest malabsorption.
5) High amounts of calcium may be lost in stool, which may create a potential problem with kidney stones (calcium oxalate stones) or osteomalacia (demineralization of bones).

MALABSORPTION SYNDROMES

CELIAC SPRUE

Sensitivity to gluten (a protein found in wheat, rye, oats and barley). This sensitivity causes the intestine to lose the villi through which nutrients are absorbed. Also, digestive enzymes are not produced in adequate amounts.

Signs and Symptoms of Celiac Sprue:

- foul-smelling diarrhea
- bloated abdomen
- anemia
- weight loss
- failure to grow

Possible Causes:

1) Usually diagnosed before the age of two. It is due to an intolerance to gluten. If a celiac patient eats foods with gluten they will damage the intestinal wall, which leads to malabsorption and eventual malnutrition.

Nutrient Applications:

1) L-glutamine
2) Lactobacillus acidophilus and bifidus
3) Slippery Elm - soothe mucus membranes
4) Aloe Vera - reduce inflammation
5) Enzyme support
6) Multi-vitamin and mineral

Dietary and Lifestyle Applications:

1) Eliminate all foods containing gluten, including wheat, rye, oats and barley. This diet, or a very restricted diet, will probably have to be followed for life.
2) A severely malnourished child may need intravenous nutrition to rebuild the body.
3) Aloe vera juice is recommended to reduce inflammation in the intestines.
4) Eat plenty of fiber, including legumes, nuts, seeds, figs, strawberries, raspberries and blackberries.
5) Avoid milk due to possible lactose intolerance.

INFLAMMATORY BOWEL DISEASE (CROHN'S DISEASE AND ULCERATIVE COLITIS)

Inflammatory Bowel Disease (IBD) is used to describe two disorders, Crohn's Disease and Ulcerative Colitis.

1. Crohn's Disease - often referred to as regional enteritis. It is a nonspecific, chronic inflammation of the intestines. It mainly involves the ileum, the lower part of the small intestine, but it can affect any part of the GI tract from the mouth to the anus. The inflammation usually involves the entire thickness of the bowel wall.

Signs and Symptoms of Crohn's Disease:

- chronic diarrhea
- abdominal tenderness, especially right lower abdomen
- fatigue
- joint pain
- weight loss
- skin lesions
- low grade fever

2. Ulcerative Colitis - is a chronic condition in which there is a nonspecific inflammatory response characterized by tiny ulcers and abscesses limited to the lining (mucosa) of the colon.

Signs and Symptoms of Ulcerative Colitis:

- bloody diarrhea
- fever
- mid-abdominal pain
- joint pains
- weight loss
- skin lesions
- painful, urgent bowel movements
- lower abdominal cramping

Possible Causes of Inflammatory Bowel Disease:

1) Heredity - several indicators suggest a genetic predisposition
2) Environmental influences and dietary factors - Crohn's Disease is increased in cultures that eat a diet high in refined sugars and decreased amounts of fruits, vegetables and fiber.
3) Infectious agents - viral, fungal, parasitic and bacterial agents have all been associated with Crohn's disease. (Burton Goldberg Group, Alternative Medicine: The Definitive Guide, Future Medicine Publishing, Inc. WA, p. 681).
4) Altered intestinal flora
5) Food allergies and chemical sensitivities have been implicated in IBD. Wheat, dairy and corn are the most common allergens.
6) Autoimmune disorders
7) Stress

Nutrient Applications:

1) Omega-3 fatty acids to aid in the inflammatory response.
2) Vitamin B-12 - especially if the distal ileum is involved, since that is where B-12 is absorbed.
3) Zinc - deficiency usually found in Crohn's disease. Zinc supplementation may normalize vitamin A metabolism problems.

4) Magnesium - deficiency is prevalent in IBD patients.

Dietary and Lifestyle Applications:

1) Decrease meat to avoid arachidonic acid consumption. Increase omega-3 oils (fish oils) to aid in inflammatory response.
2) Make sure adequate calories are consumed to prevent malnutrition.
3) Elimination diets are extremely important, since food allergies have been largely linked to IBD. Wheat, corn and dairy products are the main culprits. Carrageenan-containing foods (processed foods that contain suspending agents or stabilizers) should also be avoided.
4) A high fiber, complex carbohydrate diet is recommended to prevent IBD, but may be too harsh in patients with active IBD. Active IBD may require an elemental diet, which is a liquid diet that provides pre-digested protein and the essential nutrients.
5) Cabbage juice and juices made from green, leafy vegetables are helpful due to high chlorophyll and vitamin/mineral content. Chlorella is a good source of chlorophyll.
6) Vegetable and seaweed broths make good starters.

Considerations:

1) People with Crohn's disease can remain asymptomatic after the first bout with the disease. Other people have recurrent episodes of pain and diarrhea, accompanied by a low grade fever.
2) Crohn's and Ulcerative Colitis are associated with increased frequency of colon cancer.
3) Most often IBD occurs between the ages of 15 and 35.
4) Prostaglandin levels, especially inflammatory leukotrienes, are increased in IBD, which increases inflammation and causes intestinal cramping.

DIVERTICULOSIS/DIVERTICULITIS

A condition in which multiple small pouches form outward from the colon wall. Usually there is no pain, unless inflammation occurs around the pouches, which is termed **diverticulitis**. Inflammation is caused by waste materials becoming lodged in the pouches.

Signs and Symptoms of Diverticulosis/Diverticulitis:

- usually no symptoms are present
- if inflammation is present, symptoms include severe cramping, usually on the left side of the abdomen; sometimes accompanied by nausea and fever
- constipation

Possible Causes:

1) Low fiber diet is main culprit
2) Risk increases with age
3) Chronic constipation
4) Stress
5) Food allergies
6) Genetic history
7) Obesity
8) Gallbladder disease

Nutrient Applications:

1) High fiber diet is essential to keep colon exercised.
2) Deglycyrrhizinated licorice powder
3) Chlorophyll

4) Acidophilus and bifidus

Dietary and Lifestyle Applications:

1) High fiber diet, no refined sugars or fatty foods.
2) Regular bowel movements are a good preventative measure.
3) Avoid foods with nuts, small seeds, and foods that are hard to digest.
4) Avoid food allergies, especially dairy products.
5) A 1-3 day juice fast with broths, during acute episodes, is helpful.
6) Aloe vera juice may be helpful to prevent constipation.

IRRITABLE BOWEL SYNDROME (IBS)

A common condition in which the large intestine fails to function correctly. It is also known as mucus colitis, spastic colon and nervous indigestion. It represents 30-50% of all referrals to GI specialists and is observed more often in women.

Signs and Symptoms of Irritable Bowel Syndrome:

- abdominal pain
- excess mucus secretion in the stools
- constipation
- nausea
- diarrhea
- anorexia
- bloating
- anxiety
- flatulence (gas)
- depression

Possible Causes:

Unknown, but possible factors include:

1) Food allergies
2) Psychological factors - stress, anxiety, depression, fatigue
3) Dietary factors - including excess dietary fats and refined foods
4) Candidiasis - complicates IBS and increases food sensitivities
5) Low fiber diet
6) Laxative and antibiotic abuse

Nutrient Applications:

1) Fiber supplement - increases motility and cleanses the colon
2) L-glutamine
3) Acidophilus and Bifidus
4) Antispasmodic herbs including chamomile and valerian
5) Ginger - long history of relief for digestive problems

Dietary and Lifestyle Applications:

1) Eliminate food sensitivities. Approximately two-thirds of IBS patients have at least one food intolerance. (Murray, M. and Pizzorno, J. Encyclopedia of Natural Medicine, Prima Publishing, CA, p. 397). Most food reactions are caused by IgG reactions (delayed onset reaction; from one hour to three days), rather that the classic IgE reactions (immediate antibody reaction to an airborne allergy). For this reason, classic allergy tests (skin-scratch tests and IgE RAST (radioallergosorbent test)) are not good tests. The IgE-IgG RAST is better, but the elimination/challenge test is still the least expensive and produces the best results.
   Elimination/Challenge Test - have the patient eat only hypoallergenic foods (chicken, rice, lamb, potatoes, limited vegetables) for one week to one month. Symptoms should disappear. If not,

further evaluate the diet to make sure no allergy foods are being consumed. Re-introduce one food at a time every 3-4 days and monitor pulse. Any foods that cause a reaction need to be avoided until the body is normalized.

2) Increase dietary fiber - due to food sensitivities, obtain fiber from sources other than grains (vegetables, fruits, legumes, psyllium, and guar gum). Avoid fruits with small seeds such as raspberries and strawberries because they can irritate the gut.
3) Avoid alcohol, caffeine, spices, animal fats, dairy products, fried foods, nuts, seeds and processed foods.
4) Ginger is helpful for digestive complaints. Chamomile, valerian, rosemary and peppermint have antispasmodic effects on the colon.
5) Stress reduction techniques, including meditation, biofeedback, hypnosis, counseling and yoga are helpful.
6) Avoid smoking.
7) Exercise is helpful.

Considerations:

1) Many conditions mimic IBS including:
    1) parasites
    2) Inflammatory bowel disease
    3) Candidiasis
    4) Lactose intolerance
    5) Malabsorption syndromes
    6) Laxative abuse
    7) Diverticular disease
    8) Cancer
    9) Metabolic disorders including hyperthyroidism, diabetes and adrenal insufficiency
2) Some fiber is unaffected by digestive enzymes and passes through the stomach and intestines intact. In the colon, some forms of fiber undergo fermentation by bacteria, others are expelled in the stool unchanged. Fiber's role is to increase the size and weight of the stool and also act as a softening agent. It clears the colon of possible carcinogenic substances.

GASTRO-INTESTINAL DISTRESS

CONSTIPATION

Change in bowel movements, mainly in the number of bowel movements or a change in the consistency of bowel movements.

Signs and Symptoms of Constipation:

- unable to have regular bowel movements (1-3 bowel movements per day is typical in healthy people eating diets high in fiber)
- pain during bowel movements

Possible Causes:

1) Insufficient fluids in the diet
2) Too little fiber in the diet
3) Emotional stress
4) Excess fat and refined foods
5) Lack of exercise
6) Side effects of drugs including pain killers, anti-depressants, hypertensive medication, and drugs used to treat Parkinson's disease
7) Pregnancy
8) Iron supplements
9) Laxative or enema abuse

10) Elderly
11) Hypothyroidism
12) Bowel diseases including IBD (Inflammatory Bowel Disease), diverticulosis and IBS (Irritable Bowel Syndrome)
13) Insecticide exposure
14) Food allergies

Nutrient Applications:

1) Lactobacillus acidophilus and bifidus
2) Fiber
3) Chlorophyll
4) Magnesium

Dietary and Lifestyle Applications:

1) Drink 6-8 glasses of water per day.
2) Increase the amount of fiber in your diet. Bran, a hydrophilic fiber is specifically helpful. Corn bran is better than wheat bran and oat bran is not as irritating as both and absorbs fat better. Make sure food allergies are not present.
3) Incorporate exercise into daily routine.
4) Increase magnesium-rich foods including dark, leafy green vegetables.
5) Incorporate bananas, apples, prunes, oranges, oatmeal and flaxseeds into your diet.
6) Licorice tea is helpful in chronic constipation. **CAUTION:** Do not give to people with high blood pressure.
7) Aloe vera juice is helpful.
8) Flaxseed oil or flaxseed tea may be beneficial.
9) Epsom salt baths will increase circulation and relax a person, which may stimulate bowel movements.
10) Stomach massages may be helpful.

Considerations:

1) Breast-fed babies will have fewer bowel movements than bottle-fed babies because the breast milk is used very efficiently.
2) Functions and problems with some laxatives include:
   Castor Oil: it works by irritating the intestinal wall, thus stimulating peristalsis. It undergoes a chemical change in the colon and becomes an acid. This acid prevents the intestines from absorbing water. Prolonged use can damage the cells that line the intestines.
   Psyllium Seed: increases bulk in the intestines, initiates peristalsis and softens the stools; can cause allergies in some people.
   Milk of Magnesia: a magnesium hydroxide that draws fluid from the body into the intestines.
   Mineral Oil: coats the stool to make it easier to evacuate. Prolonged use can cause inflammation of the spleen and liver and create problems with fat-soluble vitamin absorption. It also clogs the lymph system.
   Any excessive laxative abuse will flush out necessary vitamins and minerals, decrease intestinal function and cause an excessive excretion of water, sodium, potassium and electrolytes.

DIARRHEA

Frequent, loose watery stools

Signs and Symptoms of Diarrhea:

- runny stools

- cramping
- excessive thirst
- abdominal pain
- frequent bowel movements

Possible Causes:

1) Dietary factors - excessive fresh fruit or low calorie sweeteners
2) Food allergies or sensitivities
3) Infectious agents - virus, bacteria, fungi and protozoa
4) Food poisoning
5) Reactions to medication
6) Stress and emotional distress
7) Vitamin C consumption in excess of 500 milligrams
8) Laxative abuse
9) Inflammatory bowel disease
10) Chemical toxicities/heavy metal poisoning
11) Rancid foods or contaminated water
12) Lactose intolerance
13) Malabsorption syndrome
14) Biliary or pancreatic problems
15) Hyperthyroidism

Nutrient Applications:

1) Lactobacillus acidophilus and bifidus
2) Slippery Elm bark heals and soothes the intestinal tract.
3) Goldenseal is helpful if diarrhea is due to a bacterial infection. The berberine found in goldenseal has been shown to be helpful in diarrhea that is caused by E. Coli, Salmonella paratyphi B, Shigella dysenteriae, Klebsiella, Giardia lamblia and Vibrio Cholerae.

Dietary and Lifestyle Applications:

1) Eliminate food allergies or sensitivities, especially dairy products and wheat.
2) Drink plenty of fluids to prevent dehydration.
3) Give the intestines time to heal by consuming clear broths and liquids.
4) Eliminate refined sugars and processed foods, and limit fat intake.

Considerations:

1) Mother's milk does not cause or intensify diarrhea in infants unless the baby is allergic to something the mother is eating.

COLIC

Abdominal pain caused by spasms of the intestines. It is most commonly found in infants when the infant continually cries no matter what efforts are used to console the child.

Signs and Symptoms of Colic:

- continuous crying, despite any efforts to console the child
- in infants, the abdomen may be distended and the legs are pulled into the chest
- pain in the abdomen

Possible Causes:

1) Swallowing air which can cause gas pain
2) Food allergies to formula or something the mother is eating
3) Spastic colon (hyperactive GI tract)
4) Stress in the home (anxiety or tension)
5) Overfeeding

Nutrient Applications:

1) Acidophilus and bifidus - for mother and child
2) Chamomile, fennel, licorice, ginger and peppermint

Dietary and Lifestyle Applications:

1) "Israeli researchers gave a daily dose of about ½ cup of tea made from chamomile, licorice, fennel and balm-mint to babies who were experiencing episodes of colic, and found that symptoms were eased in more than ½ the children studied" (Zand, J. Smart Medicine for a Healthier Child. 1994. Avery Publishing Group, Garden City, N.Y., p. 161).
2) A nursing mother can include chamomile, fennel and ginger tea in a daily diet to aid colicky baby.
3) Keep calm and relaxed. Emotional tension contributes to colic.
4) A stomach massage for the baby may be helpful. The massage should be done from the lower right part of the abdomen, up across the rib cage to the lower left part of the abdomen.

HEMORRHOIDS

A cluster of veins located in the anus that have become distended.

Signs and Symptoms of Hemorrhoids:

- bright red blood on toilet paper or in toilet bowl after a bowel movement
- pain or tenderness during a bowel movement
- itching, burning or inflammation around the anus

Possible Causes:

1) Straining during bowel movements (constipation)
2) Pregnancy
3) Toxic liver
4) Poor diet
5) Sitting or standing for long periods of time
6) Genetic weakness of veins or excessive venous pressure
7) Heavy lifting
8) Allergies

Nutrient Applications:

1) Vitamin C (high doses) (contraindicated in iron overload disease, gout and/or kidney stones)
2) Bioflavonoids, specifically rutin
3) Collinsonia
4) Cranes bill
5) Plaintain
6) Witch Hazel (can use as topical to alleviate symptoms)
7) Psyllium seed and guar gum - to prevent constipation
8) Vitamin A
9) B-complex

10) Folic acid

Dietary and Lifestyle Applications:

1) Increase fiber in the diet (especially millet and buckwheat) to decrease constipation. Make sure that food allergies do not exist. Also increase raw fruits, vegetables (especially asparagus, brussel sprouts, cabbage, carrots, cauliflower, corn, peas and kale) and legumes to promote peristalsis.
2) Witch hazel creme applied topically in combination with frequent warm baths may be helpful for symptomatic relief.
3) Avoid straining during bowel movements and focus on regular bowel habits.
4) Drink plenty of filtered water.
5) One tablespoon of cold pressed vegetable oil each day is beneficial to loosen stools.
6) Increase vitamin K foods in the diet, including alfalfa and dark, green leafy vegetables.
7) Consider a detoxification program to cleanse the bowel.

Considerations:

1) Any bleeding should be checked by a doctor to rule out further problems.

THE PHYSIOLOGY OF THE IMMUNE SYSTEM

DEFENSE MECHANISMS OF THE IMMUNE SYSTEM

THYMUS GLAND

The thymus gland is known as the master gland of the immune system. It is responsible for T-lymphocyte production, which controls cell-mediated immunity. Cell-mediated immunity refers to immune functions that are not controlled by antibodies. Cell-mediated immunity is important in defending against yeast, fungi, bacteria, viruses and parasites.

Thymosin, thymopoeitin and interferon are three hormones produced by the thymus gland to regulate immune function. Vitamins B-6, C and A, iron, selenium, zinc, essential amino acids and essential fatty acids have all been suggested to increase the function of these hormones and increase cell-mediated immunity. Extracts of thymus tissue have also been shown to increase immune function in several studies. (Murray, M. N.D., Encyclopedia of Natural Medicine, Prima Publishing, Rocklin, CA, 58).

The thymus gland is very susceptible to free radical attack, which can originate from environmental toxins, infections, stress and chronic illness. Antioxidants are the main defense against free radical attack, which causes thymic involution. The thymus gland shrinks with age and/or stress.

LYMPHATIC SYSTEM

The lymphatic system is a complex series of vessels that run parallel to the blood vessels and move fluid (lymph) to all parts of the body. The lymphatic system carries toxins in the lymph, from the body tissues to the lymph nodes, whose main function is to filter the lymph. The lymph nodes prevent toxins from entering the blood stream. The nodes are located in the groin, neck, armpits, intestinal tract, knees, elbows, between the ribs and along the spine. Macrophages and lymphocytes are contained in the lymph nodes and during infection the nodes may become enlarged because the body is actively fighting off foreign invaders. Regular exercise and diaphragmatic breathing are helpful in improving lymph function.

SALIVARY GLANDS, TONSILS AND ADENOIDS

The salivary glands, including the parotid, sublingual and submandibular glands, contain enzymes that aid in fighting off infection. The tonsils and adenoids are masses of lymphoid tissue in the throat that filter infections from the body. The tonsils are located at the back of the mouth; the adenoids are in the top of the throat. The tonsils and adenoids are most active in infants and children, and shrink with age.

STOMACH

The stomach produces hydrochloric acid (HCl), which destroys bacteria. Sufficient levels of HCl are necessary to prevent bacteria from entering into the body, due to improper digestion and absorption.

SPLEEN

The spleen is the largest mass of lymphoid tissue in the body. The main function of the spleen is to produce lymphocytes and destroy "worn-out red blood cells and platelets." The spleen also stores blood so that during hemorrhaging, extra blood can be released to prevent shock. Spleen tissue extract and goldenseal have been shown to enhance spleen function. (Murray, M. N.D., Encyclopedia of Natural Medicine, Prima Publishing, Rocklin, CA, 59).

LIVER

The liver is essential in immune function because it produces the majority of lymph in the body. The liver also contains Kupffer cells, which are essential macrophages that destroy foreign substances absorbed by the digestive tract. The liver and spleen also work synergistically to monitor intake and release of zinc and iron. Since bacteria require high iron concentrations to function, this regulatory function is important. (Krohn, Jacqueline, MD, The Whole Way to Allergy Relief and Prevention, Hartley and Marks, Inc., WA, 13).

MUCUS MEMBRANES OF THE DIGESTIVE, RESPIRATORY, URINARY AND REPRODUCTIVE TRACT

The mucus membranes are the body's first line of defense against foreign invaders. The membranes secrete mucus, which keeps the linings moist and trap microbes for excretion. The membranes contain white blood cells (including T-cells) and also IgA, that protect mucosal surfaces by preventing bacteria, fungi and other toxins (including food antigens) from adhering and entering through the mucosal barrier.

SMALL INTESTINE

A healthy intestinal tract is richly supplied with secretory IgA (an antibody), which provides the first line of defense in the intestinal mucosa. The small intestine also has patches of lymphocytes, known as Peyer's patches, on the mucosal wall. (Krohn, Jacqueline, MD, The Whole Way to Allergy Relief and Prevention, Hartley and Marks, Inc., WA, 13).

LARGE INTESTINE

The large intestine maintains the "good" bacteria in the gut to prevent overcolonization of harmful pathogens. The fine balance of the microflora of the gastrointestinal tract is very complex and important to the health of the individual. A human harbors more than 400 to 500 species of intestinal flora and proper regulation of this intestinal microflora is critical in preventing colonization by invading pathogens, and in regulating proper immune response. (Great Smokies Diagnostic Laboratory, Application Guide: The Digestive Tract, North Carolina, 1992).

APPENDIX

The appendix, a small appendage attached to the large intestine, contains a mass of lymphatic tissue that is important in immune function.

BONE MARROW

The bone marrow produces red blood cells, platelets and most of the white blood cells, including B-lymphocytes (responsible for antibody production), neutrophils and monocytes (important for phagocytic activity). Neutrophils seek out and ingest bacteria, foreign material and dead cells. They have been called "the first line of defense" against bacterial infections. As part of the inflammatory response, macrophages follow neutrophils into the area of infection as "the second line of defense", and consume a great quantity of bacteria.

IMMUNE SYSTEM FUNCTION

Two types of immune mechanisms:

1) **Humoral Immunity**: based on circulating **antibodies**, which are derived from **B-lymphocytes** after exposure to an antigen (a foreign invader). B-lymphocytes are a type of white blood cell (WBC) that circulate in the blood and are **produced in the bone marrow, spleen and lymphoid tissue.**
2) **Cell-mediated Immunity**: immunity based on **phagocytic (WBC) action** that engulfs and destroys yeast, fungi, bacteria, virus and parasites, rather than antibody production. Phagocytic action by neutrophils and macrophages against the antigen activate WBC's called **T-lymphocytes**, which are **derived from the thymus gland**. The T- lymphocytes include:
    1) **Helper T-cells** - main job is to increase the number of macrophages and cytotoxic T-cells and make memory T-cells. The helper T-cells interact with B-lymphocytes to aid in antibody production.
    2) **Cytotoxic T-cells** - macrophages that engulf and destroy the infectious agent directly.
    3) **Memory T-cells** - remembers the antigen so that an immune response can be quickly initiated when re-exposed to the same antigen.
    4) **Suppressor T-cells** - turns off antibody production.

When the T-cells find the antigen, they attach to it, destroy it and send out chemicals that attract other T-cells and macrophages to help destroy the foreign invader. In the meantime, the B-cells are busy producing antibodies that will further destroy the antigen. The memory cells are important in the event of re-exposure to an antigen. The memory cells speed up the immune response and are the reason for the quick reaction experienced by sensitive people who are re-exposed to certain foods, chemicals or environmental toxins.

Autoimmunity - when the body cannot identify between "self" and "non-self". The confused body misinterprets signals and produces an immune response against itself. Autoimmunity is thought to be a factor in **AIDS, rheumatoid arthritis, lupus erythematosus, Grave's disease (hyperthyroidism), diabetes mellitus and multiple sclerosis.**

WHITE BLOOD CELLS

WHITE BLOOD CELLS: also known as leukocytes; WBC's are the defense mechanism of the immune system. The WBC's are transported to areas of inflammation to destroy infectious agents, such as bacteria and viruses.

2 TYPES OF WHITE BLOOD CELLS:

1) **Granular WBC's** - develop in the bone marrow; have granules in the cytoplasm.
    1) **Neutrophils** - phagocytic action against bacteria; release lysozyme which destroys certain bacteria.
    2) **Eosinophils** - involved in allergy reactions; **release histamine**, which is a body chemical that triggers localized inflammation and irritation to combat the allergen. Histamine **causes blood vessels to dilate** causing fluid to pass from the blood to the tissues. Histamine also triggers **smooth muscle contraction.**
    3) **Basophils** - involved in allergic reactions; release histamine, heparin and serotonin. Heparin inhibits thrombin, which is needed for blood coagulation. This inhibition allows for increased blood flow to the inflamed area. Serotonin releases a chemical that causes irritation to the surrounding cells. Serotonin is found mainly in the gastrointestinal mucosa. Inflammation is the end result when histamine, heparin and serotonin are released.
        a) **Mast cells** - basophils residing in the blood vessels that release histamine, causing blood vessels to dilate.
2) **Agranular WBC's** - develop in the lymphoid tissue; have no granules.
    1) **Lymphocytes** - involved in immune mechanisms.

a) **T-cells:** processed in the thymus gland to make T-cells; activated by macrophagic activity; involved in cell-mediated immunity.

Types of T-cells:

1) **Helper T-cells:** aid B-cells in making antibodies.
2) **Cytotoxic (killer) T-cells:** attack and destroy foreign invaders; activate phagocytes to destroy pathogens.
3) **Suppressor T-cells:** inhibit WBC function (B-cells and killer T-cells) and turn off antibody production.
4) **Memory T-cells:** trigger immune response when re-exposed to the antigen.

b) **B-cells:** processed in lymphoid tissue outside the thymus gland; produce antibodies in response to an antigen.

Types of B-cells:

1) **Plasma B-cells:** secrete antibodies (approximately 2,000 antibody molecules per second for each cell) until the plasma cell dies (4-5 days).
2) **Memory B cells:** trigger immune response when re-exposed to the antigen.

2) **Monocytes** - phagocytic action; clean up cellular debris

Macrophages: large monocytes that reside in specific tissues like the spleen or liver.

NOTE: Echinacea, goldenseal, siberian and Korean ginseng and licorice possess macrophage enhancing effects. (Murray, M. N.D., Encyclopedia of Natural Medicine, Prima Publishing, Rocklin, CA, 61).

CLINICAL APPLICATION

Differential count in a blood test represents the number of each kind of WBC for every 100 WBC's. A normal differential follows these percentages. (Tortora and Anagnostakos, Principles of Anatomy and Physiology, 4th Edition. Harper and Row, New York, 44).

WBC	PERCENTAGE	IF INCREASED
Neutrophils	60 - 70 % of total	indicates bacterial infection
Eosinophils	2 - 4 % of total	indicates allergic reaction
Basophils	0.5 - 1 % of total	indicates allergic reaction
Lymphocytes	20 - 25 % of total	indicates antigen-antibody reaction
Monocytes	3 - 8 % of total	indicates chronic infection

ANTIGEN-ANTIBODY REACTION

ANTIGEN: a foreign invader to the body that is not part of the body's normal chemistry, such as yeast, fungi, bacteria, viruses and parasites.

ANTIBODIES: protein produced by the body when an antigen is present. A specific antibody fits to a specific antigen similar as a lock to a key. Antibodies are also known as immunoglobulins.

ANTIGEN-ANTIBODY REACTION: Any antigen-antibody reaction triggers an inflammatory response, including edema, tenderness, redness and heat. The inflammation is due to histamines, prostaglandins, leukotrienes and other chemicals being released from the phagocytic cells. Also, blood flow is increased to the area so that more white blood cells can be carried to the inflamed site. Once histamine levels reach a certain concentration, the mast cells release a substance to stop histamine production, since these chemicals irritate normal cells.

NOTE: Interleukin II, interferon and other chemical factors are produced by the white blood cells and are essential in destroying viruses and cancer cells. **Vitamin C, beta-carotene, zinc, manganese, echinacea and licorice** have been shown to be beneficial in increasing the production of these immune-enhancing chemical compounds. (Murray, M. N.D., Encyclopedia of Natural Medicine, Prima Publishing, Rocklin, CA, 61).

IMMUNOGLOBULINS: Antibodies are also known as immunoglobulins (Ig's). Five classes of immunoglobulins have been identified in humans.

IgA: provide localized protection on the mucus membranes and in saliva. IgA provides a first line of defense against invading pathogens. Salivary secretory IgA is used as an analysis by Great Smokies Laboratories and Diagnos-Techs, Inc. to determine the body's immune response and effectiveness. According to these laboratories, secretory IgA (sIgA) method of action is as an antibacterial, antiviral and antifungal agent, preventing colonization of invading pathogens.

Decreased Secretory IgA: indicates impaired immune performance. Low sIgA, according to these laboratories, can indicate increased susceptibility to certain conditions including autoimmune disease, food allergies, asthma, candidiasis, gastro-intestinal problems, celiac disease, recurrent infections and eczema.

Increased Secretory IgA: indicates chronic infection and immune system overload, including chronic viral infections (Epstein-Barr Virus (EBV), Human Immunodeficiency Virus (HIV)).

Adequate Secretory IgA: prevents foreign invaders from entering the body.

IgD: found in cell membranes; stimulates antibody production.

IgE: involved in allergic reactions (both food and environmental). IgE stimulates the release of histamine. Histamine is released when an allergen enters the system and triggers a variety of symptoms including redness, itching, swelling and pain.

IgG: most abundant antibody (75% of total); enhances phagocytosis and neutralizes toxins. High levels of IgG indicate a current or previous infection, specifically bacteria and viruses. IgG causes more delayed, long-term reactions.

IgM: effective against microbes (bacteria and other antigens) and is the first antibody produced after antigen exposure. If IgM levels are high, there has been a recent infection.

SUBCLINICAL AND PATHOLOGICAL CONDITIONS OF THE IMMUNE SYSTEM

IMMUNE PROBLEMS

COLDS/FLUS

Viral infections of the upper respiratory tract; a cold or flu can be the body's way of detoxifying environmental stressors and/or a poor diet.

Colds - occur any time of year; less severe than flu.

Flus - occur mainly in the late fall or winter; symptoms are more severe and more intense.

Signs and Symptoms of a Cold or Flu:

- sore throat
- coughing
- runny nose
- headache
- aching muscles
- fatigue
- swollen lymph nodes
- fever
- vomiting/nausea
- diarrhea
- head congestion
- breathing difficulties
- sneezing

Possible Causes:

1) Weakened immune system
2) Poor diet, especially simple sugars which decrease WBC function
3) Environmental toxins (chemicals and heavy metals)
4) Food allergies - wheat and cow's milk are known to be "mucus producing"
5) Airborne allergies
6) Stress - stress hormones from the adrenals decrease immune function by causing the thymus gland to shrink and decrease thymic activity
7) Poor sleep patterns
8) Thyroid problems (especially hypothyroidism)

Nutrient Applications:

1) Vitamin C - 500-1000 mg. every two hours to increase immune function (contraindicated in iron overload disease, gout and/or kidney stones).
2) Zinc Gluconate Lozenges - potent immunostimulant, antiviral activity; shown to decrease cold duration
3) Thymus extract - enhance thymus function
4) Vitamin A and beta-carotene - soothe inflamed mucus membranes and support immune system; strong antiviral activity. Beta-carotene is a potent antioxidant and offers protection for the thymus gland that is extremely susceptible to free radical attack.
5) Echinacea and goldenseal - excellent antiviral herbs for the immune system
6) Acidophilus/Bifidus - to restore healthy bacteria to the intestinal tract
7) Bioflavonoids

Dietary and Lifestyle Applications:

1) Eat a healthy, well-balanced diet. Avoid refined sugars, junk foods, additives and preservatives, dairy products and inorganic red meat.
2) Avoid food allergies.
3) Maintain a healthy immune system by decreasing environmental stressors.
4) Avoid smoking and alcohol which decrease immune function.
5) Drink plenty of filtered water, herb teas and vegetable juices. Also, sip hot liquids such as chicken broth. Keeping the mucus membranes of the respiratory tract moist aids in ridding viral infections. A vaporizer is also helpful.
6) For sore throat pain, try 1 T. slippery elm powder in boiling water with honey.
7) Do not suppress fever unless it is above 104 degrees F.
8) Get plenty of rest and sleep. Immune function is increased during sleep.
9) Orange juice and other concentrated simple sugars are not the best because they decrease WBC function. If you do drink juice, it should be diluted.
10) Raw garlic is excellent to add to the diet.
11) Pau d'arco tea has an antibiotic effect. Goldenseal and echinacea tea are also helpful.

Considerations:

1) Remember antibiotics are ineffective against viruses, therefore they are useless in treating colds.
2) Do not give aspirin in combination with a viral cold or flu to a child or a teenager. The combination of the two has been associated with a dangerous liver disease seen in children and young adults called Reye's Syndrome.

PEDIATRIC EAR INFECTION

Otherwise known as otitis media, an infection of the middle ear.

Signs and Symptoms of Pediatric Ear Infections:

- pain in the ear, often in conjunction with a cold or infection
- fever
- fullness and pressure in the ear

Possible Causes:

1) Pressure in the ear that pushes on the eardrum
2) Infection
3) Cigarette smoke exposure
4) Food allergies

Nutrient Applications:

1) Vitamin C and bioflavonoids (Vitamin C is contraindicated in iron overload disease, gout and/or kidney stones)
2) Zinc lozenges
3) Acidophilus/bifidus
4) Echinacea/Goldenseal
5) Garlic

Dietary and Lifestyle Applications:

1) Drink plenty of fluids, including water, herbal teas, soups and diluted fruit juices.
2) Eliminate dairy products and food/environmental allergies.
3) Avoid exposure to cigarette smoke.

4) Chiropractic care is very beneficial.
5) Breastfeeding protects against ear infections due to antibodies in mother's milk; cow's milk is a common allergen.
6) Antibiotics should be used sparingly and only if the ear infection moves to the mastoid bone (behind the ear) or meninges (membranes that cover the brain and spinal cord).
7) Lymphatic massage is helpful.

FEVER

Temperature at least 1-2 degrees above 98.6 F. A fever is the body's way of destroying viruses and bacteria.

Signs and Symptoms of a Fever:

- high body temperature
- pale, flushed face
- hot to the touch
- sweats/chills

Possible Causes:

1) Overexertion
2) Viral/bacterial infection
3) Dehydration
4) Bee sting/ mosquito bite
5) Allergy reaction
6) Rheumatoid arthritis

Nutrient Applications:

1) Vitamin C (Vitamin C is contraindicated in iron overload disease, gout and/or kidney stones)
2) Echinacea/Goldenseal
3) Garlic
4) Calcium

Dietary and Lifestyle Applications:

1) Caution should be used when giving aspirin in combination with a viral cold or flu to a child or a teenager. The combination of the two has been associated with a dangerous liver disease seen in children and young adults called Reye's Syndrome.
2) Drink plenty of fluids to prevent dehydration.
3) Ginger tea may be helpful for a cold, flu or stomachache that accompanies the fever.
4) Get plenty of rest and avoid getting chilled.
5) Soothing herbal baths in lukewarm water may be helpful.

VACCINATION TOXICITY

Injection of a toxin given to a person to "protect" them against certain infectious diseases such as:

1) **DPT (Diphtheria, Pertussis, Tetanus)**
   Diphtheria - potentially fatal disease that affects the kidneys, heart and upper respiratory tract. It is caused by contaminated drinking water and is very rare (2-3 cases per year in the United States).
   Pertussis - whooping cough; most dangerous factor of the DPT shot; children still get whooping cough even after the vaccination.
   Tetanus - lock jaw; dangerous infection of the central nervous system caused by improperly cleansed wounds.

2) **Measles-Mumps-Rubella (MMR)**
3) **Polio**
4) **Hepatitis B**

NOTE: In Dr. Archie Kalokerinos book **Every Second Child**, he tells the story of native Aborigines that were immunized by a vaccine program sponsored by the Australian government. Within a few days of the shots, every other child died from the vaccine. Thereafter, he gave each child 100 mg. of vitamin C per day and no child died from the shots after being immunized. (Kalokerinos, A. M.D. Every Second Child, 1981. Keats Publishing Company, New Canaan, CT). Also, in 1986, the government adopted the National Vaccination Compensation Act to collect data on the negative effects of vaccinations. Ten percent of the doctors responded and by Fall 1992 over 17,000 negative reactions to vaccines were reported, including 360 deaths. (FDA Press Release in Adverse Events Associated with Childhood Vaccines: Evidence Bearing Causality. Vienna, VA.: National Academy Press, Sept. 1993).

Nutrient Applications:

1) Vitamin C with bioflavonoids. (Vitamin C is contraindicated in iron overload disease, gout and/or kidney stones)
2) Lactobacillus acidophilus and bifidus

CHRONIC FATIGUE SYNDROME

Mysterious illness that has varied symptoms and is often brought on by a variety of problems, mainly viral infections including EBV. It feels like a flu that never heals.

Signs and Symptoms of Chronic Fatigue Syndrome:

- chronic fatigue
- headaches
- recurring infection
- muscle aches and pains
- mental confusion
- swollen lymph glands
- recurrent sore throats
- low-grade fever
- poor concentration
- food/environmental allergies
- depression/anxiety
- intestinal problems
- breathing irregularities
- irregular heartbeat
- appetite loss

Possible Causes:

1) Combined infections including yeast, parasites, bacterial and viral infections.
2) Nutrient deficiency
3) Environmental toxins (chemicals, heavy metals, alcohol and drugs)
4) Lifestyle choices, stress and poor sleep
5) Food and environmental allergies
6) Reaction to vaccinations
7) Dysbiosis
8) Thyroid imbalances (hypothyroidism)
9) Breathing problems
10) Genetic factors
11) Chronic EBV infection
12) Anemia
13) Hypoglycemia and/or hypoadrenia
14) Mercury toxicity from amalgams
15) Weak immune system

Nutrient Applications:

1) Systemic detoxification program - especially liver and lymph if EBV is suspect, since these are the primary targeted areas in EBV.
2) Liver support - methionine, carnitine, artichoke, licorice powder, milk thistle, fringe tree, etc.
3) Goldenseal, barberry or Oregon grape - contain berberine, which enhances blood flow to the spleen, which may increase the release of immune-potentiating substances from the spleen.
4) Multi-vitamin/mineral supplement including the B vitamins, zinc, selenium, chromium and manganese.
5) Beta-carotene - natural antioxidant and antiviral agent
6) Vitamin C - antiviral activity, increases WBC activity. (Vitamin C is contraindicated in iron overload disease, gout and/or kidney stones)
7) Zinc - important in thymus function and cellular immunity
8) Spleen and thymus glandular extract
9) Goldenseal and echinacea
10) Magnesium - deficiency has been shown to be a problem in CFS patients
11) Adrenal support if necessary

Dietary and Lifestyle Applications:

1) A good diet is very important. Organic foods are best. Avoid antibiotics in chicken and chemical toxicity in fish.
2) Lymphatic flow stimulation is helpful through exercise, stretching, massage and hot/cold hydrotherapy.
3) Drink plenty of filtered water.
4) Moderate exercise with passive stretching daily is suggested.
5) Relaxation/meditative exercises with deep breathing.
6) Proper sleep.
7) Stress reduction.
8) Eliminate food allergies and dysbiosis.

FOOD ALLERGIES/SENSITIVITIES

An immediate or delayed adverse reaction by the immune system to a food that most people find harmless.

ALLERGY: classic antigen-antibody response to a particular food (IgG or IgE).

FOOD SENSITIVITY: an adverse reaction to a food with no antigen-antibody response.

Types of allergy reactions:

1) **Immediate: IgE-mediated response**; immediate reaction within two hours after eating food. IgE-mediated reactions are mainly seen in airborne allergies (pollens, dusts and weeds), and are not seen as often in food allergies.
   MODE OF ACTION: IgE antibodies attach to mast cells that are mainly found in the air passages, blood and skin; when an allergen enters the body, the mast cells release substances (i.e. histamine) to ward off the allergen.
2) **Delayed: IgG-mediated response**; delayed response, usually 36-72 hours after exposure to antigen. IgG-mediated reactions are seen in most food allergies. The delayed response makes it difficult to pin down the specific food allergy.
   MODE OF ACTION: a different type of mast cell is found in the connective tissue lining the intestinal tract. A food allergy reaction starts in the digestive tract, triggered by a free-floating antibody called secretory IgA. Secretory IgA functions to protect the lining of the small intestine by secreting a thick protective coating of mucus from the mucosal lining when it comes in contact with a food allergen. If the food is eaten repeatedly, the immune system is overtaxed and the amount of secretory IgA antibodies produced is decreased. This allows the food to come in

contact with the mast cells and triggers the release of toxic chemical mediators (histamine, leukotrienes, inflammatory prostaglandins, etc.). Over the long term, the inflammatory prostaglandins decrease HCl secretion, which triggers the pancreas to underproduce bicarbonates and pancreatic enzymes. Also, the chemical mediators weaken the mucosal membrane of the intestinal wall and allow partially digested food to pass into the bloodstream. The IgG antibody attempts to clear these macromolecules from the bloodstream, but if overwhelmed, these macromolecules (immune complexes) penetrate the capillary walls and are deposited in the tissues. Inflammation is produced wherever the immune complexes are deposited. (Braly, J., M.D., Dr. Braly's Food Allergy and Nutrition Revolution. 1992. Keats Publishing, Inc., New Canaan, CT., pp. 69-72)..

Signs and Symptoms of Food Allergies and Sensitivities:

Immediate reactions: (IgE-mediated response)

- anaphylactic shock (most severe)
- eczema
- wheezing
- hives
- swelling

Delayed reactions: (IgG-mediated response)

- GI complaints including stomach pains, heartburn, excess gas, chronic diarrhea/constipation, irritable bowel syndrome, ulcers and malabsorption problems.
- dark circles under the eyes
- sinusitis
- itching
- chronic fatigue
- edema
- joint/muscle pain
- puffy eyes
- acne
- anxiety/depression
- chronic swollen glands
- eczema
- insomnia
- headaches (migraines)
- hives
- asthma
- wheezing
- hyperactivity
- bedwetting
- canker sores
- arthritis

NOTE: Offending foods can be masked because eating the food can actually make the person feel better initially. If a person stops eating the offending food, they will feel withdrawal symptoms (lasting approximately one to five days). Thus, they unconsciously crave the allergy food(s) in order to avoid the withdrawal symptoms. Frequently, a person's favorite foods are the allergy foods. Also, certain foods may work synergistically, meaning they will produce symptoms when eaten together, but not when eaten alone (i.e. eggs and apples).

Possible Causes:

1) Weakened immune system - may be due to increased T-cell levels because of constant internal battle, which causes allergic reactions to be triggered more quickly.
2) Environmental toxins (metals, chemicals, other pollutants).
3) Repetitive immunizations or antibiotic/steroidal medication that decrease immune response and disturb the normal gastrointestinal flora.
4) Dysbiosis - candida, parasites, fungi, etc. decrease efficiency of gut mucosa and increase potential for allergies.
5) Heredity - children born to parents with allergies have an increased chance of developing allergies themselves.
6) Repetitive ingestion of a small variety of foods (monotonous diet). The body becomes sensitized to the foods.
7) Genetic manipulation of foods and chemicals/pesticides added to foods.
8) Nutritional deficiencies.

9) Leaky gut syndrome - partially digested foods enter the blood and cause immune responses. Leaky gut is caused by weak digestion, NSAIDs, infections, alcohol abuse, nutritional deficiencies, drug/medication use or abuse, dysbiosis, stress, premature birth and radiation.
   NOTE: NSAIDs increase the possibility of food sensitivities because they increase the ability of food particles to cross the gut mucosa into the bloodstream.
10) Stress, physical and/or emotional trauma - due to decreased immune function, adrenal response and possibly decreased HCl production. Allergy sufferers "seem to have a significantly lowered threshold to stress, in part because of the physiological and psychological overstimulation of their adrenals" (Braly, J., M.D., Dr. Braly's Food Allergy and Nutrition Revolution. 1992. Keats Publishing, Inc., New Canaan, CT., pp. 68-69). One study showed that in solving a simple math problem, Type A personalities (tense, impatient, ambitious) have forty times as much cortisol and three times as much adrenaline circulating in the blood as Type B (more relaxed) people solving the same problem. (Ibid, pp. 68-69)
11) Lower IgA levels (IgA protects the mucosa of the intestinal tract).
12) Poor digestion (i.e. decreased HCl production, pancreatic enzyme deficiency, gallbladder problems). Food sensitivities are frequently associated with low HCl levels.
13) Poor liver function due to its role in removing foreign protein from the body and detoxifying the system.
14) Premature babies have increased risk due to underdeveloped GI tract.
15) Premature weaning of infants to solid foods when GI tract is not fully developed. Baby formulas and cow's milk contain large molecules that are difficult for the baby to digest. Also, not breastfeeding can be a trigger for potential food allergens because of decreased protective factors from mother's milk.
16) Food additives (i.e. yellow dye #5 (tartrazine) and benzoates) which have been shown to increase the number of mast cells produced in the body, which increases susceptibility to allergies.
17) Poor thyroid function.

Nutrient Applications:

1) Detoxification program is beneficial.
2) Immune support including:
   1) Vitamin C - high potency with bioflavonoids. (Vitamin C is contraindicated in iron overload disease, gout and/or kidney stones)
   2) Selenium, zinc, B-complex and vitamin A (zinc and vitamin A may increase IgA levels (gastrointestinal antibody) on mucosal surface.
   3) Thymus extract
   4) Echinacea and goldenseal
   5) Garlic - antibacterial properties
3) Bromelain, essential fatty acids and bioflavonoids for inflammatory response.
4) Glutamine - for intestinal support.
5) HCl and enzyme support if necessary.
6) Adrenal support if necessary.

Dietary and Lifestyle Applications:

1) Avoid allergy associated foods, especially dairy, wheat, citrus, eggs, chocolate and shellfish. A vegetarian diet may be helpful.
   NOTE: To find out if you are allergic to a particular food, the potentially allergic food needs to be eliminated from the diet for at least four days. When the food is re-introduced to the diet, there will be a marked increase in symptoms if that food is causing a problem. An increase in pulse rate after ingesting a food is also a good indicator that it is an allergy food.
2) After you have eliminated the allergy foods, follow a rotation diet. This means that you should only eat the same type of food every four days. This helps to avoid creating an allergy. A wide variety of non-allergenic foods should be eaten.
3) Treat any underlying infections and digestive dysfunctions.
4) Avoid non-steroidal anit-inflammatory drugs (NSAIDs).

5) Avoid smoking, toxic pollutants and petrochemicals.
6) Eliminate alcohol, sugar, tobacco and caffeine.
7) Decrease stress.
8) Garlic, ginger, onions, black pepper and cayenne may be helpful to stimulate IgA production.
9) Infants who are not breast-fed have an increased likelihood of developing allergies.
10) Check for hypothyroidism and poor adrenal function.
11) Drink plenty of filtered water.
12) Avoid food additives and preservatives.
13) Proper exercise is important to enhance oxygenation to the tissues and stimulate toxic release from the body.

ENVIRONMENTAL ALLERGIES

An immediate or delayed adverse reaction by the immune system caused by environmental factors such as pollen, house dust, molds, smoke and environmental pollutants. They can be seasonal or chronic.

Signs and Symptoms of Environmental Allergies:

- watery, red eyes
- diarrhea
- bronchitis
- runny/stuffed nose
- nausea
- chronic fatigue
- rash/hives
- digestive upset
- depression/anxiety
- ringing in the ears
- asthma
- headaches
- arthritis
- eczema
- hayfever
- sneezing
- itchy skin/eyes
- dark circles under the eyes

Common Environmental Allergens:

Mainly pollen (trees, grass, weeds, etc.), mold, house dust, smoke and environmental pollutants

Possible Causes:

1) Weakened immune system - may be due to increased T-cell levels because of constant internal battle, which causes allergic reactions to be triggered more quickly.
2) Environmental toxins (metals, chemicals, other pollutants) which weaken the immune system.
3) Repetitive immunizations or antibiotic/steroidal medication that decrease immune response and disturb the normal gastrointestinal flora.
4) Dysbiosis - candida, parasites, fungi, etc. decrease efficiency of gut mucosa and increase potential for allergies.
5) Heredity - children born to parents with allergies have an increased chance of developing allergies themselves.
6) Nutritional deficiencies.
7) Stress/physical or emotional trauma - due to decreased immune function, adrenal response and possibly decreased HCl production.
8) Poor liver function due to its role in removing foreign protein from the body and detoxifying the system.

Nutrient Applications:

1) Detoxification program is beneficial.
2) Immune support including:
    1) Vitamin C - high potency with bioflavonoids. Flavonoids are highly effective in allergy reactions. They inhibit the release of histamine from mast cells during an inflammatory response. (Vitamin C is contraindicated in iron overload disease, gout and/or kidney stones)

2) Selenium, zinc, B-complex and vitamin A (zinc and vitamin A may increase IgA levels on mucosal surface, which is a gastrointestinal antibody)
3) Thymus extract
4) Echinacea and goldenseal
5) Garlic - antibacterial properties

3) Bromelaine, essential fatty acids and bioflavonoids for inflammatory response.
4) Adrenal support if necessary.
5) Calcium and magnesium as a nerve relaxant. People with allergies usually suffer from an over reactive nervous system.
6) Pantothenic acid (vitamin B-5) may be taken during hayfever season to prevent an allergic reaction.

Dietary and Lifestyle Applications:

1) Eliminate dairy products. They increase mucus production, which creates further irritation.
2) Avoid food allergens and environmental allergens as much as possible. Allergy-proof the house.
3) Eat a healthy diet. Avoid cooked fats and oils, which compromise the digestive system.
4) Avoid non-steroidal, anit-inflammatory drugs (NSAIDs).
5) Avoid tobacco, toxic pollutants and petrochemicals.
6) Eliminate alcohol, sugar, and caffeine.
7) Decrease stress.
8) Garlic, ginger, onions, black pepper and cayenne may be helpful to stimulate IgA production.
9) Infants who are not breast-fed have an increased likelihood of developing allergies.
10) Check for hypothyroidism.
11) Drink plenty of water to thin mucus secretions.
12) Fenugreek and thyme tea may be helpful as a mild decongestant for sinus congestion sufferers. Licorice tea and Siberian ginseng strengthen the adrenal glands.

Considerations:

1) Antihistamines are common drugs used for allergies. Antihistamines are often mixed with a nasal decongestant.

Antihistamines:

Function: block the action of histamine at the receptor sites.

Side effects: most antihistamines cause drowsiness, because by blocking histamine action they block histamine function in the brain. Histamine's main function in the brain is to maintain alertness. Some antihistamines have been manufactured by drug companies which do not cause drowsiness, because they have been formulated not to affect the brain receptor sites. The drawback of antihistamines is that they have potential risks, including cardiovascular and liver problems.

CANDIDIASIS

An overgrowth of candida albicans, a yeast-like fungus in the body. Candida albicans is a yeast found in everyone and is usually kept in check by the body's good bacteria, namely lactobacillus acidophilus and bifidus. If the immune system is compromised, the yeast proliferates and transforms into a pathogenic fungus that severely compromises the immune system. Candidiasis can trigger a variety of symptoms and makes the body much more prone to allergies and infectious agents.

Signs and Symptoms of Candidiasis:

- chronic digestive complaints including gas, bloating, cramping, thrush (overgrowth of candida in the mouth) and rectal itching
- chronic fatigue
- recurrent vaginal or urinary infections
- food/environmental allergies
- low immune function

- severe PMSloss of libido
- depression/anxiety
- respiratory problems
- prostatitis
- perfumes and chemical smells aggravate the condition

Possible Causes:

1) Prolonged antibiotic use which kills the good bacteria, allowing yeast overgrowth.
2) Oral contraceptive use, estrogen-replacement therapy and/or steroidal use. **NOTE:** Yeast festers in estrogen.
3) Anti-ulcer medications including Zantac and Tagamet.
4) Immune suppression due to stress, environmental toxins, illness and infectious agents.
5) Poor dietary habits, including high sugar intake.
6) Chemical/environmental toxins.
7) Alcohol use - very toxic and feeds the yeast.
   NOTE: "Drunk disease" was first discovered in Japan when chronic candidiasis patients were tested and found to have alcohol in the blood even when they did not consume any alcohol. In these patients, it was found that they turned acetaldehyde (a toxin produced in the gut from sugar and yeast fermentation) into ethanol, which caused them to be constantly drunk. (Burton Goldberg Group, Alternative Medicine: The Definitive Guide, Future Medicine Publishing, Inc. WA. p. 589.)
8) Food and environmental allergies.
9) Hypothyroidism.
10) Diabetes (candida thrives in the presence of sugar).
11) Gallbladder problems.
12) HCL and/or enzymatic deficiencies.
13) Hypoglycemia and/or hypoadrenia.
14) Impaired liver function - liver is a key organ in fighting against candida. The liver is essential in detoxifying the toxins released when killing off yeast. If the liver is not strong enough to filter the blood, the toxins will remain in the blood and cause symptoms to become worse.
15) Mercury amalgam dental fillings.

Nutrient Applications:

1) Detoxification program is beneficial.
2) Lactobacillus acidophilus and bifidus - "good bacteria" manufacture biotin, a B-vitamin that helps control yeast.
3) Support to increase immune function - vitamins A, B, C, E and beta-carotene, goldenseal, echinacea and antioxidant support (zinc, selenium).
4) Adrenal support if necessary.
5) Essential fatty acid support.
6) HCl and pancreatic enzyme support.
7) Goldenseal (found to be an excellent anti-candida agent), Oregon grape and barberry - contain berberine which are useful anti-fungal agents.
8) Caprylic acid - natural occurring fatty acid.
9) Garlic - effective anti-fungal agent.
10) Pau d'arco - herbal fungicide
11) Grapefruit seed extract - acts as anti-fungal and antibiotic.

Dietary and Lifestyle Applications:

1) Increase immune and digestive function, especially liver.
2) Avoid sugar in all its forms including fruit juices, fruit, dairy products (contains lactose), honey, sucrose, dextrose, fructose and possibly potatoes.
3) Avoid food allergies/sensitivities.
4) Avoid alcohol, fermented and yeasty foods.

5) Eat sugar-free yogurt, vegetables, whole grains and organic meats.
6) Avoid antibiotics whenever possible.
7) Follow a Candida diet. A rotation diet may be helpful if allergies are present.
8) Avoid moldy places, chemical household products, pollutants and chlorinated water.
9) Avoid birth control pills.
10) Pau d'arco or clove tea may be helpful for the antibacterial and antifungal properties. You can alternate between the two.
11) Promote healthy intestinal flora and increase fiber to eliminate toxins in the gut.

PARASITIC INFECTIONS

A single celled organism (protozoa), worm or insect that feeds off another host organism.

Two-phase life cycle:

1) **Cyst** - closed sacs that can be transmitted easily and are resistant to destruction by digestive juices.
2) **Trophozite** - mobile and active stage of a parasite.

Types of Parasites:

A) **Protozoa** - single-celled organisms that cannot be seen by the naked eye and can destroy tissue of the host organism.
   1) **Giardia Lamblia** - leading cause of parasitic infections in the US; found in contaminated water and can cause traveler's diarrhea; correlation found with decreased secretory IgA and giardiasis.
   2) **Cryptosporidum** - found mainly in animals, but was recently identified in human stools.
   3) **Trichomonas Vaginalis** - sexually transmitted; causes foul-smelling vaginal discharge and inflammation.
   4) **Entamoeba histolytic** - transmitted by fecally contaminated food and/or water. It causes dysentery and mainly affects the lungs, liver, brain and heart.
   5) **Blastocystis hominis** - most commonly detected in the stools
B) **Nematoda:** multi-cellular organisms known as worms; they multiply by producing eggs (ova or larvae).
   1) **Roundworms** - look like earthworms.
   2) **Pinworms** - most common in US; found mainly in children. Pinworms lay eggs outside the anus.
   3) **Hookworms** - found in moist soil.
   4) **Trichinella** - contamination is due to eating partially uncooked pork.
C) **Cestoda:** tapeworms; largest parasites that attach to the intestinal wall and grow new worms. Tapeworms get their nourishment from partially digested foods from the host. Tapeworm infestation can occur by eating undercooked beef, pork or fish or by dog fleas.
D) **Trematoda** - flukes, which are flatworms.

Signs and Symptoms of Parasitic Infections:

- Diarrhea
- Constipation
- fever/chills
- high eosinophil count
- flatulence
- belching
- nausea/vomiting
- foul-smelling stools
- bloody and/or mucusy stools
- weight loss
- heartburn
- chronic fatigue
- skin problems
- headaches
- Irritable Bowel Syndrome
- Itchy
- Malabsorption
- food allergies/sensitivities
- muscle and joint pain
- arthritis
- environmental sensitivities
- anal puritus (intense anal itching)
- positive stool sample
- increased appetite
- high IgE count

Possible Causes:

1) Contaminated food and water - parasites, unlike bacteria, are not killed by chlorination.
2) Increased international travel. Drug resistant parasites are found across the world, especially in Southeast Asia, South America and Africa.
3) Mosquitoes, fleas and houseflies can be carriers of certain types of parasites.
4) Antibiotic and immune suppressive drugs, which allow opportunistic invaders to enter the body.
5) Day-care centers: "Day care centers are the source of nearly 20,000 cases of giardiasis" (Gittleman, A., Guess What Came To Dinner - Parasites and Your Health., Avery Publishing Group, NY, p. 13). Parasites spread by direct contact with feces.
6) Household pets - dogs and cats can transfer parasitic infections to their owners.
7) Raw or undercooked meats and/or fish. If the food is not cooked sufficiently, the larvae survives and infests the host organism. Microwave cooking can be a culprit if foods (fish or meat) are not cooked sufficiently.
8) Sexual contact can spread parasitic infections.
9) Certain types of parasites can be inhaled or can penetrate through the skin.
10) Immune insufficiency.
11) Dysbiosis.
12) Dietary factors and nutritional status.
13) Liver insufficiency.

Nutrient Applications:

1) A detoxification program is beneficial.
2) Sufficient pancreatic enzymes and HCl is essential. **NOTE:** The heavy metal lead binds HCl in the gut and makes HCl unavailable for digestion.
3) Effective herbs used in parasite elimination include garlic, black walnut, quassia, butternut bark, goldenseal and slippery elm (to soothe the GI mucosa). Pumpkin seeds are also helpful in parasite elimination.
4) Artemesia Annua and grapefruit seed extract for anti-parasitic effect.
5) Goldenseal contains berberine, which is active against some parasites.
6) Immune support.
7) Lactobacillus acidophilus, bifidus and bulgaricus - to recolonize the GI tract after eradication of parasites.
8) Fructooligosaccharides (FOS) - a natural carbohydrate found in Jerusalem artichoke, onions and asparagus roots that has been shown to increase bifidobacteria in the gut.

Dietary and Lifestyle Applications:

1) A good diet is essential. Avoid raw, uncooked meats and fish. Soak all vegetables in salt water (1 T. per 5 cups water) for 30 minutes and rinse well. Reduce sugar, coffee and dairy products. If dairy is reduced, substitute other calcium sources, such as broccoli.
2) Drink filtered water, especially when traveling.
3) Pomegranate juice may be helpful against tapeworms.
4) Ground pumpkin seeds aid in parasite elimination.
5) Garlic can be used as a vermifuge.
6) A healthy immune system is of primary importance in preventing parasitic infection.
7) Maintain good hygiene. Always wash hands before eating, after handling diapers, playing with pets or using the bathroom. Also, always wash your hands and utensils after handling raw meats and fish.
8) Always check ileocecal valve involvement.

Considerations:

1) Have a stool test done to verify parasitic infection.

2) Mother's milk has anti-protozoan properties. Breast feed as long as possible.
3) Parasitic infections have been associated with numerous diseases including:
    1) Crohn's Disease and Ulcerative Colitis
    2) Chronic Fatigue Syndrome and Epstein-Barr Virus
    3) Arthritis/Rheumatism
    4) Irritable Bowel Syndrome

HEAVY METAL TOXICITY

Any amount of metals which have accumulated in the body (fat cells, brain, glands, Central Nervous System, bones), that negatively affect the body's health. No amount of metals is acceptable to the body, but each person has their own tolerance level. Most common heavy metal toxicities include lead, mercury, arsenic, cadmium and nickel. Aluminum toxicity is common, but aluminum is not considered a heavy metal. Copper and nickel are essential to body function but can also be considered toxic in high amounts.

Signs and Symptoms of Heavy Metal Toxicity:

- Vary greatly depending on type of metal, extent of exposure, age and levels of protective minerals in the body to protect against heavy metal toxicity.

1) **Aluminum**
    Symptoms of toxicity - constipation, colicky pain, nausea and GI problems, anorexia, skin problems, low energy, muscle twitching, numbness, paralysis, osteomalacia, skin rashes, hyperactivity, learning disabilities, decreased liver and kidney function, headaches, ringing in the ears.
2) **Arsenic**
    Symptoms of toxicity - hair loss, dermatitis, GI problems, confusion, headaches, fatigue, muscle pains, neurologic symptoms, liver and kidney problems.
3) **Cadmium**
    Symptoms of toxicity - high blood pressure, kidney damage, increased incidence of kidney stones, depressed immune function, prostate enlargement, bone and joint aches and pains, fatigue, irritability, headaches, hair loss, liver damage, skin problems, weight loss.
4) **Copper**
    Symptoms of toxicity - anxiety, joint and muscle pains, depression, poor memory, insomnia, senility, high blood pressure, hyperactivity, PMS.
5) **Lead**
    Symptoms of toxicity - headache, fatigue, anorexia, constipation, muscle pains, anemia, agitation, poor coordination, depression, insomnia, hyperactivity, reduced immune and kidney function, high blood pressure, poor bone growth, learning disabilities, anxiety, ringing in the ears, GI problems, constipation.
6) **Mercury**
    Symptoms of toxicity - GI problems, nervous system problems, fever, chills, fatigue, headache, insomnia, loss of sex drive, irritability, depression, numbness and tingling in hands, irritability, allergy problems, asthma, may be a factor in MS.
7) **Nickel**
    Symptoms of toxicity - frontal headaches, nausea, vomiting, vertigo, lung problems, allergy reactions, fatigue, heart problems, skin rashes, psoriasis.

Possible Causes:

Methods of toxicity differ for each metal. Exposure can originate from:

1) **Aluminum**

Sources - antacids, over-the-counter drugs, douches, aluminum cookware and aluminum foil, antiperspirants, baking powders, contaminated water, food additives.

Methods of toxicity - not clear; it may interfere with magnesium function, reduce vitamin levels, or bind to DNA. Oral aluminum (antacids) can bind pepsin and weaken protein digestion. Aluminum toxicity can contribute to constipation due to astringent qualities (dries tissues and mucus linings). Underarm deodorants may clog lymphatics. Aluminum has been implicated in Alzheimer's disease. (Haas, Elson, M.D. Staying Healthy With Nutrition. 1992. Celestial Arts, Berkeley, California, 237-250).

2) **Arsenic**

Sources - soil, seafood, fuel oils and coal, weed killers, pesticides, water, laundry aids, tobacco.

Methods of toxicity - unknown

3) **Cadmium**

Sources - cigarette and pipe smoke (cadmium is found in high amounts in tobacco), refined foods, water pipes, coal burning, coffee and tea, shellfish, soft drinks, fungicides and pesticides, plastics.

Methods of toxicity - competes with zinc for binding sites, thus interferes with zinc functions. Cadmium toxicity increases with zinc deficiency May be catalyst to oxidation reactions, which can generate free radical damage. (Haas, Elson, M.D. Staying Healthy With Nutrition. 1992. Celestial Arts, Berkeley, California, pp. 237-250).

4) **Copper**

Sources - drinking water (copper pipes), cookware, oral contraceptives, copper containing supplements, most natural foods (whole grains, shellfish, liver, beans and nuts).

Methods of toxicity - copper is an essential trace mineral in the body. It is important as a catalyst in the formation of hemoglobin, and is part of the cytochrome system for cell respiration. It also converts T3 to T4 and is part of the enzymes histaminase and superoxide dismutase. Recently, however, there has been concern about excess consumption. (Haas, Elson, M.D. Staying Healthy With Nutrition. 1992 Celestial Arts, Berkeley, California ,pp. 237-250).

5) **Lead**

Sources - leaded gasoline, paint, foods, drinking water, pottery, cans, cosmetics, cigarettes, pesticides, eating lead-contaminated liver, air pollution.

Methods of toxicity - interferes with the functioning of calcium, iron, copper and zinc. It can inactivate important zinc and iron dependent enzymes It can displace calcium in the bones and is an immunosuppressant. (Haas, Elson, M.D. Staying Healthy With Nutrition. 1992. Celestial Arts, Berkeley, California, pp. 237-250).

6) **Mercury**

Sources - fungicides and pesticides, cosmetics, dental fillings, seafood, medicines, laxatives, inks used in some printing and tattoos, some types of paint.

Methods of toxicity - attacks the nervous system, interferes with some functions of selenium, acts as an immunosuppressant, and inactivates a wide range of enzyme systems. (Haas, Elson, M.D. Staying Healthy With Nutrition. 1992. Celestial Arts, Berkeley, California, pp. 237-250).

7) **Nickel**

Sources - food, dental metals, jewelry, and inhaled nickel carbonyl. Nickel carbonyl is a carcinogenic gas that results from the reaction of nickel with heated carbon monoxide, from cigarette smoke, car exhaust and some industrial wastes. Metal cooking utensils, hydrogenated fats, and fertilizers are also sources of nickel toxicity.

Methods of toxicity - nickel has been considered as an essential trace mineral for humans. Its function is unclear, but it has been found in high concentrations in RNA, and is thought to be involved in protein structure or function. Toxicity is a concern with nickel. It can accumulate in the lungs and can cause allergy reactions. (Haas, Elson, M.D. Staying Healthy With Nutrition. 1992. Celestial Arts, Berkeley, California, pp. 230-250).

Nutrient Applications:

1) A detoxification program is beneficial
2) Vitamin C to bowel tolerance. Vitamin C should not be taken in iron overload disease, gout and/or kidney stone formers.
3) Multi-mineral formula as a chelating agent
4) Liver glandular
5) Montmorillinite clay to bind toxins
6) Liver glandular
7) B vitamin complex
8) Garlic is a potent detoxifier. Kelp also aids in metal detoxification.
9) Fiber and apple pectin
10) Lecithin - protects the cell membranes

Protective nutrients for each metal:

Aluminum: calcium, magnesium, B-complex, zinc, vitamin C, garlic, kelp

Arsenic: lipoic acid, selenium, vitamin C, L-cysteine (sulfur-containing amino acid to aid in arsenic elimination), L-methionine (amino acid to protect the liver)

Cadmium: zinc, calcium, magnesium, amino acids particularly L-lysine, L-cysteine, L-methionine, L-glutathione and taurine, vitamin C and garlic

Copper: zinc, manganese, molybdenum, iron, pantothenic acid, folic acid, bioflavonoids (rutin) with vitamin C

Lead: calcium, zinc, selenium, iron, vitamin C, flavonoids, choline, amino acids (particularly L-lysine, L-cysteine, and L-methionine)

Mercury: selenium, lipoic acid, manganese, chromium, vitamin C, amino acids (particularly L-cysteine, L-cystine, L-methionine and L-glutathione)

Dietary and Lifestyle Applications:

1) Diet is important. Organic foods should be eaten whenever possible. Garlic and onions (high in sulfur to aid in detoxification), apples, fresh fruits and vegetables, beans and seeds should be emphasized.
2) Drink plenty of filtered water to flush toxins.
3) Eat plenty of fiber, including apple pectin, to bind toxins and pull out of the system.
4) Use stainless steel, iron or glass cookware.
5) Eat pumpkin seeds, which have a high zinc content.
6) Do not smoke.
7) Avoid heavy metal exposure.
8) Carrot, celery, parsley and cucumber juice is suggested.

CHEMICAL TOXICITY

Any amount of chemicals which accumulate in the body and decrease the capacity of the body to function optimally. Liver and kidney damage can occur if the body cannot get rid of the toxins.

Signs and Symptoms of Chemical Toxicity:

- Widely varied; symptomatic picture can range from skin problems and GI symptoms to liver and/or kidney damage.

Possible Causes:

1) Exposure to chemicals in the water, air or food.
2) Weak immune system
3) Liver/kidney problems

Nutrient Applications:

1) A detoxification program is suggested
2) Vitamin C to bowel tolerance. Vitamin C should not be taken in iron overload disease, gout and/or kidney stone formers.
3) L-glutathione - intracellular antioxidant; it is a key amino acid in hepatic detoxification
4) Amino acids - particularly L-cysteine, L-cystine and L-methionine
5) Multi-mineral support as a chelating agent
6) B complex with choline and inositol
7) Liver extract
8) Antioxidants
9) Garlic
10) Coenzyme Q10
11) Liver herbs - milk thistle, dandelion, licorice

Dietary and Lifestyle Applications:

1) Eat organic foods.
2) Short fasts are suggested to decrease level of toxicity.
3) High fiber diets are important to cleanse the body of toxins.
4) Epsom salt baths are helpful. Also skin brushing and saunas may be beneficial.
5) Avoid exposure to chemicals as much as possible.
6) A cleansing fast for three days every month may be helpful.
7) Drink plenty of filtered water to flush toxins.

Considerations:

1) **NOTE:** Aspartame (Nutra-Sweet) is made of phenylalanine, methanol and aspartic acid. Methanol converts to formaldehyde and formic acid, which is highly toxic to the thymus gland.

THE PHYSIOLOGY OF THE MUSCULOSKELETAL SYSTEM

The musculoskeletal system of the body is composed of the skeletal system (bones, cartilage and joints), muscles, ligaments, tendons, and connective tissue, which act in concert together to supply humans with a wide range of movement.

BONES

The 206 bones of the body make up a framework, or skeleton, that give it its structure and shape. They serve to:

1) protect the soft tissues and organs.
2) act as a reservoir of minerals.
3) generate the cells of the blood (including some of the infection-fighting white blood cells).

1) **Protection** - the bony structure of the skeletal system encases vulnerable organs, such as the skull around the brain, and the ribcage around the heart and lungs.
2) **Mineral Reservoir** - Bones are composed of inorganic salts, including calcium and phosphate, which are embedded into collagen. The homeostasis of the blood calcium concentration, necessary for maintaining health, depends on the changes of calcium movement between the blood and the bones. When blood calcium is low, parathyroid hormone works to take calcium out of the "storagehouse" and put it into the blood. If blood calcium is high, the direction of movement would be higher in the other direction, (i.e. into the bone).
3) **Cell Formation** - Red bone marrow is the site for blood cell formation. This includes red blood cells, which perform their function in the blood vessels (their main function is to control hemostasis and blood clotting after injury), and also white blood cells, which perform their function in the tissues (their main function is to phagocytize bacteria and infectious organisms). White blood cells formed from bone marrow include neutrophils, eosinophils, basophils, and some lymphocytes and monocytes.

The intercellular substance of bone makes up the matrix, and contains many fibers of collagen. In the developing fetus, the complex process of ossification changes cartilage and fibrous membranes to bone. Bone-forming cells (osteoblasts) secrete carbohydrate and collagen. The collagen gets embedded in the carbohydrate, or cementing substance, and constitutes the matrix.

Bones grow by the combined action of osteoblasts and osteoclasts. **Osteoclasts** enlarge the area of the bone cavity by eating away at the bone of the cavity walls, and **osteoblasts** build new bone around the perimeter. In childhood and adolescent years, this ossification (bone-building) process exceeds bone destruction; the process evens out in later years, however, and after the age of 35-40, bone loss exceeds bone gain. As thickness of bone decreases, and the size of the cavity increases, bones are less apt to resist compression and bending. Vertebrae collapse, to some extent, causing the decreased height seen in old age. Regular exercise, which subjects bone to a form of stress, forces the bone to lay down more mineral salts and collagen fibers, thereby strengthening the bone.

The difference between the collagen fibers of bone, and that of other connective tissue, is that they are tough and rigid - mainly due to deposits of calcium salts. Bones are living structures, and so must receive food and oxygen, and eliminate metabolic wastes. For this reason, bone is well-perfused with blood vessels.

BONE DISORDERS

Osteoporosis: Osteoporosis involves a loss of calcium and phosphate salts, resulting in bone that is weak, porous, brittle, and very susceptible to breakage. It is characterized by low bone mass, however, the composition of the remaining bone is chemically normal. In other words, there is normal mineralization, but abnormal remodeling, hence lower bone mass. When it occurs in the spine, the vertebrae may get compressed and cause deformities of the spine. Risk factors include a low calcium intake, hormonal changes associated with aging/menopause, amenorrhea, alcoholism, smoking, lactose intolerance, overactive thyroid, and impaired calcium absorption.

Osteomalacia, on the other hand, is characterized by bone that is abnormal, due to impaired mineralization. While it also results in lower bone mass, the remaining bone is not chemically normal. For instance, the mineralization of bone requires phosphorous as well as calcium, and in one type of osteomalacia (Oncogenic osteomalacia), phosphorus and vitamin D are both inhibited. Chronic consumption of phosphate-binding antacids can cause hypophosphatemic osteomalacia (Shils and Young, pp. 864, 878). **Rickets** is a form of osteomalacia defined as defective mineralization, which happens at the epiphyseal plate (of growing bones).

CARTILAGE

Cartilage is very similar to bone, in that it is made up of many collagenous fibers. However, in cartilage, the fibers are embedded in a firm gel, instead of the hard, cement-like substance of bone. This is why cartilage is firm but flexible, while bone is tough and rigid. Oxygen and nutrients have to diffuse into cartilage, because it is not perfused with blood vessels like bone. There are three types of cartilage:

1) **Hyaline -** Hyaline cartilage is the most abundant cartilage, covering the articular surfaces of bones and helping to cushion them from injury.
2) **Fibrous** - Fibrocartilage has the most collagenous fibers in its matrix, and is therefore the strongest. Fibrocartilage is between the disks of the vertebrae, and helps to cushion the spine against jolts.
3) **Elastic** - Elastic cartilage has elastic as well as collagenous fibers, so it is flexible as well as being firm. The external ear and Eustachian tube are composed of elastic connective tissue.

JOINTS

Joints occur between the bones, and hold the bones together, while allowing movement between them. For the most part, people are generally unaware of their joints, unless a tissue dysfunction causes painful awareness. On the basis of structure, there are three main types of joints:

1) **Fibrous** - Fibrous joints are between the articulating surfaces of bones, binding extremely close together and preventing movement, such as skull bones.
2) **Cartilagenous Joints** - Cartilagenous joints are connected by cartilage that allows a minimum amount of movement, such as the vertebrae.
3) **Synovial Joints** - Synovial Joints are freely movable, abundant, and complex joints. They can be characterized by: a joint capsule, a synovial membrane (secretes lubricating synovial fluid), articular cartilage (to cushion the surface of the bones), a joint cavity, menisci (pads of fibrocartilage; the knee has several menisci), and/or ligaments (fibrous connective tissue which holds bone to bone).

JOINT DISORDERS

In a normal joint, the bones are lubricated at their junction by synovial fluid secreted by the synovium, which is a thin membrane on the inside of the ligaments that covers the joint. The ligaments, along with the synovial lining, encapsulate the joint and protect it. In addition, a layer of cartilage also cushions the ends of both bones. In **rheumatoid arthritis**, the synovium becomes inflamed and swollen. This damages the joint capsule and the cushion of cartilage. Without the protective cushion, the ends of the bones start to degrade. Rheumatoid arthritis affects more than 2 million people, most of them women. In **osteoarthritis**, the disease begins with the degeneration of the cushion of cartilage between the joints. As it degrades, the synovium and the ends of the bones thicken, resulting in the pain and stiffness associated with arthritis. Osteoarthritis is the most common form of arthritis, affecting almost 16 million Americans, most of whom are over the age of 45. **Ankylosing spondylitis, or spinal arthritis**, means, "fused spine", and results in rigidity of the spinal column. Inflammation gradually degrades the flexible joints in the lower spine, and can be the cause of low back pain. This disease affects over 300,000 people, most of whom are males.

MUSCLES

There are three types of muscle tissue: **smooth muscle, cardiac muscle, and skeletal muscle.** Smooth muscle lines the arteries and some of the viscera. Cardiac muscle lines the heart. Skeletal muscle, however, is the muscle involved in the framework of the body, in the structural sense. Skeletal muscle accounts for 40-50% of body weight. The skeletal muscles are important in **movement, heat production, and posture.** Because they are so numerous and active, the skeletal muscle cells contract to furnish body heat. Shivering, which is the body's response to cold, generates needed heat. The partial contracted state of some of the skeletal muscles makes sitting, standing, and other positions possible.

Skeletal muscle is made up of lots of fibers, which in turn are made up of smaller fibers called myofibrils. The myofibrils in turn are made up of thick myofilaments (**myosin** molecules), and thin myofilaments (**actin** molecules). Nerve impulses release **calcium** from the **sarcoplasmic reticulum** (a network of tubules and sacs, analogous to the endoplasmic reticulum of other cells) into the **sarcoplasm** (the cytoplasm of the sarcoplasmic reticulum), and calcium binds to the protein **troponin**, allowing myosin to interact with actin. This interaction pulls the thin myofilaments toward the center, shortening the muscle fibers. In short, this is what is called a muscle contraction. Calcium is only available for a few seconds before it firmly binds again to the sarcoplasmic reticulum, which has a high affinity for calcium. This binding process allows for the relaxed state of the muscle.

LIGAMENTS AND TENDONS

Ligaments are strong cords of dense fibrous connective tissue that **connect bone to bone** at most of the synovial joints. While allowing movement, such as at the knee, ligaments provide sturdy support for the joint. **Tendons** are also bands of connective tissue, however, the **connective tissue that surrounds a muscle extends out in a continuous manner until it attaches to bone or another muscle**. Some tendons are encased by a fibrous connective tissue called tendon sheaths, which contain the placement of the tendon. The cavity between the sheath and the tendon contains synovial fluid, permitting easy movement.

CONNECTIVE TISSUE

When **collagen fibers** are laid down, they form a connective tissue which is an essential "body glue". As we have seen, connective tissue, along with carbohydrate and minerals, is a component of bone. Connective tissue embedded in a firm gel is a component of cartilage. **Fascia** is a term that describes the broad band of fibrous connective tissue beneath the skin, or surrounding muscle and various organs. The **superficial fascia** directly under the skin also consists of adipose tissue along with the connective tissue. This superficial fascia serves four important functions:

1) Serves as a storehouse for water and fat.
2) Provides a layer of insulation to shelter from heat loss.
3) Offers mechanical protection from injury.
4) Provides a pathway for nerves and vessels.

Deep fascia is a dense connective tissue that lines the body wall and extremities, holds the muscles together, and separates the muscles into functioning groups. It also carries nerves and blood vessels.

Note: Low back pain is one of the most common ailments reported. Affecting four out of five people at some time, it can result from any combination of the above mentioned structural components: bones (mostly vertebrae), muscles, ligaments - and also the spinal cord and nerves. **Scoliosis**, and also **spondylolithesis** (vertebrae slipping onto other vertebrae) can initiate lower back pain. Additionally, the **disks** of the lower back can **rupture** or **herniate**. The center of the ring may rupture through the outside ring of the disk and impinge on nerves or the spinal cord.

SUBCLINICAL AND PATHOLOGICAL CONDITIONS OF THE MUSCULOSKELETAL AND NERVOUS SYSTEM

MUSCULOSKELETAL PROBLEMS

MUSCLE CRAMPS/SPASMS

Involuntary contraction of the skeletal muscles causing sudden and intense pain; sometimes called a "charley horse".

Signs and Symptoms of Muscle Cramps/Spasms:

- sudden and sharp pain and muscle discomfort
- tightness and/or lump of muscle tissue beneath the skin
- burning sensation in the muscle

Possible Causes:

1) Overuse or injury of the muscle; can occur in athletes who are overfatigued and dehydrated
2) Inactivity or lack of exercise
3) Hypothyroidism
4) Inadequate diet, low in calcium and magnesium or high in foods that decrease calcium availability, such as refined sugars, caffeine, high-phosphate foods, soft drinks and high amounts of meat. Vitamin E deficiency also aggravates muscle cramping.
5) Poor circulation; arteriosclerosis
6) Anemia
7) Heavy coffee consumption
8) Diuretic drugs for heart problems and high blood pressure may also contribute to muscle cramps because they increase mineral loss of key nutrients, including potassium, calcium and magnesium.
9) Stress
10) Diabetes or arthritis
11) Spinal misalignment or residue from past injury
12) Poor posture and/or poor fitting shoes
13) Food allergies/sensitivities
14) Hypoglycemia
15) Growing children
16) Pregnancy

Nutrient Applications:

1) Magnesium - high amounts can be taken, but may cause diarrhea if taken in excess
2) Calcium - popular nutrient for muscle cramps
3) Vitamin E - found to be beneficial for restless leg syndrome (Ayres, S. Jr., Mihan, R. Leg Cramps and Restless Leg Syndrome. A Progress Report on Response to Vitamin E (tocopherol). South Med J. 1974; 67 (11): 1300-12).
4) Potassium - aids in calcium and magnesium metabolism

Dietary and Lifestyle Applications:

1) Diet is important. Eliminate sugar and caffeine from the diet. Increase fiber and protein and enjoy healthy snacks to avoid hypoglycemic symptoms. Increase calcium and magnesium rich foods including green leafy vegetables, fruits (avoid citrus), alfalfa, millet, yogurt, brewer's yeast, kelp, chlorophyll and cornmeal. An alkaline diet is suggested, which includes a high consumption of fruits and vegetables. An alkaline diet will decrease calcium loss. Vitamin E foods including whole grains, raw nuts and seeds are important. High potassium foods may also be helpful.
2) Stretching and strengthening exercises and massage may be beneficial to alleviate spasms.
3) Hot epsom salt baths followed by stretching is suggested. Cold packs may decrease spasm and relax a tensed muscle.
4) Carrot, celery, beet and cucumber juice is suggested.
5) Avoid dehydration. Drink plenty of filtered water.

NOTE: If cramping is due to walking, and stops when you stand still, see your doctor. Impaired circulation (claudication) may be suspect.

BACK PAIN

ACUTE - sudden or immediate pain brought on by quick movement or injury from an accident, fall or by lifting a heavy object.

CHRONIC - pain that develops over time and lasts for a long period of time.

Signs and Symptoms of Back Pain:

- acute or chronic pain in the back area

Possible Causes:

1) Poor posture and movement
2) Poor fitting shoes
3) Poor muscle strength in the back, abdomen, legs or buttocks
4) Spinal misalignment; also foot, knee and leg misalignment
5) Chronic ileo-cecal valve (ICV), due to valves direct association with the lumbar vertebrae
6) Improper lifting
7) Pregnancy or "beer bellies"
8) Kidney/bladder problems, gallstones, adrenal problems, or uterine/ovarian cysts
9) Pelvic disorders
10) Arthritis/rheumatism
11) Abnormal curvature of the spine
12) Stress - physical and/or emotional
13) Bone disease
14) Disc problems

Nutrient Applications:

1) Calcium and magnesium for muscle relaxation
2) Herbal relaxants such as passion flower, valerian, skullcap and feverfew
3) White willow bark - as a natural pain reliever
4) Vitamin C and bioflavonoids to strengthen connective tissues, especially important in smokers who deplete their vitamin C levels
5) Manganese - aid in ligament/cartilage repair
6) Proteolytic enzymes - for inflammation

Dietary and Lifestyle Applications:

1) Prevention is the best medicine. Regular chiropractic care, moderate exercise, stretching and strengthening exercises and a healthy diet are all key to preventing back pain.
2) Bodywork, including massage, may be very beneficial.
3) Yoga, biofeedback, acupuncture and relaxation exercises have all been helpful in relieving or decreasing back pain.
4) Orthotics may be necessary.
5) In acute situations, apply ice for 10 minutes, heat for 5 minutes, ice, heat and ice for same appropriate amount of time, as often as needed. (Burton Goldberg Group, Alternative Medicine: The Definitive Guide, Future Medicine Publishing, Inc. WA, p. 552).
6) Detoxification may be needed.
7) Avoid certain sports that aggravate your condition. Golf, tennis, bowling, baseball and weightlifting all place strains on the back due to twisting motion or heavy lifting. Contact sports such as basketball and football are dangerous to the back.
8) Avoid heavy lifting. Always bend your knees and keep the back straight when lifting, so that you use your leg muscles, not your back.
9) Sleep on a firm mattress and avoid sleeping on your stomach.

ARTHRITIS

Inflammation of the joints surrounding ligaments, tendons or cartilage.that can affect any part of the body. Three most common types of arthritis include **osteoarthritis, rheumatoid arthritis and gout**. Each one will be discussed separately. Other forms of arthritis include systemic lupus (immune system malfunction) and ankylosing spondylitis (affects the joints in the spine which inflame, stiffen up and fuse together).

OSTEOARTHRITIS

Degenerative joint disease that primarily affects the large, weight bearing joints and the joints in the hands. It is seen mainly in the elderly and is the most common form of arthritis.

Disease process - slow, progressive cartilage deterioration is followed by "hardening of the joints" due to calcification and bone spur formation. The "joint cushion" deteriorates, which leads to pain and limited movement of the joint.

Signs and Symptoms of Osteoarthritis:

- early morning joint stiffness
- loss or restriction of joint mobility
- pain that is worse after use
- stiffness after periods of rest
- creaking/cracking of joints after movement
- tenderness and swelling in certain areas
- restricted mobility
- pain in the joint before or during changes in the weather

Possible Causes:

1) Age - Osteoarthritis probability increases with age. In the US, over 80% of the population over 50 shows signs of osteoarthritis. This is due to the decreased ability of the collagen matrix to repair itself, and also from general wear and tear.
2) Obesity
3) Poor diet and exercise regime over a long period of time
4) Genetic predisposition
5) Skeletal defects
6) Hormonal imbalances. **NOTE:** Osteoarthritis increases after menopause.

7) Nutritional imbalances
8) Injury - increases risk of developing osteoarthritis in the injured area
9) Food allergies and sensitivities - NSAIDs increase problem of food sensitivities by creating "leaky gut syndrome". Food elimination/rotation diet is suggested.

Nutrient Applications:

1) Calcium and magnesium - essential for bone/ligament and muscle health
2) Glucosamine sulfate - glucosamine plus sulfur; glucosamine works differently than NSAIDs; NSAIDs inhibit proteoglycan synthesis (cartilage is made from proteoglycans), whereas glucosamine prevents proteoglycan degradation, thus enhancing cartilage production.
3) Antioxidants:
   1. **Vitamin C** - high potency vitamin C aids in collagen formation and cartilage growth; supplementation in guinea pigs was shown to inhibit osteoarthritis progression (Schwartz, E.R. The Modulation of Osteoarthritic Development by Vitamin C and E. Int J Vit Nutr Res. Supple 26: 141-46, 1984). (Vitamin C is contraindicated in iron overload disease, gout and/or kidney stones)
   2. **Vitamin E** - may work like vitamin C to inhibit osteoarthritis progression. Also acts as antioxidant and inhibits the prostaglandins that promote inflammation.
   3. **Selenium and zinc**
4) Proteolytic enzymes (eg. bromelaine) - catalyze oxidative reactions and decrease inflammation.
5) Boron - osteoarthritis patients have shown improvement when supplemented with boron; boron decreases urinary excretion of calcium and magnesium and increases estradiol levels. **NOTE:** The parathyroid gland contains more boron than any other tissue. Boron enhances parahormone activity and the parathyroid gland is the primary organ controlling mineralization of bone. (Burton Goldberg Group, Alternative Medicine: The Definitive Guide, Future Medicine Publishing, Inc. WA, p. 533). Boron may be irritating to premenopausal women.
6) Superoxide Dismutase (SOD) - effective antioxidant, especially in combination with catalase. Manganese enhances SOD activity because it is part of the SOD enzyme.
7) Yucca and Devil's Claw - anti-inflammatory herbs .
8) Shark Cartilage - aids in decreasing joint inflammation and pain. Shark cartilage contains mucopolysaccharides which are carbohydrates that combine with water to stimulate immune function. Supplementation with shark cartilage is thought to repair damaged cartilage. It is also known to have properties that inhibit angiogenesis, which is invasion of new blood vessels in cartilage. **NOTE:** Cartilage does not have a blood supply.
9) Niacinamide - shown to improve joint flexibility.
10) Bee pollen (propolis) and black currant seed oil may also be helpful.
11) Feverfew - decreases inflammation by inhibiting compounds that cause inflammation.
12) Pantothenic Acid - deficiency in rats caused osteoarthritis lesions.
13) Green lipped Mussel Extract - in a New England study, green lipped mussel extract was shown to be beneficial for severe osteoarthritis patients who did not respond to medication. (Werbach, M., M.D., Healing Through Nutrition, Harper Collins Publishers, NY, p. 286).
14) Proanthocyanidins - aid in collagen metabolism and decreasing joint inflammation.

Dietary and Lifestyle Applications:

1) A detoxification program is beneficial.
2) Stress reduction is essential.
3) Proper diet is important. A vegetarian diet is best.
   A. Avoid dairy products, refined foods, meat, citrus fruits and nightshade foods (tomatoes, white potatoes, eggplant, peppers (not black pepper) and margarine.
   NOTE: The nightshade foods are alkaloids that increase inflammation and inhibit collagen repair. They also contain a toxic substance called solanine that triggers reactions in people.
   B. Increase complex carbohydrates, dietary fiber, fruits, vegetables and nuts. Increase cold water fish for an essential fatty acid source (Omega-3) including salmon, mackerel, sardines and

herring. Avoid saturated fats and follow a low-fat diet proportionately rich in polyunsaturated fatty acids (PUFA's).

C. Increase boron-rich foods including alfalfa, lettuce, peas, cabbage, apples, dates, prunes, raisins, almonds and hazelnuts.

D. Sulfur and methionine-containing foods such as legumes, cabbage, brussel sprouts, garlic and onions are also beneficial.

NOTE: Sulfur is an important mineral needed by cartilage tissue. Methionine has shown positive results against rheumatoid arthritis. (di Padova, C. S-adenosylmethionine in the treatment of osteoarthritis. Review of the clinical studies. *Am J Med. 1987;* 83(5A): 60-65).

4) Avoid caffeine, alcohol and tobacco.
5) It is important to avoid allergy foods, since these foods have been associated with osteoarthritis. An elimination/rotation diet is recommended. Avoid environmental toxins as much as possible.
6) Regular chiropractic care is beneficial to address structural/postural problems.
7) Maintain normal weight to avoid added weight bearing stress to the joints.
8) Supplemental cod liver oil may be helpful to decrease inflammation.
9) Drink 6-8 8-ounce glasses of filtered water per day to flush toxins and avoid dehydration. Chronic pain is often associated with chronic dehydration.
10) A half pound of fresh cherries or blueberries per day may be beneficial. They contain proanthocyanidins that aid in collagen metabolism and decrease joint inflammation.
11) Hot baths and hot pads may provide some relief.
12) Avoid smoking.
13) Juicing is good. Pineapple juice, due to its bromelain content, may be helpful. Ginger is also beneficial as an anti-inflammatory agent.
14) Do not take an iron supplement. It may be involved in joint destruction in arthritis due to pro-oxidant effect.
15) Deep massage, such as rolfing, has been shown to be beneficial.

Considerations:

1) Non-steroidal anti-inflammatory drugs (NSAIDs) are the primary drug used to treat osteoarthritis and rheumatoid arthritis. Aspirin is the most common NSAID used. NSAIDs provide temporary relief, but in the long-term they accelerate joint destruction.

   NSAID action: prevent prostaglandin formation in order to decrease inflammation; they also inhibit cartilage synthesis and increase cartilage destruction, thus actually accelerating osteoarthritis progression.

   Side effects: damage to the gastro-intestinal tract and increased ulcer risk. (**NOTE:** "More people die each year as a result of peptic ulcers caused by NSAIDs than from cocaine abuse" (Murray, M. Natural Alternatives to Over-the-Counter and Prescription Drugs, William Morrow and Company, Inc., NY, p. 68). NSAIDs also increase allergies/sensitivities, edema and possibly liver and kidney damage.

RHEUMATOID ARTHRITIS

Degenerative joint disease that primarily affects the synovial tissue (the membranes around the joints that secretes lubricating fluid to allow bones to move easily against each other). Rheumatoid arthritis is an autoimmune disease in which the body attacks its own tissue and causes the joints to become swollen, tender and possibly deformed. Women are most often affected (3:1 ratio) and the disease begins between 20 and 50 years of age. Rheumatoid arthritis can affect any part of the body, including the heart, lungs and eyes and is a very debilitating disease. It is a chronic disease, but does have flare-ups where symptoms are more intense, and then is followed with periods of remission.

Signs and Symptoms of Rheumatoid Arthritis:

- chronic fatigue and weakness
- low grade fever
- joint stiffness and pain

- painful, swollen joints
- inflamed joints
- skin over joint has a purplish color

Possible Causes:

1) Genetic susceptibility
2) Food allergies/sensitivities due to leaky gut problems - theory is that the undigested foods that pass through the intestinal wall deposit in the joints, cause inflammation and the body attacks the joint with the allergy-producing food particles.
3) Poor diet
4) Nutritional imbalance
5) Poor bowel function
6) Dysbiosis
7) Stress that triggers hormonal imbalances
8) Infectious agents

Nutrient Applications:

1) Proteolytic enzymes - anti-inflammatory enzymes; shown to decrease swelling and improve joint mobility.
2) Omega-3 fatty acids (i.e. EPA, DHA) - fish oil source shown to decrease inflammation
3) Antioxidants - free radical scavengers
   1. **Proanthocyanidins (flavonoids)** - grape seed and pine bark extract - powerful antioxidants and collagen protectors.
   2. **Vitamin C with bioflavonoids** - Rheumatoid arthritis patients have decreased vitamin C levels; deficiency can cause spontaneous bruising. (Vitamin C is contraindicated in iron overload disease, gout and/or kidney stones)
   3. **Vitamin E and Selenium** - the two together have been shown to improve rheumatoid arthritis (Munthe, E. and Aseth, J. Treatment of Rheumatoid Arthritis with Selenium and Vitamin E. Scandinavian Journal of Rheumatology, 1984; 53: 103)..
   4. **Zinc** - zinc is decreased in rheumatoid patients.
4) Copper - copper in the serum and in the joints is increased in rheumatoid arthritis, but decreased in the liver. Copper supplementation has been shown to be beneficial for inflammation.
5) Green lipped Mussel Extract - in a New England study, green lipped mussel was shown to be beneficial for severe osteoarthritis patients who did not respond to medication. It may also be helpful in rheumatoid arthritis. (Werbach, M., M.D., Healing Through Nutrition, Harper Collins Publishers, NY, 286).
6) Herbs such as feverfew and devil's claw may be beneficial.

Dietary and Lifestyle Applications:

1) A detoxification program is beneficial.
2) Stress reduction is essential.
3) Proper diet is important. A vegetarian diet is best.
   A. Avoid dairy products, refined foods, meat, citrus fruits, nightshade foods (tomatoes, white potatoes, eggplant, peppers (not black pepper) and margarine.
   NOTE: The nightshade foods are alkaloids that increase inflammation and inhibit collagen repair. They also contain a toxic substance called sotanine that triggers reactions in people.
   B. Increase complex carbohydrates, dietary fiber, fruits, vegetables and nuts. Increase cold water fish for an essential fatty acid source (Omega-3) including salmon, mackerel, sardines and herring. Avoid saturated fats and follow a low-fat diet rich in PUFA's.
   C. Increase boron-rich foods including alfalfa, lettuce, peas, cabbage, apples, dates, prunes, raisins, almonds and hazelnuts.

D. Sulfur and methionine-containing foods such as legumes, cabbage, brussel sprouts, garlic and onions are also beneficial.

NOTE: Sulfur is an important mineral needed by cartilage tissue. Methionine has shown positive results against rheumatoid arthritis. (di Padova, C. S-adenosylmethionine in the treatment of osteoarthritis. Review of the clinical studies. Am J Med. 1987; 83(5A): 60-65).

4) Avoid caffeine, alcohol and tobacco.
5) It is important to avoid allergy foods, since these foods have been associated with osteoarthritis. An elimination/rotation diet is recommended. Avoid environmental toxins as much as possible.
6) Regular chiropractic care is beneficial to address structural/postural problems.
7) Maintain normal weight to avoid added weight bearing stress on the joints.
8) Supplemental cod liver oil may be helpful to decrease inflammation.
9) Drink 6-8 8-ounce glasses of filtered water per day to flush toxins and avoid dehydration. Chronic pain is often associated with chronic dehydration.
10) A half pound of fresh cherries or blueberries per day may be beneficial. They contain proanthocyanidins that aid in collagen metabolism and decrease joint inflammation.
11) Hot baths and hot pads may provide some relief.
12) Avoid smoking.
13) Juicing is good. Pineapple juice, due to its bromelain content, may be helpful. Ginger is also beneficial as an anti-inflammatory agent.
14) Do not take an iron supplement. It may be involved in joint destruction in arthritis due to pro-oxidant effect.
15) Deep massage, such as rolfing, has been shown to be beneficial.

Considerations:

1) Non-steroidal anti-inflammatory drugs (NSAIDs) are the primary drug used to treat osteoarthritis and rheumatoid arthritis. Aspirin is the most common NSAID used. NSAIDs provide temporary relief, but in the long-term they accelerate joint destruction.

   NSAID action: prevent prostaglandin formation in order to decrease inflammation; they also inhibit cartilage synthesis and increase cartilage destruction, thus actually accelerating osteoarthritis progression.

   Side effects: damage to the gastro-intestinal tract and increased ulcer risk. NSAIDs also increase allergies/sensitivities, edema and possibly liver and kidney damage.
2) Blood tests to confirm rheumatoid arthritis include:
   a) Erythrocyte sedimentation rate - determines how fast red blood cells settle to the bottom of a container.
      Too fast = can suggest rheumatoid arthritis (also can suggest anemia, infection, inflammation, rheumatic fever or cancer)
   b) blood test to check for rheumatoid factor (an antibody formed in rheumatoid arthritis)

GOUT

A type of arthritis caused when uric acid crystals accumulate in the joints. Uric acid is a by-product of purine metabolism. Purines can be eaten in foods (mainly meat) or made by the body. Ninety percent of gout sufferers are men over 30. Most first attacks of gout occur at night and involve the joint of the big toe.

Signs and Symptoms of Gout:

- severe pain in the first joint of the big toe
- fever/chills
- constipation/indigestion
- headaches
- heart and/or kidney problems

Possible Causes:

1) Obesity
2) Poor diet
3) Hypertension
4) Metabolic or renal problems - increased production or decreased excretion of uric acid
5) Chronic anemia - causes an increased production of purines
6) Certain types of medications - drugs to treat high blood pressure (i.e. thiazide diuretics) may provoke gout by decreasing water content of the body and increasing uric acid levels.
7) Stress
8) Lead toxicity - has been shown to cause gout. Certain foods such as artichokes, dandelion, carrots, beets, cabbage, grains and beans aid in lead detoxification. (See section on heavy metal toxicity (lead)).

Nutrient Applications:

1) Proteolytic enzymes - anti-inflammatory enzymes; shown to decrease swelling and improve joint mobility.
2) Omega-3 fatty acids (i.e. EPA, DHA) - fish oil source shown to decrease inflammation.
3) Antioxidants - free radical scavengers
   1. **Proanthocyanidins (flavonoids)** - grape seed and pine bark extract - powerful antioxidants and collagen protectors.
   2. **Bioflavonoids** - Rheumatoid arthritis patients have decreased vitamin C levels, and deficiency can cause spontaneous bruising, which can be helped with bioflavonoid supplementation. (Vitamin C is contraindicated in iron overload disease, gout and/or kidney stones). Vitamin C may increase uric acid levels, however adequate serum levels must be obtained.
   3. **Vitamin E and Selenium** - the two together have been shown to improve rheumatoid arthritis (Munthe, E. and Aseth, J. Treatment of Rheumatoid Arthritis with Selenium and Vitamin E. Scandinavian Journal of Rheumatology, 1984, 53: 103).
   4. **Zinc** - zinc is decreased in rheumatoid patients.
4) Folic acid - aids in inhibition of xanthine oxidase, an enzyme which produces uric acid.
5) Devil's Claw - shown to decrease uric acid levels and reduce joint pain.

Dietary and Lifestyle Applications:

1) A detoxification program is beneficial.
2) Proper diet is essential. Eat plenty of fresh fruits and vegetables, grains, nuts and seeds. Cherry juice is excellent. Cherries, strawberries and blueberries contain high amounts of proanthocyanidins, which are powerful flavonoid substances. A low-purine diet is recommended. Purine-rich foods include all meats, herring, asparagus, shellfish, anchovies, sardines, mushrooms, meat-based gravies and broths, yeast and mackerel. Cold water fish is especially high in Omega 3 fatty acids. Avoid refined carbohydrates and saturated fats because sugars increase production of uric acid, while saturated fats decrease excretion of uric acid.
3) Avoid alcohol because alcohol increases uric acid production and decreases excretion. Alcohol also stresses kidney function.
4) Decrease weight if obese. Uric acid levels have been shown to significantly decrease after losing excess weight.
5) Drink plenty of filtered water to promote uric acid excretion and prevent kidney stone formation.
6) Avoid environmental pollutants as much as possible.

Considerations:

1) NSAIDs and a drug called cochicine are used to treat gout.
   A) **Non Steroidal Anti-Inflammatory Drugs (NSAIDs)**

NSAID Action: prevent prostaglandin formation in order to decrease inflammation; they also inhibit cartilage synthesis and increase cartilage destruction, thus actually accelerating osteoarthritis progression.

Side Effects: damage to the gastro-intestinal tract and increased ulcer risk. NSAIDs also increase allergies/sensitivities, edema and possibly liver and kidney damage.

B) **Colchicine** - anti-inflammatory drug that does not affect uric acid levels in the body.

Colchicine Action: works by decreasing joint acidity and dissolving the crystals.

Side Effects: gastro-intestinal problems, fatigue, anemia, hair loss, allergic reactions, numbing, liver damage.

OSTEOPOROSIS

Progressive decrease in bone density, which develops when bone breaks down faster than it can be rebuilt. Women and the elderly are at a high risk. Twenty million Americans are affected with osteoporosis.

Osteoporosis - disease characterized by **quantitatively** low bone mass, but the composition of the remaining bone is chemically normal. (Shils, M. and Young, V. Modern Nutrition in Health and Disease, Lea & Febiger, PA, p. 864).

Osteomalacia - disease characterized by bone that is **qualitatively** abnormal owing to an impaired state of mineralization. When the defective mineralization of cartilage is at the epiphyseal plate of growing bones, it is termed rickets. (Shils, M. and Young, V. Modern Nutrition in Health and Disease, Lea & Febiger, PA, p. 864). Osteomalacia is also known as a "softening of bones."

NOTE:

Osteoblasts - bone cells that build new bones

Osteoclasts - bone cells that break down bone

Signs and Symptoms of Osteoporosis:

- usually symptoms are not present
- spontaneous bone fractures
- painful bones
- severe backache
- curvature of the spine

Possible Causes:

1) Hormonal imbalance (i.e. menopause)
   A) Decreased estrogen and progesterone levels; these hormones play a key role in building bone.
      Estrogen - some control over osteoclasts; aids in decreasing bone loss by slowing bone resorption (bone break down), but does nothing to build bone.
      Progesterone - stimulates osteoblasts to build bones.
2) Poor diet - refined foods, soft drinks, caffeine, excess salt and high amounts of protein all increase risk of osteoarthritis by increasing loss of calcium. A vegetarian diet is best. High protein diets increase ammonia production in the gut, which prevents the kidneys from reabsorbing calcium, thus increasing urinary excretion of calcium.
   NOTE: The blood maintains equal levels of both calcium and phosphorus. For example, if soft drinks, which are high in phosphorus, are ingested, the body will leech calcium from the bones to maintain a balanced level of calcium and phosphorus in the blood.
3) Insufficient weight-bearing exercise. Weight bearing exercises aid in building bone mass.
4) Poor absorption of calcium in the gut due to decreased digestive function (i.e. decreased HCl or pancreatic enzymes) or inadequate levels of vitamin D. Both are required for calcium absorption and vitamin D aids in calcium utilization.
5) Environmental toxins - leech calcium in order to bind toxins.

NOTE: Fluoride, found in our drinking water, has been "shown to increase bone mass, but the resulting bone is abnormal and lacks strength." (Burton Goldberg Group, Alternative Medicine: The Definitive Guide, Future Medicine Publishing, Inc. WA, p. 775). Lead and cadmium toxicity can imbalance mineral content.

6) Dysbiosis or antibiotic use, which decrease good bacteria in the gut. Vitamin K is produced by the "good bacteria" and is needed in building bone.
7) Medications (i.e. corticosteroids, which are similar in function and structure to the adrenal gland hormones) decrease calcium absorption and inhibit osteoblasts (bone building cells). Birth control pills can also create a problem in osteoporosis.
8) Hyperthyroidism or excess thyroid medication - excess thyroxin (thyroid hormone) decreases bone mass by pulling excess minerals out of the bones.

   NOTE: Endocrine problems with the parathyroid or thyroid can effect osteoporosis.

   1. **Parathyroid Gland** - increases blood calcium levels by secreting parathyroid hormone (PTH):

   PTH Functions:
   1) Stimulate osteoclasts, which break down bone.
   2) Decrease urinary excretion of calcium.
   3) Increase calcium absorption in the gut.
   4) Increase vitamin D conversion in the kidneys (vitamin D is needed for calcium absorption in the gut).

   2. **Thyroid Gland** - decreases blood calcium levels by secreting calcitonin.

   Calcitonin Functions:
   1) Stimulate osteoblasts, which build bone.
   2) inhibit osteoclasts and parathyroid hormone (PTH).

   Calcitonin and PTH are controlled by blood calcium levels.

9) Anorexia or decreased body fat - decreases progesterone, which is needed to stimulate osteoblasts.
10) Cigarette smoking - shown to decrease blood estrogen levels, which mediates control over osteoclasts. Decreased estrogen will increase osteoclast activity and enhance bone loss.
11) Trace mineral deficiency
12) Kidney stones/kidney disorders
13) Parathyroid problems
14) Food allergies
15) Excess alcohol consumption

Nutrient Applications:

1) Calcium - excess calcium supplementation (suggested dosage is 800-1000 mg./day) should not be taken without combining with other minerals, especially magnesium, in order to avoid calcium from depositing in the soft tissues, possibly causing kidney stones, arthritis, arteriosclerosis and other problems. Also, an acidifying calcium is the suggested form of calcium to prevent this problem.
2) Magnesium - osteoporosis patients have decreased magnesium levels.

   NOTE: Vitamin D conversion is dependent on a magnesium-containing enzyme. Also, magnesium plays a role in PTH and calcitonin secretion and in activating alkaline phosphatase, the enzyme which aids in forming calcium crystals in bones.
3) Boron - decreases urinary excretion of calcium and magnesium and increases estradiol levels to aid in preventing bone loss. Boron also aids in activating vitamin D to aid in calcium absorption and utilization.
4) Microcrystalline Hydroxyapatite (MCHC) - a veal bone meal that contains calcium, magnesium, phosphorus and other nutrients necessary for bone growth.
5) HCl and enzyme support, if necessary, to absorb nutrients.
6) Vitamin D to aid in calcium absorption and utilization.
7) Vitamin C to aid in collagen synthesis. (Vitamin C is contraindicated in iron overload disease, gout and/or kidney stones)

8) Herbs such as dong quai, licorice root and black cohosh have estrogenic activity (contraindicated in pregnancy). The sterols from wild yam are used as a natural progesterone.
9) Vitamin B-12, folic acid and B-6 have been recommended for osteoporosis.

Dietary and Lifestyle Applications:

1) A vegetarian diet (i.e. low protein, low sugar and low phosphorus diet) is beneficial, possibly due to decreased bone loss in the later years. Avoid refined foods, high protein foods, soft drinks, sugar, dairy products and fried foods. Fatty foods contain fatty acids that form calcium soaps in the gut that interfere with calcium absorption. (Werbach, M., M.D., Healing Through Nutrition, Harper Collins Publishers, NY, p. 286). Alcohol and caffeine should be avoided.
2) Boron-rich foods include whole grains, fruits, vegetables, nuts and seeds. Calcium-rich foods include leafy green vegetables, fish, tofu, yogurt, beans and fish.
3) Drink filtered water that contains no fluoride.
4) Avoid aluminum-containing antacids.
5) Avoid smoking.
6) Be cautious of glucocorticoid medications (i.e. Prednisone).
7) Weight-bearing exercise aids in the building of bone mass.
8) Eat deep red/blue berries such as blueberries, raspberries, cherries, etc., which are high in proanthocyanidins and anthocyanidins. These substances are flavonoids that aid in collagen stabilization.
9) Phytoestrogenic foods, which have weak estrogenic activity, such as papaya, soybean foods, apples, carrots, brown rice, whole wheat and sesame seeds may be helpful.
10) Adequate exposure to sunshine (without burning - sunscreen will minimize risk of skin cancer), to aid in vitamin D production.

Considerations:

1) Many menopausal women take estrogen to prevent osteoporosis. Estrogen has been shown to slow bone loss, but has no effect on building new bone. Long-term use of estrogen does not seem to be the answer since many potential risks accompany long term estrogen use. The risks include salt and water retention, increased fat production, liver problems, heart disease and increased risk of certain types of cancer (uterine and breast).
2) There are two types of bone:
   1) cortical bone - compact bone found mainly in the limbs.
   2) trabecular bone - spongy bone found mainly in the spine and a small amount in the limbs.

   Trabecular bone has a higher osteoporetic tendency because 40% is broken down and rebuilt every year, compared to 10% in cortical bone.
3) Blood test possibly indicating osteoporosis would look as follows:

   Serum calcium - decreased
   Alkaline Phosphatase - normal to decreased
   Serum Phosphorus - increased
   Uric Acid - increased
   TSH (Thyroid Stimulating Hormone) - decreased

FRACTURES/BROKEN BONES

A break in a bone

Signs and Symptoms of a Fracture:

- Can range from no symptoms to severe pain, bruising, inflammation and breakage of the skin
- pain intensified by touching the affected area
- loss of function in the injured area

NOTE: In any fracture a doctor should be consulted immediately.

Possible Causes:

1) Injury
2) Osteoporosis
3) Thyroid or parathyroid problems
4) Bone cancer

Types of Fractures:

1) Closed/Simple fracture - bone does not break through the skin.
2) Open/Compound fracture - bone breaks through the skin.
3) Comminuted fracture - bone is shattered into several pieces.
4) Stress fracture- hairline crack on the bone that is often invisible on an X-ray for up to six weeks.

Nutrient Applications:

1) Raw veal bone (bone meal) - contains necessary nutrients to rebuild bone
2) Calcium and magnesium
3) Vitamin D
4) Parathyroid
5) Vitamin C with bioflavonoids - for bone/muscle trauma and collagen formation (Vitamin C is contraindicated in iron overload disease, gout and/or kidney stones)
6) Proteolytic enzymes - for inflammation
   NOTE: Do not use enzymes directly after surgery, so that necessary scar tissue can form. Start one week to ten days after surgery to aid in breaking up adhesions.

Dietary and Lifestyle Applications:

1) Avoid refined foods, high protein foods, soft drinks, sugar, dairy products and fried foods. Alcohol and caffeine should be avoided.
2) Boron-rich foods include whole grains, fruits, vegetables, nuts and seeds. Calcium-rich foods include leafy green vegetables, fish, tofu, yogurt, beans and fish.
3) Drink filtered water that contains no fluoride.
4) Avoid aluminum-containing antacids.
5) Avoid smoking.
6) Be cautious of glucocorticoid medications (i.e. Prednisone).
7) Eat deep red/blue berries such as blueberries, raspberries, cherries, etc., which are high in proanthocyanidins and anthocyanidins. These substances are flavonoids that aid in collagen stabilization and are powerful antioxidants.
8) Adequate exposure to sunshine (without burning - sunscreen will minimize risk of skin cancer), to aid in vitamin D production.

BONE SPURS

A growth on a bone, usually located in the heel

Signs and Symptoms of Bone Spurs:

- painful, bony growth, usually on the heel

Possible Causes:

1) Tendency to form calcium deposits, as in arthritics

2) Parasympathetic tendency - systemic alkalinity
3) Overweight
4) Calcium metabolism problems

Nutrient Applications:

1) Acidifying calcium - calcium plus HCl
2) Magnesium - balanced ratio of calcium and magnesium
3) Proteolytic enzymes - for inflammation
4) Vitamin C and bioflavonoids - collagen and connective tissue repair (Vitamin C is contraindicated in iron overload disease, gout and/or kidney stones)

Dietary and Lifestyle Applications:

1) A detoxification program is beneficial.
2) Wear proper shoes.
3) Alternating hot and cold foot baths may be helpful. Add chamomile tea to water.
4) Avoid weight-bearing exercises - try swimming or biking.
5) Eat a healthy diet free of refined foods. Keep citrus fruits (alkaline-ash foods) intake to a minimum. Both may alter the mineral balance in the body.

STRAINS, SPRAINS AND OTHER INJURIES

STRAINS - pulled muscle, ligament or tendon caused by overworking or overstretching. If it is a bad strain, muscle fibers actually tear, causing muscle contraction and internal bleeding. Common muscle strains include the hamstrings and the groin area.

Signs and Symptoms of Strains:

- localized pain in area of injury
- tenderness and swelling
- stiffness after 24 hours following injury
- muscle spasms

SPRAINS - damage to the ligaments, which connect bone to muscle, caused by overstretching or overworking the joint. Common joint sprains include the ankles, knees and foot arches.

Signs and Symptoms of Sprains:

- sprains vary in degree from minimal sprains with no ligament tears and mild tenderness to complete tearing of the ligaments and extreme bruising
- rapid swelling
- bruising
- pain and tenderness
- joint dysfunction

Possible Causes:

1) Due to an injury during a sports event and/or any type of exercise.
2) Poor muscle tone and/or poor physical shape.
3) Inadequate stretching and/or warm-up before physical activity.
4) Poor nutritional status.
5) Lifting heavy objects.

6) Prolonged periods of activity without proper rest.
7) Unexpected twisting or other type of movement.
8) HCl and/or pancreatic enzyme deficiency due to decreased nutrient absorption.
9) Hormonal problems.

Nutrient Applications:

1) Proteolytic enzymes - to aid in inflammation
2) Calcium and magnesium
3) Vitamin C with bioflavonoids (Vitamin C is contraindicated in iron overload disease, gout and/or kidney stones)
4) Valerian, passion flower, skullcap and chamomile - natural herbal muscle relaxers
5) White willow bark - natural herbal pain reliever
6) Multiple vitamin/mineral supplement to aid in all aspects of healing

Dietary and Lifestyle Applications:

1) Use the RICE method - REST, ICE, COMPRESSION, ELEVATION for initial stages of injury (first 24-36 hours following injury). Ice for 20 minutes out of every hour. After the initial stage, you can ice for twenty minutes and then alternate ice with moist heat (20 minutes each), ending with ice treatment. This will aid in increasing circulation for healing.
2) With a serious strain/sprain, it is important to see a doctor immediately.
3) A healthy diet is beneficial.
4) Drink plenty of filtered water. Avoid dehydration.
5) Avoid heavy lifting or exercise, especially until fully healed.
6) **PREVENTION:** Always incorporate proper stretching, strengthening and warm-up/cool down exercises when participating in any type of exercise regime to aid overall flexibility and muscle strength.
7) Skilled massage therapy may be very beneficial.

INFLAMMATION

Swelling, heat or pain due to injury, trauma, infection or toxins.

Signs and Symptoms of Inflammation:

- swelling
- redness
- heat
- pain

Possible Causes:

1) Injury/trauma (i.e. sprain/strain)
2) Infection (i.e. bacterial)

Nutrient Applications:

1) Proteolytic enzymes - to aid in inflammation
2) High potency vitamin C with bioflavonoids - Vitamin C should not be taken in iron overload disease and/or kidney stone formers.
3) Beta-carotene
4) Zinc
5) Garlic - anti-infectious agent
6) Vitamin A and E emulsion

7) Essential fatty acids

Dietary and Lifestyle Applications:

1) Use the RICE method - REST, ICE, COMPRESSION, ELEVATION for initial stages of injury (first 24-36 hours following injury). Ice for 20 minutes out of every hour. After the initial stage, you can ice for twenty minutes and then alternate ice with moist heat (20 minutes each), ending with ice treatment. This will aid in increasing circulation for healing.
2) Diet is important. Avoid meat and animal fats to decrease arachidonic acid (pro-inflammatory). Eat fish for EPA source, which decreases leukotriene (pro-inflammatory) production. Eat organic fruits and vegetables. Avoid all refined foods, sugar, soft drinks and white flour products.
3) Increase garlic consumption, which is an anti-infectious agent.
4) Drink plenty of filtered water.

BURSITIS/TENDONITIS

Bursitis: inflammation of the bursa, a sac-like membrane found in the joints. The bursa contains fluid that acts as a cushion between the bones and the muscles. The fluid lubricates the joints.

Signs and Symptoms of Bursitis:

- pain and swelling in the affected joint, especially on movement
- restricted range of motion
- most often affects the joints of the elbow, hip, knee and shoulder

Tendonitis: inflammation of the tendon, which is a type of connective tissue that attaches muscle to bone. It usually affects the synovial membrane at the joint and therefore may be called tenosynovitis.

Signs and Symptoms of Tendonitis:

- pain and tenderness at the affected tendon
- restricted range of motion
- most often affects the elbow (i.e. tennis elbow), shoulder, thumb, knee and Achilles tendon

Possible Causes:

1) Injury or repeated trauma
2) Excessive use or strain
3) Calcium deposits
4) Allergies (food and/or environmental)
5) Certain diseases have an increased tendency to develop tendonitis including autoimmune disorders (rheumatoid arthritis), gout and people with high cholesterol levels.

Nutrient Applications:

1) Proteolytic enzymes - to aid inflammation
2) High potency vitamin C - to aid in collagen formation. Collagen is the main constituent of connective tissue. (Vitamin C is contraindicated in iron overload disease, gout and/or kidney stones)
3) Flavonoids - to decrease inflammation and for collagen-stabilizing effect
4) Acidifying calcium - to mobilize calcium deposits

Dietary and Lifestyle Applications:

1) Rest is essential. Follow the RICE method. REST, ICE, COMPRESSION, ELEVATION for initial stages of injury (first 24-36 hours following injury). Ice for 20 minutes out of every hour. After the initial stage, you can ice for twenty minutes and then alternate ice with moist heat (20 minutes each), ending with ice treatment. This will aid in increasing circulation for healing.
2) Consult a chiropractor to facilitate healing.
3) Avoid the nightshade foods (tomatoes, white potatoes, eggplant, peppers (not black pepper).
4) Avoid food allergies. Follow an elimination/rotation diet.
5) After acute stage, flexibility exercises (gentle range of motion exercises) are important to prevent joint stiffness and/or frozen shoulders and other joints.
6) To prevent reoccurrence, always warm up and cool down after exercising. Stretching and strengthening exercises are helpful.
7) Ultrasound (sound vibrations that are directed with heat into the injured area to increase blood flow and lymphatic drainage) is helpful to aid in recovery or remove adhesions or calcification. A TENS (Transcutaneous Electrical Nerve Stimulation) unit is beneficial to relieve pain.

CARPAL TUNNEL SYNDROME

Compression of the median nerve in the wrist that is very painful. The "carpal tunnel" is a passageway through the wrist which is comprised of bones and ligaments that protect the nerves and tendons extending into the hand. If the tissue in the tunnel becomes inflamed, the median nerve is compressed, resulting in pain.

Signs and Symptoms of Carpal Tunnel Syndrome:

- numbness and tingling sensation in the hands and fingers
- wrist pain that shoots up the forearm or into the hands and fingers
- "pins and needles" sensation in the hands
- symptoms usually worse in the evening
- occurs in one or both hands

Possible Causes:

1) Repetitive stress and strain to the wrists due to particular occupation or sport (i.e. typists, carpenters, blacksmiths, factory workers, grocery clerks, golfers, etc.)
2) Edema which can create pressure on the nerve as in pregnancy
3) Endocrine disorders such as hypothyroidism and diabetes
4) Misalignment of the spine, mainly the sixth cervical
5) Rheumatism or osteoarthritis
6) Nutrient deficiencies, mainly vitamin B-6
7) Trauma/injury
8) Muscle spasms
9) Known side effect of lithium therapy

Nutrient Applications:

1) Vitamin B-6 (pyridoxine) - people with carpal tunnel syndrome have been noted to exhibit marginal B-6 deficiencies. Vitamin B-6 should be combined with magnesium to enhance effect. **NOTE:** High dosages of B-6 (>250 mg. daily) for long periods of time can create a nerve disorder called sensory neuropathy.
2) B-complex - high potency to provide B vitamin support
3) Proteolytic enzymes - to aid inflammation
4) Relaxing/pain relieving herbs including valerian, passion flower, skullcap, chamomile and white willow bark.

Dietary and Lifestyle Applications:

1) A whole foods diet is important. Limit protein intake to 50 grams per day. Avoid foods containing yellow dyes, as both inhibit metabolism of B-6. Also avoid processed, refined foods such as sugar, caffeine and soda pop that deplete the body of essential nutrients, especially B vitamins.
2) Rest the joint when possible.
3) Avoid antidepressant drugs because, in some cases, carpal tunnel is a known side effect of this type of therapy.

Considerations:

1) Carpal tunnel syndrome is more common in women 35 and over, especially if they are menopausal or taking oral contraceptives.

HEADACHES

Pain in the head due to a variety of different reasons. The intensity, location and frequency of the headache varies greatly from person to person. Headaches are a very common health complaint and are triggered from outside the brain tissue, since the brain itself does not have any sensory nerves. Only certain areas of the head actually feel pain and these include the skin and tissues directly beneath the skin, the arteries, veins, cranial and cervical nerves.

Types of Headaches:

1) **Muscle Contraction Headaches** - caused by a muscle contraction.
   A) **Tension Headaches** - most common; thought to be caused by "a spastic contraction of the cranial and cervical muscles on the outside of the skull and blood vessel enlargement in the scalp" (Larson, D., M.D. Mayo Clinic Family Healthbook, William Morrow and Company, Inc., NY, p. 547). This contraction can be due to subluxations of the spine, stress and anxiety, poor posture, metabolic/digestive problems, or a poor diet.

   #### *Signs and Symptoms of Tension Headaches:*

   - dull pain in the back of the neck, temples and scalp

2) **Vascular Headaches** - caused by vascular irregularities
   A) **Migraine Headaches** - intense, sharp pain associated with altered dilation and constriction of the blood vessels in the head. Migraines affect more females than males due to hormonal changes. There are three types of clinical patterns associated with migraines:
      1) **Classic Migraines** - "auras" accompany the migraine which include blurred vision, flashes of light, dizziness, numbness on one side of the body and muddled thinking that occurs 20 minutes before the headache pains start.
      2) **Common Migraines** - no warning signs or "auras" before the headache.
      3) **Complicated Migraines** - neurological symptoms that last even after the headache disappears, such as numbness, tingling, speech problems, etc.

   B) **Cluster Headaches** - most painful; affects mostly men who are Type A personalities and heavy smokers. Some believe that cluster headaches are related to a chemical in the brain that causes blood vessels to enlarge and cause pain.

   #### *Signs and Symptoms of Cluster Headaches:*

   - intense burning pain located usually around the eyes and temples that usually occurs in episodes at the same time every day for several days and then returns every few months
   - watery eyes

- ➢ nasal congestion
- ➢ no warning signs

C) **Caffeine Withdrawal Headaches** - dull, throbbing head pain due to caffeine withdrawal

Possible Causes:

1) Food allergies/sensitivities - usually favorite foods; this is a major cause of most headaches
2) Chemical/environmental allergies - i.e. MSG, sulfites, pollution, perfumes, etc.
3) Stress/anxiety
4) Hormonal imbalances
5) Genetic predisposition - over half of migraine sufferers have a history of migraines in their family
6) Head trauma
7) Candidiasis
8) Dental problems - a dentist should be consulted if this cause is suspect
9) Smoking - nicotine causes blood vessels to constrict, while carbon monoxide causes them to dilate, setting up a scenario for migraines and cluster headaches
10) Spinal misalignments, pelvic or foot problems - chiropractic care is recommended
11) Poor posture - creates muscular tension that could trigger a headache
12) Toxic colon - bad bacteria can convert tyrosine in the gut to tyramine, which increases blood pressure and can cause headaches
13) Toxic liver
14) Eye strain - eyeglasses will eliminate this problem
15) Excess salt intake, aspartame (NutraSweet) or MSG
16) Platelet aggregation - blood clotting which constricts the arteries and decreases blood to the brain
    NOTE: Migraine sufferers have increased serotonin levels (a vasoconstrictive neurotransmitter) that enhances artery constriction; serotonin is released when catecholamine (adrenaline and noradrenaline) levels rise due to stress.
17) Poor diet and nutrient deficiencies
18) Heavy metal toxicity
19) Anemia
20) Reactive hypoglycemia - need to stabilize blood sugar to avoid headache stimulus
21) Hypertension
22) TMJ (Temporomandibular Joint)
23) Alcohol abuse
24) Weather changes
25) Caffeine or other drug withdrawal

Nutrient Applications:

1) Essential fatty acids including EPA (Omega-3 fish oil), and black currant seed oil to decrease platelet aggregation and provide anti-inflammatory substances to prevent vasoconstriction. (McCarron et al. Ameliorations of Severe Migraines by Fish Oil (Omega-3) Fatty Acids. AJCN 1986; 43:710).
2) Herbs to aid in headache relief:
    A) Feverfew - shown to decrease intensity and frequency of migraine attacks. Feverfew inhibits serotonin secretion, inhibits the production of pro-inflammatory substances such as prostaglandins, leukotrienes and thromboxane and decreases vasoconstriction.
    B) Valerian - relaxing, sedative, anti-spasmodic herb
    C) Skullcap and passion flower - natural herbal relaxants for tension
    D) Turmeric - natural anti-inflammatory
    E) Ginger - decreases inflammation in the liver and stomach
    F) White Willow Bark - natural pain reliever; contains salicylic acid, which is a natural forerunner of aspirin
3) Niacin - beneficial due to vasodilating effects; do not use with cluster headaches or in high amounts

4) Magnesium (Mg) - low levels are found in migraine sufferers; Mg maintains blood vessel tone and prevents muscle spasm; it also aids in people with mitral valve prolapse, which is a common problem associated with migraines.
5) Vitamin C with bioflavonoids (Vitamin C is contraindicated in iron overload disease, gout and/or kidney stones)
6) Goldenseal - to prevent tyrosine conversion in the bowel to tyramine. Tyramine is structurally similar to the catecholamines, but has weaker action.

Dietary and Lifestyle Applications:

1) Avoid food allergies. An elimination/rotation diet is suggested.
2) A detoxification program is suggested. This may make symptoms worse for the first few days.
3) Avoid environmental pollutants and chemical additives as much as possible.
4) A whole foods diet is suggested. Eat non-allergenic whole grains, organic poultry and fish, fresh fruits and vegetables. Avoid refined foods including caffeine, soda pop, chocolate, all food additives, dairy products, red meats and alcohol. If reducing dairy products, substitute other calcium sources. (**NOTE:** Cheese, sour cream, chocolate and alcohol contain vasoactive amines (i.e. tyramine) that trigger vasoconstriction). Partially hydrogenated oils (margarine, shortenings and fast foods) should be avoided. Red wine has been known to trigger migraine attacks, possibly by inhibiting an enzyme that breaks down these vasoactive amines. Chocolate alters copper metabolism, which is necessary for normal blood flow.
5) Chiropractic care is essential. Spinal manipulation is important for headache sufferers to eliminate the nerve impingement and postural imbalance.
6) Stress reduction is important. Meditation, biofeedback, massage, yoga and any other form of stress relief is beneficial to decrease the frequency and intensity of the headaches. Progressive relaxation exercises, where every part of the body is tightened then released in succession, is a good idea. Acupuncture treatment is also highly recommended.
7) Hot baths, steam rooms and saunas are helpful to relieve stress and increase circulation, which aids in removal of toxic metabolites. Cold pack applications to the head, in conjunction with hot foot baths may be beneficial.
8) A TENS (Transcutaneous Electrical Nerve Stimulation) unit has been shown to be beneficial.
9) Cayenne pepper may be helpful due to its major ingredient, capsaicin. Capsaicin aids in pain relief and inhibits platelet aggregation.
10) Avoid Nutra-Sweet, Equal, Accent, MSG and nitrites (salami, pepperoni, hot dogs and sausage). Most contain tyramine and phenylalanine, which are amino acids that may trigger headaches. Tyramine has been shown to increase blood pressure, causing dull aches in the head.
    NOTE: Dysbiosis can cause the amino acid tyrosine to be converted to tyramine by the bad bacteria in the gut. Berberine, found in goldenseal, prevents this conversion (Murray, M. and Pizzorno, J. Encyclopedia of Natural Medicine, Prima Publishing, CA, p. 420).

Considerations:

1) Drugs used to treat headaches include NSAIDs (i.e. aspirin and ibuprofen) and acetaminophen (i.e. Tylenol). Ergotamine is a drug commonly used to treat migraines.
    A) **Non Steroidal Anti-Inflammatory Drugs (NSAIDs)** - Aspirin and Ibuprofen (i.e. Advil)
    NSAID Action: prevent prostaglandin formation in order to decrease inflammation.
    Side Effects: damage to the gastro-intestinal tract and increased ulcer risk. NSAIDs also increase allergies/sensitivities, edema and possibly liver and kidney damage.
    B) **Acetaminophen (i.e. Tylenol)**
    Action: affects hypothalamus to inhibit pain messages.
    Side effects: easier on the stomach than most NSAIDs because acetaminophens do not inhibit mucus-producing prostaglandins. They can cause liver/kidney damage, allergic reactions, vomiting, indigestion and shortness of breath.
    C) **Ergotamine** - a commonly used drug for migraines.

Action: constricts blood vessels in the head preventing the pain caused from overdilation of the vessels during a migraine.

Side effects: diarrhea, vomiting, dizziness, nausea, foot and ankle edema; can increase the frequency or severity of headaches.

2) Serotonin is made from the amino acid tryptophan. Serotonin decreases pain sensations, but increased levels have been shown to initiate migraines in some people.

NERVE PROBLEMS

SCIATICA

Inflammation and pain radiating down the sciatic nerve, from the back into the buttocks and down the leg, usually on the posterior (back), lateral (outward) side of the leg.

NOTE:

Sciatic Neuritis - sciatic pain due to inflammation; best treated with manipulation and diet.

Sciatic Neuralgia - sciatic pain due to irritation from a herniated disk or other outside mechanism (bone pain, muscle spasm, etc.).

Signs and Symptoms of Sciatica:

- severe pain along the sciatic nerve (back, buttocks and down the outside of the leg)

Possible Causes:

1) Herniated (slipped) disk
2) Back injuries
3) Pressure on the nerve due to injury or over-exertion
4) Osteoarthritis
5) Chronic injuries
6) Can be associated with diabetes or gout
7) Nutrient deficiencies
8) Referred pain from malfunction of internal organs
9) Stress (physical and/or emotional)
10) Liver stress
11) Low thyroid function
12) Obesity
13) Build up of lactic and pyruvic acid along the nerves, which irritate the nerve endings. May be due to metabolism problems.

Nutrient Applications:

1) Proteolytic enzymes - to relieve inflammation
2) Calcium and magnesium - natural muscle relaxants
3) Valerian, passion flower, skullcap and chamomile - natural herbal muscle relaxers
4) White willow bark - natural herbal pain reliever
5) Vitamin B complex - to aid metabolism and relieve stress

Dietary and Lifestyle Applications:

1) Chiropractic care is essential to remove sciatic nerve interference. Sciatic pain can be due to subluxation of the spine, pelvis, etc., herniated disk, muscle spasms, nerve irritation or injury.
2) To prevent chronic musculoskeletal problems, proper stretching and strengthening exercises are important to avoid weak muscles, which imbalance the body and create problems.
3) Eat a healthy diet. Avoid sugar, caffeine and soda pop, which rob the body of essential nutrients.

4) Decrease weight if necessary.

NEURITIS/NEURALGIA

Neuritis: inflammation of a nerve or group of nerves.
Neuralgia: spasms and pain along the length of a nerve.

Signs and Symptoms of Neuritis/Neuralgia:

- mild to severe pain, tingling and loss of feeling in a nerve area
- redness and inflammation along the nerve
- burning pain

Possible Causes:

1) Nutrient deficiency, specifically B vitamins and/or calcium/magnesium imbalance
2) Thyroid imbalance
3) Infection along the nerve
4) Injury or irritation of the nerve
5) Herpes simplex virus or shingles
6) Heavy metal toxicity (i.e. lead, mercury)
7) Associated diseases such as gout, leukemia or diabetes
8) Alcohol abuse
9) Bone fractures
10) Acid/alkaline imbalance (i.e. acidosis - excess lactic and pyruvic acid on the nerve endings)

Nutrient Applications:

1) B complex, especially thiamine, folic acid, B-12 and niacin
2) Lecithin - aids in nerve support
3) Calcium and magnesium - important for nerve conduction and as muscle relaxants
4) Proteolytic enzymes - may be beneficial in neuritis for the inflammation
5) Natural herbal remedies including: passion flower, valerian, chamomile, skullcap, white willow bark, and prickly ash bark

Dietary and Lifestyle Applications:

1) Eat a healthy diet. Avoid foods that stimulate the nervous system such as caffeine, chocolate, refined sugars, soda pop and cigarettes.
2) Drink plenty of filtered water.
3) Chiropractic care is beneficial to remove nerve irritation.

SHINGLES

Acute infection of the central nervous system that is caused by the herpes zoster virus. It affects the nerve endings in the skin. The virus can lay dormant in the spine and nerve ganglia for years until it is reactivated later in life due to a stress or trauma. **NOTE:** The herpes zoster virus also causes chicken pox.

Signs and Symptoms of Shingles:

- intense pain in the affected area for 3-4 days, followed by an outbreak of excruciatingly painful, itchy blisters
- usually occurs in the waist area under the ribs
- blisters heal within 1-2 weeks and form scabs that fall off

Possible Causes:

1) Weak immune system, especially due to HIV, Hodgkin's disease and other types of cancer, severe trauma and high levels of stress
2) Anti-cancer medications
3) Long-term corticosteroid use
4) Chicken pox virus that lies dormant until reactivated by a major stressor

Nutrient Applications:

1) Immune support including vitamin C with bioflavonoids, B-complex, vitamins A and E, zinc, selenium, echinacea, goldenseal and thymus support. (Vitamin C is contraindicated in iron overload disease, gout and/or kidney stones)
2) L-lysine - amino acid that aids in herpes virus
3) Calcium and magnesium - for nerve function and relief as antistressors
4) Proteolytic enzymes - aids in pain relief due to swelling or inflamed nerve endings

Dietary and Lifestyle Applications:

1) A detoxification program is beneficial.
2) A TENS (Transcutaneous Electrical Nerve Stimulation) unit may be effective in relieving the pain.
3) Eat a healthy diet including raw fruits and vegetables, whole grains, brewer's yeast and brown rice. Avoid refined carbohydrates.
4) Add cayenne to foods. An ingredient found in cayenne, capsaicin, has been shown to offer relief of pain.
5) Avoid scratching or itching the blisters.
6) Baths at body temperature are helpful.
7) Red pepper ointment, applied topically, can be helpful for the pain. Exhibit caution, as sensitivities may exist.

THE PHYSIOLOGY OF THE CARDIORESPIRATORY SYSTEM

Every cell in the body depends on the cardiorespiratory system for delivery of life-giving oxygen. Without oxygen, cells cannot metabolize, and eventual death of the cell results. The lungs and tissues of the respiratory system must first draw the ambient air into the body. A control center in the brain regulates the reflex to breathe, and a concerted effort with the muscular action of the diaphragm causes the inflation of the lungs and entry of oxygen into the body. The heart and the rest of the cardiovascular system are responsible for pumping that oxygen to every living cell in the body. The oxygen diffuses into blood from the lungs. The blood/oxygen travels by way of vessels (left pulmonary artery) to the left side of the heart, where it is pumped out to the tissues. The blood picks up the carbon dioxide and metabolic wastes from the cells, returns to the right side of the heart, gets pumped to the lungs, where it can get reoxygenated to start the cycle again.

THE RESPIRATORY SYSTEM

UPPER RESPIRATORY SYSTEM: Air is taken in through the **nose** and **mouth**, where it meets in a common passageway of the **pharynx.** The nose is equipped to warm, moisten, and filter the air. It then passes through the **larynx**, which connects the pharynx to the **trachea,** or windpipe.

LOWER RESPIRATORY SYSTEM: The trachea consists of a mucosa, submucosa, cartilaginous layer, and adventitia. The epithelium lining the trachea protects it from dust. The cartilaginous layer consists of incomplete rings of hyaline cartilage. Smooth muscle and elastic connective tissue provide a firm support so that air is not obstructed. The trachea terminates in the chest and then divides into two **bronchi**: the **right primary bronchus**, and the **left primary bronchus**. The right bronchus connects to the right lung, while the left bronchus connects to the left lung.

The **lungs** are the two organs which are set in the **thoracic (chest) cavity**. The medial surface of each lung has a vertical slit, called the **hilus**, which is where the **bronchi, pulmonary vessels, lymphatics, and nerves** enter and exit. These various structures are all held together by the **pleura** (a layered membrane whose outer layer lines the thoracic cavity, and whose inner layer lines the lungs) and **connective tissue.** The **pleural cavity** is between the two layers of membrane, and is filled with a fluid secreted by the membranes, which allows for easy movement during the breathing process.

The bronchi divide again after entering the lungs, to form smaller bronchi (**secondary bronchi**), which branch to even smaller bronchi (**tertiary bronchi**), which branch into smaller **bronchioles**, and finally into **terminal bronchioles**. With the continual branching of the bronchi to eventual bronchioles, it is no surprise that it is sometimes referred to as the, "bronchial tree". Terminal bronchioles gradually branch into tiny **respiratory bronchioles**. Consequently, the respiratory bronchioles divide again into several **alveolar ducts**. Surrounding the alveolar ducts are the **alveoli**, which are thin, elastic pouches. When two or more of these pouches share the same opening, they are referred to as an **alveolar sac.**

The important exchange of gases between the lungs and the heart occurs across a membrane between the alveoli and the blood capillaries. This membrane is called the **alveolar-capillary membrane.** When fresh air comes into the lungs, it travels all the way to the alveolar sacs, crosses the membrane into the blood, reoxygenates the blood returning from tissues, and gets delivered to the **heart** (via the pulmonary veins), which then pumps the life-giving oxygen throughout the body. While the heart has long been used as the symbol of life and love, the lungs, as we have seen, are equally important in their role of oxygen delivery.

RESPIRATORY DISORDERS

As the branching of the bronchioles continues, the appearance of cartilage lessens, and the appearance of smooth muscle increases. This becomes important in a clinical sense, because the smooth muscle goes into spasm during an **asthma attack**, which is usually triggered by an allergic reaction. With no cartilage to support the airways, the spasms can shut off the passageway. The alveoli sometimes remain inflated during exhalation. The mucus membranes secrete excess mucus, clogging the passageway further.

Bronchitis arises from an infection, which causes inflammation of the bronchioles and results in oversecretion of mucus from the mucus lining of the respiratory tract. A cough usually develops that rids the body of the thick sputum that is created. Smoking is the biggest risk factor for bronchitis; other factors include family history, air pollution, respiratory infections, and a deficiency in antibodies, especially IgA antibodies.

Emphysema literally means, "full of air". The walls of the alveoli lose their elastic quality, and cannot force the air out during expiration. This can damage alveoli, and interfere with gas exchange. The waste from metabolizing cells, ie carbon dioxide, cannot easily cross the barrier, which becomes tough, fibrous connective tissue. This causes resistance to the blood flow, and the heart gets overworked trying to push blood through the capillaries. Emphysema is usually a result of an irritation that has been present for some time. Cigarette smoke, air pollution, and industrial dust are the worst offenders. The disease can be prevented/halted by elimination of the offenders.

Bronchial asthma, bronchitis, and emphysema are similar diseases, in that they all involve an interference of the air passageways. For this reason, they are referred to by the general definition of **chronic obstructive pulmonary disease (COPD).**

Pneumonia is a bacterial infection which causes inflammation of the alveoli. The dead white blood cells from fighting the infection, along with fluid, fill the alveolar sacs. Oxygen cannot pass through the inflamed sacs easily and therefore cannot get to the tissues.

THE CARDIOVASCULAR SYSTEM

The cardiovascular system is composed of the **heart**, the **blood vessels,** and the **blood.** The cardiovascular system is responsible for delivery of oxygen to the cells of the body. The **blood** carries the oxygen, the **vessels** provide the passageway, and the **heart** provides the pump to ensure that living cells, especially brain cells, do not suffer from a lack of this elemental gas.

The **blood** can be thought of as a transportation fluid; the fluid part of the blood is called **plasma,** while the solid part is made up of cells: **red blood cells, white blood cells**, and **platelets.** The red blood cells have **hemoglobin** in them, which binds to the oxygen, allowing for transportation of the oxygen through the **blood vessels**. The blood vessels can be thought of as a conduit system, which delivers fresh oxygen from the lungs to the heart/tissues, and also returns blood (with carbon dioxide) to the heart, so that the heart can pump the deoxygenated blood back to the lungs in order to pick up more oxygen. In addition to carrying oxygen and carbon dioxide, the blood carries water, nutrients, hormones, enzymes, vitamins, antibodies, and other proteins. For instance, the blood is important in temperature regulation and plays an important role in eliminating metabolic wastes through excretory pathways; it also delivers substances in need of detoxification to the liver.

The conduit system consists of three types of blood vessels: **arteries, veins,** and **capillaries.** The arteries carry blood away from the heart, and branch into tinier **arterioles.** The veins carry blood back to the heart, and branch into smaller little **venules**. The capillaries are so tiny that they are microscopic; they connect the arterioles to the venules, and allow for gaseous exchange. The arteries are composed of three layers:

1) **Outer layer** (tunica **adventitia**) is made up of fibrous connective tissue, and provides support for the rest of the vessel, similar to the outside tubing of a hose. Vessels receive their own blood supply on the outside of the adventitia.

2) **Middle layer** (tunica **media)** is made up of smooth muscle tissue, so it is mostly elastic. The smooth muscle tissue controls the constriction and dilation of the arteries.
3) **Innermost layer** (tunica **intima**) is next to the blood, and is composed of endothelial cells. It is this innermost lining of the arteries that is affected by fatty plaque formation, which obstructs circulation through the arteries.

Veins have the same three layers, however, these layers are much thinner in the veins. Since there is not as much smooth muscle, the veins rely partially on skeletal muscle contraction to help return blood to the heart. **Semilunar valves** are present at intervals in the veins, and they prevent a backflow of blood. Stretching of the walls in the veins, particularly around these valves, can result in **varicose veins.**

As the veins bring deoxygenated blood back from the tissues, they dump into the **right atrium** of the heart, which is one of the heart's **four chambers**. Blood from the upper body comes into the atrium through the **superior vena cava,** and blood from the lower body comes through the **inferior vena cava.** The blood then passes through a valve (the **atrioventricular (AV) valve, or tricuspid valve**) into the right ventricle, another chamber of the heart. It is then pumped through a **semilunar valve** up to the lungs by way of the pulmonary artery, to get reoxygenated.

Once the blood picks up fresh oxygen, it returns to the heart via the pulmonary vein, and dumps into the left atrium, a third chamber of the heart. It then passes through a **left AV valve, or bicuspid valve** into the **left ventricle,** a fourth chamber of the heart. Blood passes through a **semilunar valve** into the main **aorta,** and the blood is then perfused throughout the body. The conduction system of the heart allows for **contraction and relaxation.** During **contraction**, the right side of the heart is pumping blood to the lungs, and the left side of the heart is pumping blood to the tissues. During **relaxation**, the right side of the heart is filling with blood from the veins, and the left side is filling with freshly oxygenated blood returning from the lungs.

The heart is living tissue which must have its own constant blood supply. The **coronary arteries** are the arteries which feed the heart. When these coronary arteries are obstructed, by a thrombus or plaque formation, it can interrupt the oxygen supply to the heart and cause tissue death (**myocardial infarction).** "It has recently been learned that under some conditions most tissue damage occurs when blood flow is restored (reperfusion) to an area, not when it is interrupted. When blood supply is interrupted, the affected tissue produces an enzyme called xanthine oxidase. When blood is restored, the enzyme reacts with oxygen in the blood to produce superoxide free radicals, which cause the tissue damage. Attempts are now underway to restore oxygen-starved tissue by preventing the formation of superoxide free radicals using drugs such as superoxide dismutase..." (Tortora, GJ & Anagnostakos, NP. 1987. Principles of Anatomy and Physiology, Harper and Row, NY, NY., p. 469).

SUBCLINICAL AND PATHOLOGICAL CONDITIONS OF THE CARDIOVASCULAR SYSTEM

HEART PROBLEMS

HEART DISEASE

Heart disease accounts for over 50% of all deaths in the United States and over 50 billion dollars per year in medical expenses. It is the leading cause of death in the United States even though it is one of the most preventable degenerative diseases we face. Heart disease includes such problems as angina (chest pain), arteriosclerosis (hardening of the arteries), myocardial infarction (heart attack) and stroke (brain deprived of oxygen).

1) **Angina** - chest pain caused by lesions in the coronary arteries, valves or heart wall, which temporarily block the blood/oxygen supply to the heart.

   Signs and Symptoms of Angina:

   - chest pain radiating to left arm and/or left neck
   - discomfort/heaviness in the chest or throat
   - exercise causes increased discomfort

2) **Arteriosclerosis** - fatty deposits (mainly cholesterol plus calcium) that accumulate in the inner arterial walls, causing the walls to harden and thicken. These arterial lesions cause the arteries to narrow, inhibiting circulation. These lesions can form as early as one year of age.

   Signs and Symptoms of Arteriosclerosis:

   - no symptoms present until lesions are big enough to inhibit circulation; most vessels have to be greater than 90% occluded before symptoms occur
   - angina
   - frequent leg cramps
   - dizziness
   - minor exercise causes exhaustion

3) **Strokes** - can be caused by atherosclerosis of the arteries, which blocks the supply of blood to the brain. Strokes can also be caused by a blood clot that forms in the cerebral arteries or an embolus (a blood clot that forms in another part of the body and is carried by the blood to the brain). Blood vessel ruptures and hemorrhaging of the brain can also cause a stroke. Strokes are the third leading cause of death in the United States.

   Signs and Symptoms of Strokes:

   - paralysis of limbs
   - loss of speech
   - loss of eyesight

4) **Myocardial Infarction** - heart attack; caused by a lack of oxygen to the heart usually due to atherosclerosis in the coronary arteries.

5) **High Cholesterol** - high levels of cholesterol in the blood; influenced by hereditary factors and diet (mostly saturated fat).

   Cholesterol: found naturally in the body including the liver, blood, brain, nerves and bile. It is produced mainly in the liver and is used for digestion (bile acids), membrane integrity and as a sex hormone precursor. If cholesterol is not used up by the body, it remains in the blood where it can become oxidized and form plaques or lesions on the arterial walls.

   Two types of cholesterol:

   1) **LDL (Low Density Lipoprotein)** - the "bad cholesterol" that picks up cholesterol and deposits it in the arteries and tissues. It appears that LDL cholesterol may only become harmful when it is oxidized.
   2) **HDL (High Density Lipoprotein)** - the "good cholesterol" that picks up cholesterol and transports it back to the liver for elimination.

Triglycerides: blood fats composed of three fatty acids attached to a glycerol backbone.

Averages:

Total Cholesterol:
Average = 200 mg/dl
Borderline High = 200 - 239 mg/dl
High Risk = 240 mg/dl and above

HDL:
Average = Men: 45-50 mg/dl
Women: 50-60 mg/dl
Higher Protection = 70-80 mg/dl
High Risk = < 35 mg/dl

LDL:
Recommended level = < 130 mg/dl

Triglycerides:
Recommended level = 50-150 mg/dl

6) **Circulatory Problems:** many factors contribute to circulation problems. Hypertension, atherosclerosis, Raynaud's Disease, varicose veins and hypothyroidism all need to be considered in circulation problems.

Possible Causes:

1) Poor diet consisting of refined, fatty or nutrient-deficient foods. "Excess amounts of animal protein in the absence of the micronutrients (specifically B-6) promotes the accumulation of homocysteine, which is a potent smooth muscle cell and arterial endothelial poison derived from incomplete degradation of sulfur-containing amino acids" (Linder, M., Nutritional Biochemistry and Metabolism with Clinical Applications, Appleton and Lange, CT, p. 456). Homocysteine is found in high amounts in red meat and dairy products.
2) Oxidized cholesterol in the blood. Oxidized cholesterol enters the blood through a variety of ways. Processed foods, environmental pollutants, trauma, infection, metabolism of animal products and stress can all trigger the formation of oxidized cholesterol. Two chemicals, fluoride and chlorine,

which are both found in our drinking water can affect the arteries (chlorine) and lower thyroid function (fluoride).

3) Stress - increases free radical production and stimulates adrenaline production, which causes platelet aggregation and thickening of the blood.
4) Lack of exercise
5) Environmental pollutants
6) Trauma
7) Infection
8) Hereditary factors
9) Smoking
10) Obesity (20-30% overweight)
11) Alcohol abuse
12) Fat metabolism problems (gallbladder/liver)
13) Diabetes - LDL glycation (LDL alteration) may occur in diabetes
14) Hypertension (Normal = 120 / 80 mmHg)
    Systolic > 135 mmHg (borderline high)
    > 150 mmHg (high)
    Diastolic > 90 mmHg (borderline high)
    > 100 mmHg (high)
15) Long-term birth control use; the pill has been shown to increase cholesterol levels
16) Drug use (especially steroids) diuretics and L-Dopa (a drug used for Parkinson's Disease) all increase cholesterol levels.

Dietary and Lifestyle Applications:

1) A detoxification program is beneficial.
2) Good dietary habits are essential. A **vegetarian based diet**, high in vegetables, fruits and grains and low in fat and cholesterol is best. Vegetarians demonstrate lower cholesterol levels than meat-eaters. Also, vegetarian diets are **low in methionine and homocysteine**. Homocysteine comes from methionine. Methionine is not necessarily a "bad amino acid" to have around, especially in the presence of enough B-6.

NOTE: High levels of homocysteine have been shown to increase free radical production, which in turn oxidizes cholesterol. Studies have shown that men with increased homocysteine in their blood have a three time greater risk of having a heart attack. (Peng, S.K. and Taylor, C.B. "Cholesterol Autooxidation, Health and Arteriosclerosis. World Reviews of Nutrition and Diet. 1984; 44:117-154).

Gamma linolenic acid found in black currant seed oil and evening primrose oil decrease stickiness of platelets. Fish oils (**omega-3 fatty acids - EPA/DHA**) found in salmon, mackerel and herring decrease triglyceride levels.

NOTE: EPA/DHA (fish oils) have been shown to:
1) decrease VLDL production.
2) decrease blood pressure.
3) increase prostaglandins (namely PGI3) that favor vasodilation..
4) lower blood cholesterol.
5) decrease triglyceride levels.

These are the same effects that are reported with aspirin ingestion, but without the added risks, including ulcers (PG's control stomach acid production) and increased risk of stroke. A study done in the Netherlands suggested that two fish meals per week would lower risk of fatal heart attacks by 50%.

Avoid chemical preservatives and additives. Crushed garlic and onions may also be helpful. They have been shown to lower triglyceride levels and decrease platelet aggregation. Garlic contains alline, the substance partially responsible for garlic's potent odor. When garlic is crushed, allinase (an enzyme), is released that combines with alline to form ajoene. The ajoene is the isolated fraction of garlic responsible for prevention of the platelet aggregation. Garlic per day seems to be effective in reducing risk for heart disease. **Ginger** may also be effective in protecting against heart disease.

Fiber is very important, since fiber binds cholesterol and bile acids and promotes their excretion. Oat bran and brown rice bran are excellent sources of fiber due to decreased risk of allergies. **Avoid saturated fats and hydrogenated fats**, which raise cholesterol. Also **avoid trans fatty acids**. On the other hand, **monounsaturated fats (olive oil) and polyunsaturated fats (vegetable oils)** have been shown to lower cholesterol levels.

3) Stress reduction is beneficial, including meditation, massage, biofeedback, yoga and any other forms of relaxation. Stress increases the production of cholesterol that is made by the body.
4) Obtain optimal weight. Reduce weight if necessary.
5) Avoid smoking.
6) Acupuncture and chelation therapy may be beneficial in heart disease.
7) Moderate exercise is important. Exercise has been shown to increase HDL and decrease total cholesterol.
8) Avoid alcohol. Moderate amounts of alcohol have been associated with increased HDL levels, but this study has been refuted by other researchers. Sugar and alcohol have been shown to increase natural cholesterol production by the body.
9) Avoid coffee. Epidemiological studies believe that coffee consumption increases cholesterol levels. In a recent nine week study, roasted, ground coffee showed a strong correlation to hypercholesterolemia. The drip filter method, made by boiling and steeping, did not show this correlation (Bak, AA and Grobbee, DE: New England Journal of Medicine 321: 1132. 1989).
10) A dry brush massage will aid in increasing circulation.

Nutrient Applications:

Many nutrients are called for in the prevention of heart disease:

1) **Antioxidants:** to prevent oxidation of LDL

a) **Vitamin C:** antioxidant; aids in collagen synthesis, which is important for arterial wall integrity. (Vitamin C is contraindicated in iron overload disease, gout and/or kidney stones).

NOTE: In one study, the RDA amount of vitamin C (60 mg.) showed no protection against heart disease, but when that amount was increased to approximately 3,000 mg. for a 154 pound human, arterial damage was reversed (Burton Goldberg Group, Alternative Medicine: The Definitive Guide, Future Medicine Publishing, Inc. WA, p. 716).

It has been suggested that vitamin C in combination with lysine aids in dissolving blood clots and may increase HDL while decreasing LDL. (Burton Goldberg Group, Alternative Medicine: The Definitive Guide, Future Medicine Publishing, Inc. WA, p. 716).

b) **Vitamin E:** aids in prevention of lipid peroxidation and inhibits platelet aggregation. Vitamin E helps to repair the arterial walls.

NOTE: At the American Heart Association Annual Meeting in 1992, studies were presented. They suggested that a daily intake of 100 IU's of vitamin E for two years decreased the risk of heart disease in a group of 87,000 female nurses by 41%. Males decreased their risk by 37%. The higher the dose, the better the results. (Newsweek, May 31, 1993,p. 62).

c) **Selenium:** reduced levels of selenium decrease the levels of glutathione peroxidase, a powerful antioxidant enzyme.

d) **Beta-carotene:** powerful antioxidant

e) **Coenzyme Q10:** antioxidant known to strengthen the heart; CoQ10 aids in energy production because it is one of the main components in the Krebs Cycle.

2) **Homocysteine metabolizers:** homocysteine comes from methionine, which is found in high amounts in animal protein.
   a) **Vitamin B-6:** needed to convert homocysteine (free radical precursor) to cystathionine, a harmless end product. It may also inhibit platelet aggregation.
   b) **Vitamin B-12:** needed to aid in the breakdown of homocysteine.
   c) **Folic Acid:** aids in the metabolism of homocysteine by converting homocysteine back to methionine.
3) **Niacin:** very effective at decreasing LDL and triglyceride levels while increasing HDL levels; high potency for long periods of time does have side effects including flushing, liver inflammation and increased uric acid levels.
4) **Pantothene:** active form of pantothenic acid; shown to decrease cholesterol and triglyceride levels.
5) **Magnesium:** magnesium levels are repeatedly decreased in people with coronary heart disease. Magnesium deficiency also leads to low levels of potassium because without magnesium the heart muscle cannot retain potassium. Magnesium is effective for artery dilation, and aids in decreasing total blood cholesterol levels while increasing HDL cholesterol. Magnesium also inhibits platelet aggregation and prevents irregular heartbeats (arrhythmias).
   NOTE: Excess vitamin D intensifies magnesium deficiency.
6) **Calcium:** decreases cholesterol levels and is protective against coronary heart disease.
7) **Chromium:** decreases LDL and triglyceride levels in the blood and increases HDL cholesterol.
8) **Carnitine:** an amino acid found in food or made by the liver or kidneys from lysine and methionine. It transports long chain fatty acids across the membrane into the mitochondria (the energy center of the cells). Decreased carnitine levels lead to decreased energy production by the cells.
   NOTE: Deficiency of L-carnitine has been implicated in angina and severe confusion. L-carnitine aids in decreasing blood lipids (mainly triglycerides) and increasing HDL.
9) **Bromelain:** it has been suggested that bromelain may be effective in dissolving blood clots and has worked in relieving angina pains.
10) **Essential Fatty Acids:**
    1) **Omega-3 Fatty Acids:** EPA-DHA is converted into the 3-series prostaglandins; found in fish oils. Increased intake of fish oils (as in the Eskimos) has been shown to decrease risk of atherosclerosis, decrease angina pain and decrease triglyceride levels.
    2) **Omega-6 Fatty Acids:** Linoleic acid is an essential omega-6 fatty acid which is necessary to produce arachidonic acid (AA). Arachidonic acid makes the 2-series of prostaglandins. While the 2-series is necessary for proper functioning of the immune system, an overabundance without balance of the omega-3's, and/or gamma-linolenic acid, can have detrimental effects, mainly inflammation. Some of the omega-6's (e.g. gamma-linolenic), are converted into the 1-series of prostaglandins; found in black currant seed oil and evening primrose oil; anti-inflammatory; also decrease risk of atherosclerosis.

    NOTE: Saturated/hydrogenated fats, refined foods, B-6 and zinc deficiency, excess alcohol consumption, infections and chemicals all decrease the 1-series of prostaglandins in the body.
11) **Proper zinc to copper ratio:** a high intake of zinc (>160 mg. per day) may decrease HDL levels and increase risk of atherosclerosis, while copper deficiency increases cholesterol levels. Copper is needed for fat metabolism and connective tissue production (Murray, M. and Pizzorno, J. Encyclopedia of Natural Medicine, Prima Publishing, CA, p. 166).
12) **Lecithin:** also known as phosphatidyl choline (choline plus phosphorus, glycerol and fatty acids). Lecithin and choline are known for their cholesterol lowering effects, and as protectors against heart disease. They help to alleviate fatty livers in animals.
13) **Inositol:** aids in cholesterol and triglyceride reduction and as a protective factor in coronary heart disease.
14) **Herbal and Food Support:**
    a) **Hawthorn Berries:** they have many functions including peripheral vasodilation (dilating vessels away from the heart) in order to decrease blood pressure, and allowing the heart to function with increased ease. Hawthorn berries also dilate the coronary vessels and increase oxygen utilization by the heart.

b) **Cayenne:** in combination with hawthorn berries they, "produce a special kind of synergism that augments the cardiotonic activity of both" (Mowrey, D.B., Scientific Validation of Herbal Medicine, Keats Publishing, CT, p. 136).

c) **Garlic:** contains sulfur compounds that work as an antioxidant and aid in dissolving blood clots. (Burton Goldberg Group, Alternative Medicine: The Definitive Guide, Future Medicine Publishing, Inc. WA, p. 718). It also decreases cholesterol and triglyceride levels, and increases HDL levels.

d) **Ginger:** decreases platelet aggregation and cholesterol levels.

e) **Kelp:** hypotensive and cardiotonic properties.

f) **Onions:** inhibit platelet aggregation and fibrin formation (fibrin is a major component of blood clots).

Considerations:

1) Several studies, including the Framingham study, found no correlation between cholesterol levels and the amount of eggs a person consumed.
2) Over 80 - 90% of the cholesterol in the body is manufactured by the body, mainly the liver. Only 10-20% is actually ingested from food. Saturated fat raises cholesterol more so than dietary cholesterol by upregulating synthesis. Evidence suggests that the real culprit is oxidized LDL cholesterol from the blood, or the inability to down regulate endogenous production of cholesterol. Since cholesterol may not be harmful until it is oxidized, the main focus is on the factors that trigger oxidation of LDL.

MITRAL VALVE PROLAPSE

A defect of the heart valve (mitral valve) that allows oxygenated blood to flow from the left ventricle to the left atrium. In mitral valve prolapse, the valve falls back into the atrium during systole.

Signs and Symptoms of Mitral Valve Prolapse:

- usually no symptoms are present
- sometimes palpitations or chest pains

Possible Causes:

1) Spasm and latent tetany, in which the muscles are continually irritated.
2) Poor heart function due to varied causes (discussed under heart disease).
3) More common in women who have scoliosis or other skeletal problems.

Nutrient Applications:

1) Magnesium - aids in muscle spasm (latent tetany)
2) Carnitine - patients with mitral valve prolapse have been shown to have low blood and urine levels of carnitine.
3) See Heart Disease for further applications.

Dietary and Lifestyle Applications:

1) See Heart Disease.

RAYNAUD'S DISEASE

Named after a French physician; it is a circulatory problem that affects the hands and feet and makes them hypersensitive to the cold. Women are four to five times more likely than men to have the problem.

Signs and Symptoms of Raynaud's Disease:

- fingers and toes turn white or bluish hue when exposed to the cold
- stinging pain in hands
- affected area may turn red or blue before circulation returns to normal

Possible Causes:

1) Exposure to the cold.
2) Certain medications that affect the blood vessels including calcium channel blockers for hypertension, heart medications, birth control pills and migraine headache medications (i.e. ergotamine).
3) Smoking - decreases blood flow to the skin, constricting the arterioles.
4) Buerger's Disease - a rare disorder that causes disease in the blood vessels of the hands and feet. There is a direct link between both tobacco chewing and smoking, and Buerger's Disease.
5) Poor diet and nutrient deficiency.

Nutrient Applications:

1) Vitamin E - aids in circulation (400 IU daily)
2) Coenzyme Q10 - improves oxygenation to the tissues
3) Magnesium - nutritional vasodilator
4) B Complex - aids in fat and cholesterol metabolism. Niacin is a potent vasodilator.
5) EPA (Omega-3 fish oil) - improves circulation by decreasing blood viscosity

Dietary and Lifestyle Applications:

1) Avoid cold exposure. Dress warmly, especially the hands and feet.
2) Eat a good diet. Foods high in magnesium (vasodilating effect) and vitamin E (raw seeds and nuts) are recommended.
3) Avoid smoking and coffee (both constrict the blood vessels).
4) Be careful of medications.
5) Deep breathing, massage, spinal manipulation and biofeedback may be helpful to increase circulation to the extremities.
6) Moving the arms and legs rapidly will aid circulation.

HYPERTENSION

High Blood Pressure (Normal = 120 / 80 mmHg)
Systolic > 135 mmHg (borderline high)
> 150 mmHg (high)
Diastolic > 90 mmHg (borderline high)
> 100 mmHg (high)

Essential hypertension: no known medical cause (90-95%)

Secondary hypertension: caused by another disease (5-10%)

Blood pressure is defined as the force exerted by the blood against the vessel wall. Normal blood pressure is 120/80 mmHg. The systolic reading (120) is the maximum pressure the heart is exerting during contraction. The diastolic reading (80) is the pressure when the heart is between pumps and is at rest. The diameter of the arteries and the amount of blood pumped through the arteries determines the blood pressure. The kidneys are responsible for the amount of water circulating in the body and the level of salt retained by the body. Increased salt levels cause more water to be retained and can cause blood pressure to increase.

Signs and Symptoms of Hypertension:

- usually no symptoms are present (hypertension is sometimes referred to as the "silent killer")
- could include dizziness, fatigue, nosebleeds, breathing problems, insomnia and GI problems

Possible Causes:

1) Dietary habits including high salt and dietary fat intake (there is a subpopulation exhibiting salt-sensitive hypertension), and low magnesium and potassium levels. High blood pressure has been termed the "Westerner's disease" since the Western diet seems to precipitate the problem.
2) Atherosclerosis - plaque builds up in the arteries and creates increased pressure
3) Obesity
4) Alcohol and coffee consumption
5) Smoking - stimulates the adrenal glands, which secrete adrenaline and can increase blood pressure; also cigarettes lead to toxic metal exposure (cadmium and lead). Decreased vitamin C levels are a problem with cigarette smokers. One puff on a cigarette can decrease vitamin C as much as 50%.
6) Stress
7) Food allergies/sensitivities
8) Heavy metal exposure, specifically cadmium and lead
9) Drug abuse or contraceptive use
10) Secondary hypertension can be caused by kidney problems (kidneys control fluid balance), adrenal problems (adrenaline has a blood vessel constricting effect), oral contraceptive use or pregnancy.

Nutrient Applications:

1) Magnesium - intracellular levels of magnesium are consistently low in hypertensives; it is a potent vasodilator.
2) Calcium - has been shown to decrease blood pressure
3) Vitamin C - current studies definitely reveal an inverse relationship with vitamin C consumption and blood pressure. (Vitamin C is contraindicated in iron overload disease, gout and/or kidney stones).
4) Coenzyme Q10 - aids in energy metabolism, heart function and blood pressure
5) Garlic - hypotensive effect
6) Kidney - glandular kidney support
7) Potassium - counterbalances increased sodium levels
8) Hawthorn berries - high in anthocyanidins and proanthocyanidins (powerful flavonoids); known for hypotensive and cardiotonic effect.

Dietary and Lifestyle Applications:

1) A detoxification program is beneficial. Detoxing the liver and lymphatic system is very helpful. Mini tramps, dry brushing and deep breathing aid in lymphatic detoxification.
2) Eat a healthy diet low in salt, fat and sugar. Increase essential fatty acids (vegetable oils) and fish (organic sources). Increase foods that contain potassium (bananas, melons, oranges, avocados, broccoli, cabbage, cauliflower, potatoes and squash), magnesium (nuts (especially almonds), potatoes, kidney beans, green leafy vegetables, wheat germ, whole grains and soybeans) and calcium (green, leafy vegetables, nuts and yogurt). Increase fiber intake, and liberally include onions and garlic, which have been shown to decrease blood pressure. A vegetarian diet is beneficial.
3) Cayenne mixed with lemon juice or vegetable juice aids in detoxification and has shown success in decreasing blood pressure (Burton Goldberg Group, Alternative Medicine: The Definitive Guide, Future Medicine Publishing, Inc. WA, p. 728) .
4) A weight reduction program should be followed, if necessary.
5) Practice relaxation exercises including meditation, yoga, massage and biofeedback.
6) A moderate exercise program is recommended.
7) Avoid smoking and caffeine.
8) Avoid environmental pollutants and drink filtered water.

9) If you are taking MAO inhibitors (drugs used to lower blood pressure and fight depression) do not take tyrosine. It may increase blood pressure.

SUBCLINICAL AND PATHOLOGICAL CONDITIONS OF THE RESPIRATORY SYSTEM

RESPIRATORY PROBLEMS

ASTHMA

A respiratory reaction in which the bronchial tubes spasm and excessive mucus is secreted into the lungs, inhibiting breathing and creating a variety of symptoms.

Two types of asthma:

1) **Extrinsic** - allergy-induced reaction in which serum IgE (an immunoglobulin) increases.
2) **Intrinsic** - bronchial reaction triggered by stress, cold, exercise, environmental pollutants or an infection.

Signs and Symptoms of Asthma:

- wheezing
- difficulty in breathing
- coughing up mucus
- tightness in the chest
- increased eosinophil count in the blood
- increased levels of IgE

Possible Causes:

1) Allergens including mold, dust, pollen and animal dander. These allergens increase IgE levels from mast cells, producing histamine and other chemicals that trigger asthmatic symptoms.
2) Respiratory infections
3) Emotional distress
4) Exercise-induced asthma
5) Exposure to cold, dry air
6) Environmental pollutants and chemicals (sulfur dioxide, formaldehyde, nitrogen dioxide, ozone, perfume, solvents, paints, plastics, etc.)
7) Smoke
8) Food allergies, especially wheat, milk and eggs. Food additives (tantrazine, sodium benzoate, sulphites) and preservatives can also trigger asthmatic symptoms
9) Low hydrochloric acid
10) Hypoglycemia
11) Medications - NSAIDs (aspirin, ibuprofen, etc.), beta blockers
12) Alcohol abuse
13) Liver toxicity
14) Poor gastro-intestinal function
15) Heavy metal toxicity
16) Candida/parasites

Nutrient Applications:

1) Vitamin A - tissue repair and immune support

2) Vitamin B-6 (pyridoxine) - after three months of B-6 supplementation, asthmatics have shown a decrease in frequency and severity of asthmatic attacks (Reynolds, R.D. and Natta, C.L., Depressed plasma pyridoxal phosphate concentrations in adult asthmatics, AJCN, 1985, 41:684-688).
3) Vitamin C - aids in immune support and has been shown to decrease asthmatic attacks; it aids in decreasing histamine secretion and is a powerful antioxidant (Werbach, M., M.D., Healing Through Nutrition, Harper Collins Publishers, NY, p. 37). (Vitamin C is contraindicated in iron overload disease, gout and/or kidney stones).
4) Vitamin B-12 - most effective when injected intramuscularly in high amounts; especially effective when given after sulfite ingestion to prevent an asthmatic attack (Murray, M. and Pizzorno, J. Encyclopedia of Natural Medicine, Prima Publishing, CA, p. 152).
5) Magnesium - magnesium deficiency is observed in the blood in one of every four asthmatics; Mg is a potent vasodilator and relaxes bronchial smooth muscle (Werbach, M., M.D., Healing Through Nutrition, Harper Collins Publishers, NY, p. 37).
6) Flavonoids - powerful antioxidants
7) HCl - if HCl deficiency is suspect

Dietary and Lifestyle Applications:

1) Strengthen the immune system to prevent infection.
2) Eat a healthy diet. An elimination/rotation diet is suggested. Avoid food additives and preservatives, especially sulfites, BHA, BHT, tantrazine (F,D & C yellow dye #5), MSG, etc.. One tablespoon of olive oil two times daily is suggested for essential fatty acid support. A vegetarian diet is highly suggested. Be careful of potatoes in the diet due to high sulfite content.
3) Eliminate and/or avoid food allergies and environmental pollutants when possible.
4) Avoid caffeine, chlorinated water, refined sugar, excess salt and chocolate.
   NOTE: It has been found that the greater the intake of dietary salt, the more reactive the bronchial tubes are to histamine. (Werbach, M., M.D., Healing Through Nutrition, Harper Collins Publishers, NY, p. 35).
5) Decrease stress levels. Practice relaxation exercises.
6) Avoid wine and beer due to high sulfite content. Sulfites can trigger an attack.
   NOTE: Some asthma medication contains sulfites, which could be aggravating the problem.
7) Avoid NSAIDs (aspirin and ibuprofen) when possible. Many asthmatics have sensitivities to acetylsalicylic acid (aspirin).
8) Avoid smoking or smoke of any kind, including fireplace smoke.
9) Drink plenty of filtered water to prevent mucus buildup. Warm fluids are very soothing to asthmatics. They act as natural bronchodilators.
10) If you must go out in cold weather wear a scarf or facemask.
11) Air filters may be helpful.
12) Mild exercise is suggested, but never exercise to exhaustion.

Considerations:

1) Asthma medications are excellent for short-term relief, but may have long-term detrimental effects:
   a) **Bronchodilators** (Albuterol, Bitolterol, Ephedrine, Isoproterenol, Metaproterenol, Pirbuterol, Terbutaline)
      Action: Bronchodilators effectively relax the bronchial muscles, open the bronchial passages and prevent histamine release in order to rapidly relieve breathing problems during an asthmatic attack. They come in pill form or as aerosols (inhalers). The inhaler is preferred because it does not have as many side effects.

      Side Effects: nervousness, headaches, rapid heartbeat, pallor, dry mouth, insomnia, increased blood pressure, anxiety, chest pain, dizziness, vomiting.
   b) **Corticosteroids** (most common is Prednisone)
      Action: decreases inflammatory response; aids in preventing asthmatic attacks, but not useful during an attack. Again the inhaled form is best to decrease side effects.

Side Effects: rashes, hives, itching, faintness, acne, headaches, indigestion, cough, nausea, vomiting, yeast overgrowth (candida albicans), hoarseness, dry mouth, decreased immune response, prolonged use increases risk of infection.

2) **Ephedra (Ma Huang in Chinese)** has been used for asthma conditions due to its natural source of ephedrine. Ephedrine is a potent bronchodilator, but ephedrine or ephedra can create side effects including anxiety, increased blood pressure, insomnia and increased heartrate. Patients with thyroid problems, heart disease, diabetes, prostate problems or high blood pressure need to avoid ephedrine. Long term use can cause adrenal gland exhaustion due to chronic stimulation. For these reasons, ephedra use is not suggested by the authors.
3) **Tryptophan Warning:** In the case of asthmatics, tryptophan could be potentially harmful. Tryptophan is an essential amino acid that is the precursor for serotonin (a neurotransmitter). Serotonin may trigger constriction of the bronchial tubes in asthmatics. B-6 supplementation "may be helpful in asthmatics because it corrects the metabolic defect in tryptophan metabolism commonly found in asthmatics, who often have high levels of serotonin in both blood and saliva." (Werbach, M., M.D., Healing Through Nutrition, Harper Collins Publishers, NY, p. 39).

HAYFEVER

Also known as allergic rhinitis; allergic reaction to inhaled allergens including pollens, dust and animal dander that affects the mucus membranes of the eyes, nose and airways.

Signs and Symptoms of Hayfever:

- stuffy, runny nose (usually clear mucus)
- ear pain and pressure
- watery, itchy eyes
- body aches
- frequent sneezing
- fatigue
- nervousness
- sore throats
- coughing/wheezing

Possible Causes:

1) Weakened immune system that is more susceptible to allergens
2) Airborne allergens including pollens, dust, molds and animal dander
3) Food allergies/sensitivities can make inhalant allergies worse
4) Environmental pollutants and/or chemicals that weaken immune response
5) Early weaning as an infant
6) Smoke exposure
7) Emotional stress
8) Liver toxicity
9) Poor gastro-intestinal function
10) Candida/parasites
11) Heavy metal toxicity
12) Alcohol - causes bronchial tissues to swell

Dietary and Lifestyle Applications:

1) A detoxification program is highly suggested.
2) Avoid the allergen when possible.
3) Strengthen the immune system.
4) Eat a healthy diet. An elimination/rotation diet is suggested. Avoid food additives and preservatives, especially sulfites, BHA, BHT, tantrazine (F,D & C yellow dye #5), MSG, etc.. A vegetarian diet is suggested. Eat plenty of fiber.
5) Eliminate and/or avoid food allergies and environmental pollutants when possible.

6) Avoid caffeine, chlorinated water, refined sugar, excess salt and chocolate.
7) Avoid smoking.
8) Drink plenty of filtered water.
9) "A simple way to consume bioflavonoids is to cut orange and/or lemon peels into strips and cook them with honey until soft. Eat 1-2 teaspoonfuls daily" (Giller, R., and Matthews, K., Natural Prescriptions, Ballantine Books, NY, p. 169).
10) Avoid salicylates found in aspirin and certain foods (almonds, berries, grapes, pickles, apples, beer, wine, tea and soft drinks).

Nutrient Applications:

1) Vitamin C - natural antihistamine and immune builder; take in large doses (2-3 grams) during allergy season.
   NOTE: Vitamin C is contraindicated in iron overload disease and people prone to kidney stones.
2) Bioflavonoids - potent antioxidants and anti-inflammatory agents
3) B-complex, especially pantothenic acid - pantothenic acid has been shown to relieve hayfever symptoms when taken daily (Giller, R., and Matthews, K., Natural Prescriptions, Ballantine Books, NY, p. 169).
4) Immune support including vitamin A, B, C, E, zinc, selenium, glandular support, echinacea, goldenseal, etc.
5) Omega-3 fish oils and gamma-linolenic acid (i.e. black currant seed oil and evening primrose oil) - for anti-inflammatory effect

SINUS INFECTION (Sinusitis)

An inflammation and/or infection of the nasal sinus cavities including:

1) **Frontal sinus:** in the forehead.
2) **Ethemoid sinus:** between the eyes at the bridge of the nose.
3) **Sphenoid sinus:** behind the eyes deeper into the head.
4) **Maxillary sinus:** in the cheek bones.

Signs and Symptoms of Sinus Infections:

- nasal congestion and discharge
- headaches
- pain and swelling around the eyes and/or cheeks
- postnasal drip
- difficulty breathing
- toothache
- fever/chills

Possible Causes:

1) Bacterial, viral or fungal infection (usually precipitated by the common cold)
2) Chronic hayfever or repeated acute infections
3) Chronic allergies, especially to dairy products
4) Poor diet
5) Suppressed immune function
6) Environmental pollutants, chemicals, heavy metal toxicity
7) Dental abscess or other dental problems
8) Deviated septum
9) Hypoadrenia

Nutrient Applications:

1) Vitamin A - promotes health of the mucus membranes
2) Vitamin C - strengthens the immune system. (Vitamin C is contraindicated in iron overload disease, gout and/or kidney stones).

3) Proteolytic enzymes - aids in inflammation
4) Goldenseal - effective for acute bacterial sinus infections (Murray, M. and Pizzorno, J. Encyclopedia of Natural Medicine, Prima Publishing, CA, p. 508).
5) Thymus extract - immune support
6) Liver extract - antihistamine effect
7) Bioflavonoids - anti-inflammatory agent

Dietary and Lifestyle Applications:

1) Make sure to strengthen the immune system and treat for hayfever or cold if necessary.
2) Eat a healthy diet. Avoid refined sugars, saturated fats and dairy products (they increase mucus formation). Increase fresh fruits and vegetables and whole grains. Avoid food additives and preservatives. An elimination/rotation diet is suggested.
3) Avoid food allergies and environmental pollutants.
4) Drink plenty of filtered water. Warm fluids are very soothing.
5) A humidifier may be helpful. A hot facecloth placed over the sinuses may help to relieve congestion.
6) Be careful of medications, especially antihistamines as they will eventually dry nasal secretions with long-term use and cause increased congestion.
7) Get plenty of rest during an acute infection.

COUGHS

A protective reflex by the body to clear the breathing passage of different secretions or foreign items.

Signs and Symptoms of a Cough:

- Different types of coughs can represent different problems:
  1) **Cough with clear or white phlegm** - caused by a viral infection (usually cold or flu); should dissipate in a few days.
  2) **Cough with yellow or green phlegm** - chronic infection is involved and may need more intense treatment.
  3) **Blood with cough** - consult physician immediately (may be pneumonia).
  4) Severe coughing with thick mucus - may indicate bronchitis.
  5) **Dry coughs worse in the evening** - may be due to asthma or allergy.
  6) **Coughing due to cold weather** - may be due to asthma.

Possible Causes:

1) Infection
2) Smoking
3) Asthma, bronchitis, pneumonia, laryngitis, sinusitis
4) Allergies and/or hayfever
5) Trachea problems
6) Environmental pollutants and chemicals and inhaled irritants
7) Medications, especially blood pressure medications
8) Heartburn - persistent acid regurgitation could be causing a cough

Nutrient Applications:

1) Vitamin C with bioflavonoids - immune support. (Vitamin C is contraindicated in iron overload disease, gout and/or kidney stones).
2) Vitamin A - promote health of the mucus membranes
3) Zinc lozenges - aids a sore, irritated throat
4) Mullein - used in India for upper respiratory problems; contains mucilage and antibiotic properties
5) Plantago (plaintain) - provides good relief of coughing, wheezing and irritation

Dietary and Lifestyle Applications:

1) Do not smoke. If smoking, and then stopping, the coughing could increase temporarily as the bronchial passages and lungs attempt to clean out the toxins.
2) Avoid food allergies.
3) Avoid environmental pollutants and irritating agents.
4) Treat infection or chronic problem associated with the cough.
5) Gargling with salt water can be quite effective.
6) Eat a healthy diet. Avoid dairy products, refined foods and salt.
7) Warm tea with lemon and honey is helpful.
8) A humidifier is beneficial.
9) Natural throat lozenges from the health food store are recommended to soothe irritation.

BRONCHITIS

Inflammation of the bronchial tubes due to infection or irritation. Bronchitis, if left untreated, can lead to pneumonia.

Acute - short, symptomatic attack associated with bacterial infection.

Chronic - constant inflammation due to irritation of the bronchial tubes without infection present.

Signs and Symptoms of Bronchitis:

- Coughing
- fatigue
- chills/shaking
- difficulty breathing
- fever
- sore throat
- pain and soreness in the chest

Possible Causes:

1) Infection (usually follows a cold)
2) Environmental pollutants and/or chemical toxins
3) Food allergies or chemical sensitivities
4) Smoking
5) Hospital stay that makes you susceptible to bronchitis
6) Cancer
7) Weak immune function

Nutrient Applications:

1) Vitamin C - high potency, especially important during first few days of infection
   NOTE: Vitamin C is contraindicated in iron overload disease, gout and people prone to kidney stones.
2) Bioflavonoids - powerful antioxidants and anti-inflammatory agents
3) Propolis - natural antibiotic
4) Beta Carotene - potent antioxidant; protects lung tissue
5) Vitamin A - promotes healthy mucus membranes
6) Proteolytic enzymes - aid inflammation
7) Thymus gland - immune support
8) Echinacea/Goldenseal - herbal immune enhancers
9) Vitamin E - antioxidant; aids in tissue healing
10) Zinc - aids in tissue healing
11) Garlic - potent immune stimulator

Dietary and Lifestyle Applications:

1) Mucous-producing foods such as dairy products, sugar, eggs and starches should be avoided. Hot, spicy foods may be added to the diet to help open the bronchial passages. These foods include onions, garlic, chili peppers, jalapenos, horseradish and cayenne pepper.
2) Drink plenty of filtered water.
3) Get plenty of rest.
4) Place a hot pack on the chest for 15-30 minutes to relieve congestion.
5) Humidifiers are beneficial.
6) Avoid smoke.

PNEUMONIA

Inflammation of the lungs due to infection or irritation. Pneumonia is the fifth leading cause of death in the United States and is especially prevalent in the elderly. It is much more common in the winter.

Signs and Symptoms of Pneumonia:

- cough with possible blood in the sputum
- chest pain
- fever
- chills
- shallow breathing

Possible Causes:

1) Weak immune function, especially due to common cold, HIV, drug and alcohol abuse
2) Immunosuppressive drugs
3) Chronic infections (i.e. pneumococcus, staph, streptococous, fungus, E. Coli, klebsiella, etc.)
4) Drug and alcohol abuse
5) Smoking
6) Environmental pollutants and/or chemical toxins that suppress immune function
7) HIV (Human Immunodeficiency Virus)
8) Kidney failure
9) Malnutrition
10) Allergies

Nutrient Applications:

1) Vitamin C - high potency, especially important during first few days of infection
   NOTE: Vitamin C is contraindicated in iron overload disease and people prone to kidney stones.
2) Bioflavonoids - powerful antioxidants and anti-inflammatory agents
3) Propolis - natural antibiotic
4) Beta Carotene - potent antioxidant; protects lung tissue
5) Vitamin A - promotes healthy mucus membranes
6) Proteolytic enzymes - aid inflammation
7) Thymus gland - immune support
8) Echinacea/Goldenseal - herbal immune enhancers
9) Vitamin E - antioxidant; aids in tissue healing
10) Zinc - aids in tissue healing
11) Garlic - potent immune stimulator

Dietary and Lifestyle Applications:

NOTE: See physician immediately! Chest X-ray verifies pneumonia.

1) Mucous-producing foods such as dairy products, sugar, eggs and starches should be avoided. Hot, spicy foods may be added to the diet to help open the bronchial passages. These foods include onions, garlic, chili peppers, jalapenos, horseradish and cayenne pepper.
2) Drink plenty of filtered water.
3) Get plenty of rest.
4) Place a hot pack on the chest for 15-30 minutes to relieve congestion.
5) Humidifiers are beneficial.
6) Avoid smoke.

THE PHYSIOLOGY OF THE URINARY SYSTEM

The urinary system is an intricate system of organs which helps regulate homeostasis by routing such substances as metabolic wastes, toxins, electrolytes, and water out of the body in a fluid composition called, "**urine**". These organs include two **kidneys,** two **ureters,** one **bladder,** and one **urethra.**

THE KIDNEYS

The kidneys are bean-shaped organs which lie on either side of the vertebral column just above the waist. The role of the kidneys in maintaining metabolic homeostasis cannot be underestimated, and as H.W. Smith put it, "The composition of the blood (and internal environment) is determined not by what the mouth ingests but by what the kidney keeps" (Smith, HW. Lectures on the kidney. 1943, Univ. of Kansas, Lawrence, Kansas, p. 3). The kidneys maintain fluid, electrolyte, and acid-base balance. They control the secretion rate of ADH (antidiuretic hormone) and aldosterone, two hormones which regulate sodium retention (and therefore blood pressure), they synthesize the hormone erythropoietin (stimulates red blood cell formation), and synthesize prostaglandins of the E series.

The kidney has an outer portion, or **cortex,** and an inner portion, or **medulla.** The functional units of the kidney are **nephrons.** The kidney has over a million nephron units in it. The parts of a nephron are: **Bowman's capsule, proximal tubule, distal tubule** (all located in the cortex)**, loop of Henle and collecting tubule** (both located in the medulla).

The kidney performs its function of urine formation by three processes: **1) filtration, 2) reabsorption, and 3) secretion.**

1). **Filtration**. As blood enters the **glomerular capillaries** of the kidney, water and solutes are filtered out into structures called **Bowman's capsules.** The rate at which this occurs is known as the **glomerular filtration rate.** Each network of capillaries is known as a **glomerulus.**

2). **Reabsorption**. The majority of water, electrolytes, and all nutrients are reabsorbed from **proximal convoluted tubules.** The regulation of sodium, glucose, and amino acids are among the most important of the substances reabsorbed. As the tubules descend, they become **loops of Henle**, which are basically responsible for either concentrating or diluting the urine. If, for instance, blood volume decreases drastically in hemorrhage, the water-conserving property of the loop of Henle could be life-saving. As the tubule becomes the **distal tubule,** it reabsorbs sodium (not as much as the proximal tubule), and water (when ADH is present).

3). **Secretion.** Tubular secretion refers to the movement of substances from the blood into the tubular fluid. Distal and **collecting tubules** secrete potassium, hydrogen, and ammonium ions. When blood aldosterone increases, potassium secretion increases. This is also where certain drugs, such as penicillin, are secreted into the tubular fluid for excretion.

Extracellular fluid (ECF) volume regulates urine volume by acting on the hormones which affect urine concentration, ADH and aldosterone. ADH increases water absorption in the distal and collecting tubules, which decreases urine volume. Aldosterone increases absorption of sodium and other ions in the distal tubule, which pulls water along with them, and decreases urine output. When **ECF volume increases**, the **sodium** content will be **lower**, and this **inhibits ADH**, which **increases urine** volume. In other words, increased intake of water naturally results in increased output!

THE URETERS

The two ureters are tubes that extend from the kidneys to the bladder. Ureters collect urine and direct it down the tubes to the bladder. Peristaltic waves help move the urine down the ureters for excretion. At their widest point, the ureters are only ½ inch in diameter. This is one of the reasons that kidney stones, which can lodge in the ureters and distend its walls, can cause excruciating pain.

THE BLADDER

The bladder is a bag-shaped structure, covered by smooth muscle, which collects the urine that drains into it from the ureters. It is lined with a mucus membrane, with some elastic tissue which allows for its distensibility in holding urine.

THE URETHRA

The urethra is another tube, however, this one connects the bladder to the outside of the body so that the urine can be excreted. The name for this opening to the outside is the **urinary meatus.**

SUBCLINICAL AND PATHOLOGICAL CONDITIONS OF THE URINARY SYSTEM

KIDNEY AND BLADDER PROBLEMS

URINARY TRACT INFECTIONS

Urinary tract infections include any infections along the urinary tract, including both the bladder and kidneys.

1) **Cystitis (Bladder Infection):** inflammation of the bladder usually caused by some type of bacterial infection; very common in women because the bladder and urethra are very close to the vagina and anus.

   Signs and Symptoms of Cystitis:

   - painful urination (burning or itching)
   - frequent urination, especially at night
   - foul-smelling urine
   - cloudy, dark urine
   - slight fever
   - lower abdominal pain

2) **Pyelonephritis -** infection of the kidney; very serious; see physician immediately.

   Signs and Symptoms of Pyelonephritis:

   - high fever
   - low back pain
   - shaking/chills
   - nausea/vomiting
   - burning on urination
   - increased frequency of urination
   - possible blood in urine

Possible Causes:

1) Bacterial infection, especially E. Coli in the bowel
2) Not urinating frequently enough or not emptying the bladder completely. Urine retained in the bladder precipitates bacteria, especially if retained much longer than needed.
3) Poor hygiene - genitals must be kept dry and clean
4) Frequent intercourse
5) Yeast infection, especially if taking antibiotics for repeated infections
6) Allergies, mainly from foods
7) Stress and anxiety
8) Heavy metal toxicity
9) Poor kidney function

Nutrient Applications:

1) Vitamin C - for immune support. Vitamin C is contraindicated in iron overload disease and people prone to kidney stones.
2) Bioflavonoids - potent antioxidants and anti-inflammatory agents
3) Vitamin A - immune support; antibacterial effect; vitamin A deficiency causes a variety of metabolic changes conducive to bladder-stone formation (Nutr Rev 49 (8): 249-50,1991).
4) Zinc - promotes tissue healing
5) Propolis - natural antibiotic
6) Proteolytic enzymes - aid inflammation
7) Uva Ursi (bearberry) - diuretic and urinary antiseptic properties
8) Juniper berries - diuretic and urinary antiseptic properties
9) Goldenseal - excellent antimicrobial agent
10) Lactobacillus - replenishes the beneficial intestinal flora when on antibiotic therapy

Dietary and Lifestyle Applications:

1) Drink plenty of filtered water.
2) Urinate frequently and immediately when you feel the need.
3) Practice good hygiene.
4) Empty bladder after intercourse and clean the genital area thoroughly.
5) Drink natural cranberry juice to aid in preventing cystitis. Cranberry juice contains hippuric acid, which prevents bacterial growth by acidifying the urine. During active bladder infections, the hippuric acid in cranberry juice may increase burning. If this happens, try ¼ teaspoon of baking soda in water. This may help relieve the burning. **NOTE:** It has been suggested that the cranberry juice also prevents bacteria from adhering to the bladder wall.
6) Avoid feminine hygiene sprays, douches, tampons and bubble baths.
7) Avoid nylons and nylon underwear. Cotton underwear is best.
8) Avoid refined foods, caffeine, soft drinks, chocolate, alcohol and citrus fruits. Citrus fruits actually make the urine more alkaline, which precipitates bacterial growth. Increase onion and garlic consumption. Vegetarian diets are best. Low protein diets are suggested because the liver and kidneys breakdown protein and remove toxins. The lighter the load on the kidneys the better. Dandelion (diuretic and liver cleanser) and uva ursi (diuretic and urinary antiseptic) herb teas may be helpful.
9) Natural diuretics, such as watermelon and celery, are suggested.
10) If on or taking antibiotics, include acidophilus in the treatment program.
11) Check for yeast. Treat for yeast and follow yeast diet if needed.
12) Avoid food allergies. An elimination/rotation diet is suggested.
13) Hot sitz baths may be helpful.
14) Avoid high oxalate foods such as meat, fish, spinach, rhubarb, chocolate, swiss chard, eggs and beet tops, which can precipitate kidney stones.
15) Check for heavy metal toxicity.

KIDNEY STONES

Accumulation of mineral salts, mainly calcium; blockage occurs anywhere along the urinary tract, including the kidneys, ureter or bladder. Kidney stones form when the urine becomes too concentrated with calcium salts, uric acid and other substances, and does not stay in solution. They form hard mineral deposits called stones. The types of kidney stones include:

1) **Calcium stones** - most common (75-85%); more common in men; calcium combines with oxalate (most common), phosphate or carbonate.
2) **Uric Acid stones** - 8% of stones formed; usually found in people with gout; stones are made up of uric acid.
3) **Cystine stones** - 1% of stones formed; hereditary problem called cystinuria in which excess cystine is excreted in the urine.

4) **Struvite stones** - mainly found in women due to urinary tract infections. The bacteria produces an enzyme that triggers the stone formation that may block the urinary tract and damage the kidneys.

Kidney stones are becoming increasingly common in the United States. Approximately 20-25% of the US population is expected to have a kidney stone in their lifetime. It is also expected that 60% of the people who have had a stone have another one within seven years. The main culprit is the western diet.

Signs and Symptoms of Kidney Stones:

- no symptoms until stone blocks the urinary tract
- intense radiating pain starting in the mid back and moving to the lower abdomen
- blood in the urine
- chills and fever
- nausea/vomiting

Possible Causes:

1) The western diet including refined carbohydrates, simple sugars and high oxalate foods (spinach, rhubarb, coffee, swiss chard, chocolate). High sugar consumption stimulates insulin release from the pancreas, which in turn increases calcium excretion in the urine. High protein diets with low levels of fruits and vegetables, coffee, soft drinks and excess salt consumption increase calcium excretion in the urine, adding to the problem.
2) Not enough fluid intake; especially common in summer when people need more fluids.
3) Heavy metal toxicity - high cadmium levels have been associated with kidney stone formers
4) Stress
5) Low magnesium levels - magnesium keeps calcium in solution
6) Heredity
7) Gout - uric acid stones
8) Cystinuria - cystine stones
9) Hyperparathyroidism - poor calcium metabolism
10) Excess vitamin D - vitamin D is needed for calcium absorption
11) Alcohol abuse - the more alcohol consumed, the greater the risk
12) Obesity
13) Vitamin C – vitamin C does not cause kidney stones, but may increase the risk in those with a propensity to form stones.

Nutrient Applications:

1) Magnesium - very important in preventing stones - magnesium helps keep calcium in solution, and allows oxalate to bind to it (magnesium oxalate) rather than calcium. Magnesium oxalate does not crystallize, thereby preventing stones.
2) Vitamin B-6 (pyridoxine) - needed to break down oxalic acid; vitamin B-6 deficiency increases oxalic acid levels and decreases glutamic acid levels. Glutamic acid decreases the precipitation of calcium oxalate and prevents stone formation.
3) Proteolytic enzymes - aid in inflammation
4) Kidney glandular - kidney support
5) Potassium - decreases urine calcium levels and aids in preventing stone formation

Dietary and Lifestyle Applications:

1) A detoxification program, especially for heavy metals is suggested.
2) Increase fluid intake to a minimum of eight glasses of filtered water each day.
3) Eat a healthy diet. Avoid refined carbohydrates, sugar and high oxalate foods (spinach, rhubarb, meat, chocolate, beet tops, eggs and swiss chard). Also avoid high protein foods, coffee, soft drinks, dairy products and excess salt. Protein increases the excretion of calcium, uric acid and oxalate in the urine. The others increase calcium excretion. Caffeine ingestion increases the amount of

calcium and salt in the urine. Urinary calcium levels increase as salt levels increase. Increase fresh fruits and vegetables. A vegetarian diet is suggested. Increase fiber intake, magnesium-rich foods (green, leafy vegetables), cranberries, rice bran, black cherries, whole grains and asparagus. Asparagus, "contains asparagine that helps in breaking up oxalate crystals" (Burton Goldberg Group, Alternative Medicine: The Definitive Guide, Future Medicine Publishing, Inc. WA, p. 943).

Cranberry juice is helpful for stone formers because it has been shown to decrease urinary calcium levels up to fifty percent. (Werbach, M., M.D., Healing Through Nutrition, Harper Collins Publishers, NY, p. 238). Rice bran contains phytin, a substance that binds calcium in the intestines. High fat diets should be avoided. Undigested fat binds to calcium in the gut and prevents the calcium from binding to oxalate in the gut. Eventually these oxalates end up in the urine and encourage kidney stone formation.

4) Do not supplement with high doses of vitamin C, as this may increase oxalate levels in the urine. If taking a calcium supplement, make sure it is an acidifying calcium, do not take more than 600 mg/day, and balance with magnesium. Acidifying calcium helps keep calcium in solution. **NOTE:** Mineral water originates from limestone, which is high in calcium.
5) Avoid alcohol.
6) Reduce weight if necessary. Obesity can lead to hypercalciuria (excess calcium in the urine).
7) Avoid antacid use. Antacids contain aluminum (toxic metal) and calcium carbonate, which is an alkalizing calcium.
8) Check for heavy metals since they are all toxic to the kidneys, especially cadmium. Cadmium causes kidney damage and encourages stone formation. Zinc and calcium compete against cadmium for absorption in the gut.
9) Watermelon can be eaten as a natural diuretic.

THE PHYSIOLOGY OF THE EYE

Light enters the eye through the **pupil,** which is a hole in the center of the **iris,** or the colored part of the eye. The **cornea,** a fibrous connective tissue layer, covers and protects the iris. The inner coat of the eye, the **retina,** is a layer of light-sensitive nerve cells, called **rods and cones**. In the center of the retina in the back of the eye is a yellow spot called the **macula.** The macula consists primarily of cones. This area distinguishes fine detail at the center of this vision field. The 125 million rods and 7 million cones transform light into nerve impulses, which are transmitted via the optic nerve and read by the brain.

The **lens,** located right behind the pupil and iris, divides the eye into two cavities. The anterior cavity, in front of the lens, is filled with a clear, watery fluid called **aqueous humor.** In between the cornea and sclera (white part of the eye), is a **canal of Schlemm**, where aqueous humor is drained off into the blood.

A jelly-like substance called **vitreous humor** fills the posterior cavity, between the lens and retina. The pressure in the eye, called the **intraocular pressure**, is due mostly to aqueous humor, but partially to vitreous humor.

EYE DISORDERS

The functions of the eye demand fluidity of cellular membranes. Since unsaturated fatty acids provide for this fluidity, whereas saturated fatty acids account for rigidity, it is not surprising that the eye has the highest percentage of unsaturated fatty acids incorporated into its membranes of any tissue in the body. Ironically, the double bond in the unsaturated fatty acid that accounts for membrane fluidity, is more susceptible to **free radical attack.**

Free radicals, which are increased by UV light, carry a single electron in their outer shell, making them highly reactive. The double bond in the fatty acid is in a vulnerable position for the free radical to steal an electron. The loss of the electron converts the fatty acid into a radical, which in turn converts the next fatty acid into a radical, and so on, known as the "**chain reaction**" of lipid peroxidation. With the change to a radical, the composition of the fatty acid is drastically affected. Since every cell membrane is composed of a phospholipid bilayer which includes these fatty acids, the disruption eventually ends in membrane rupture and cell death. Because of the rapid turnover of phospholipids in the eye, it is a site of high mitochondrial activity in the body. Incompletely reduced oxygen from the mitochondrial electron transport system is another source of free radicals. For these reasons, the eye experiences a high incidence of free radicals/lipid peroxidation. **Antioxidants,** which stabilize radicals and halt the chain reaction, prevent that damage and maintain the integrity of cell membranes.

Macular Degeneration: The macula requires a healthy supply of blood, however, when the small vessels of the eye become constricted and hardened, the blood deficiency promotes degeneration of the area with resulting blurred vision. Reading and other activities requiring sharp vision become increasingly difficult, and ultimately central vision disappears. Although macular degeneration is generally regarded by the medical community as untreatable, accumulated research shows that antioxidants are therapeutic in its prevention and treatment. The antioxidants combat free radicals responsible for the cellular damage and degeneration. In addition, they help increase circulation and cell growth, which aids in restoring the eye to a healthy state.

Cataracts: The eye lens must remain clear to focus light on the retina. Dysfunction of the lens due to partial or complete opacification is called cataract. A major health concern, approximately 50 million people in the world are blind from cataracts. Altered proteins accumulate and aggregate in lens opacities. The free radicals, formed from the UV light, alter proteins, and the accumulation of damaged proteins indicates that protective systems are not keeping pace with oxidative insults. "Primary defenses (against photooxidative damage) include protection of proteins and other constituents by lens antioxidants" (Annals NY Acad Sci., Beyond Deficiency, 1992, 669:113).

Glaucoma: When normal drainage of aqueous humor through the canal of Schlemm is blocked, intraocular pressure rises to a high level. As the pressure rises, it can push the iris forward, completely blocking the canal from drainage; this can result in degeneration of the retina and blindness.

SUBCLINICAL AND PATHOLOGICAL CONDITIONS OF THE EYES

VISION PROBLEMS

EYE PROBLEMS -

1) **Eye infections:** an inflammation or infection of the mucus membranes that line the eye (conjunctiva (conjunctivitis - "pink eye"), the iris, or other parts of the eye.

Signs and Symptoms of Eye Infections:

- pain and swelling around the eye
- redness and itching of the eye
- discharge from the eye
- blurred vision
- light sensitivity

Possible Causes:

1) Bacterial or viral infection
2) Allergies
3) Nutrient deficiencies
4) Stress
5) Eye injury
6) Environmental pollutants and chemical toxins
7) In newborns - incomplete opened tear duct

2) **Macular Degeneration:** deterioration of the macula, the central portion of the retina; it is one of the leading causes of blindness in the United States and Great Britain.

Signs and Symptoms of Macular Degeneration:

- loss of vision
- progressively blurred vision

Possible Causes:

1) Prolonged exposure to free radicals and ultraviolet light
2) Nutrient deficiencies - especially decreased antioxidant levels
3) Poor dietary habits - high refined food intake
4) Environmental pollutants and chemical exposure
5) Aging, high blood pressure, and atherosclerosis are all risk factors for macular degeneration

3) **Cataracts:** clouding of the clear lens of the eye; major cause of blindness; cataracts can sometimes be removed surgically.

Signs and Symptoms of Cataracts:

- blurred vision

- impaired night vision
- halos shining around lights

Possible Causes:

1) Aging
2) Prolonged exposure to free radicals and ultraviolet light
3) Eye disorders
4) Injury to the eye
5) Medications (i.e. steroids)
6) Nutrient deficiencies
7) Diseases such as diabetes
8) Hereditary factors

4) **Diabetic Retinopathy:** decreased oxygen supply to the retina due to deterioration of the retinal blood vessels as a result of diabetes. It is a major cause of blindness in diabetics.

Signs and Symptoms of Diabetic Retinopathy:

- vision impairment
- diagnosis of diabetes

Possible Causes:

1) Diabetes
2) Blood sugar handling problems
3) Poor diet
4) Nutrient deficiencies
5) Stress
6) Hypertension

5) **Glaucoma:** a group of several diseases characterized by "progressive damage to the optic nerve due to increased pressure within the eyeball" (Larson, D., Mayo Clinic Family Health Book, William Morrow and Company, Inc., p. 765).

Signs and Symptoms of Glaucoma:

- blurred vision
- eye pain
- red eyes
- blind spots in the eye
- gradual loss of peripheral vision

Possible Causes:

1) Aging
2) Nutrient deficiencies
3) Environmental toxins and pollutants
4) Eye injury
5) Medication (i.e. corticosteroids) - corticosteroids destroy the collagen ın the eye
6) Eye tumors
7) Allergies (food and environmental)
8) Hereditary factors

Nutrient Applications:

1) Eyebright - herb to support the eye
2) Antioxidants - to combat free radical damage (Gaby, A.R., M.D. and Wright, J.V., M.D. Nutritional Factors in Degenerative Eye Disorders: Cataract and Macular Degeneration." Jnl of Adv Med 6(1) Spg, 1993: 27-39).
   A) **Vitamin C** - very important antioxidant of the eye; aids in collagen integrity; shown to be helpful in glaucoma by lowering inner eye pressure; also shown to halt cataract progression. contraindicated in iron overload disease and people prone to kidney stones.
   B) **Vitamin E** - shown to be helpful in cataracts and macular degeneration.
   C) **Selenium** - shown to improve visual acuity; glutathione peroxidase is a selenium-dependent enzyme, which combats free radicals.
   D) **Zinc** - needed for proper visual function.
   E) **Bioflavonoids** - antioxidant and anti-inflammatory properties; proanthocyanidins (grape seed and pine bark extract) and quercetin are potent bioflavonoids. Bioflavonoids are beneficial in capillary integrity. **NOTE:** Bilberry is rich in flavonoids, specifically proanthocyanidin compounds.
   F) **Glutathione** - very high amounts of glutathione are found in the lens of the eye. Glutathione is made up of three amino acids - cysteine, glycine and glutamic acid; glutathione is very helpful against toxins. It is the substance needed for glutathione peroxidase to scavenge free radicals.
   G) SOD (Superoxide Dismutase) and Catalase - important antioxidant enzymes.
   H) **Beta-carotene and vitamin A** - necessary for proper lens function.
   I) **Taurine** - protects the eyes from ultraviolet light.
   J) **Ginkgo Biloba -** antioxidant properties; promotes vasodilation and improved cellular metabolism.
   K) **N-acetyl cysteine -** a stable derivative of cysteine, which has antioxidant properties and makes up part of the tripeptide glutathione.
3) Riboflavin - is a cofactor for glutathione peroxidase, which is a potent antioxidant enzyme for the eye.
4) Proteolytic enzymes - aid in inflammation and provide necessary components for all cells to function.
5) Gymnema Sylvestra - anti-diabetic effects.
6) Chromium - glucose tolerance factor.
7) Siberian Ginseng - may be helpful in patients with color blindness.
8) Amino Acids (free form) - may be helpful to ensure proper nutrition.

Dietary and Lifestyle Applications:

1) Eat a healthy diet. Include fresh fruits and vegetables, especially carrots, broccoli, yams, squash, green leafy vegetables and cantaloupe. Carrot juice is beneficial. Increase legume consumption because of high amounts of sulphur-containing amino acids. Increase berry consumption including blueberries, cherries, etc. They are high in proanthocyanidins (potent bioflavonoids). Avoid rancid foods and hydrogenated oils. Avoid refined foods such as sugar, refined flour, caffeine and chocolate.
2) Avoid environmental pollutants and toxins whenever possible. Avoid direct exposure of sunlight to the eyes and electromagnetic stress when possible.
3) Avoid smoking and alcohol.
4) Be careful of medications, especially steroids which can damage the optic nerve.
5) Eye exercises may be helpful. Consult an eye specialist.
6) Make sure to rest the eyes sufficiently. Do not strain the eyes or read by dim light.
7) If eyes are tired or inflamed, a cold compress placed over closed eyes may help soothe irritation.
8) See an optometrist/opthamologist for further medical attention when needed.
9) Check for liver congestion, thyroid problems, hypertension, diabetes, candida/parasites and pineal function. All can affect vision.

THE PHYSIOLOGY OF THE EAR, NOSE, & THROAT

THE EAR

The organ referred to as the ear presents an image of the cup-shaped body of tissue on either side of the head. The ear actually contains many parts, that make up an intricate system which allows for the sense of hearing. The flappy piece of flesh and cartilage on the outside is the **outer ear,** and includes the beginning of the **auditory canal.** The auditory canal is a tunnel that directs sound to the **eardrum.**

The **middle ear** refers to the inner surface of this eardrum, along with three small **ossicles** (tiny bone structures). Rather than listing the Latin names of the ossicles, the common names are much more interesting, and describe each one's shape - the **hammer,** the **anvil**, and the **stirrup**. These small bones vibrate in response to the vibrations of air in the tunnel, and then transmit these vibrations to the **inner ear.** The **inner ear** contains the actual receptors for hearing, and the beginning of the **auditory nerve,** which connects to the brain to translate signals.

The **Eustachian tube** is a tunnel which goes from the middle ear to the back of the nasal cavity (pharynx), and connects the two. It equalizes air pressure. If this tunnel becomes clogged, the eardrum could be in danger of bursting.

Although the ear is usually associated with the sense of hearing, it is also responsible for the sense of balance. At the beginning of the inner ear are three fluid-filled **semicircular canals**. Movement of the fluid is detected by tiny, hairlike nerve endings on the inside of the canal. The nerve endings transmit the message as a nerve impulse by way of the **vestibular nerve** to the brain. The brain can then send messages to the muscles to correct the imbalance.

THE NOSE

The organ referred to as the **nose** usually presents an image of the bulbous form of tissue in the middle of the face. The nose, like the ear, also contains many parts. The parts make up an intricate system which allows for the sense of smell. The **cilia,** which are tiny hairlike structures lining the **nasal cavity,** send nerve impulses to the brain in response to air, and the brain interprets smell. The nose also allows for an important passageway of air to the lungs. Air reaching the lungs has been warmed, moistened, and filtered for particulate matter by the rich blood supply and mucus secretions.

The roof of the nasal cavity is the site for the **olfactory epithelium**, which contains most of the nerves for smell. Four pairs of **paranasal sinuses** (spaces containing air which drain into the nasal cavity), like the nasal cavity, are lined with mucus-producing cells. Sinusitis may develop if the sinus passages are obstructed, and infected mucus cannot drain properly into the **pharynx.** Pain usually accompanies the infection near the sinus cavity involved. The nasal cavity connects to the pharynx, which is the beginning of the throat.

THE THROAT

Sometimes the **pharynx** is referred to as the throat, however, the **throat** actually consists of the **pharynx,** the **larynx,** and the **epiglottis.** The pharynx serves as a common passageway for both food and air; food travels from the pharynx down the esophagus, and air travels down the pharynx to the trachea. The pharynx also plays an important role in sound formation - for instance, the different vowel sounds can only be made by changing the shape of the pharyx. The pharynx is composed mainly of muscle, and is lined with a mucus membrane.

The larynx **(voice box)** opens into the trachea from the pharynx. It is composed mostly of cartilage that is joined together, with some fibrous/elastic connective tissue, and is also lined by a mucus membrane. The lower part of the larynx is where the vocal cords reside. The vibration of these vocal cords is what produces voice. Swelling of the mucosa surrounding the vocal cords is a dangerous condition; even moderate swelling can interfere with air passage, resulting in asphyxiation.

The **epiglottis** is a band of connective tissue which closes over the trachea during the swallowing reflex, so that food doesn't enter the trachea and lungs. When the expression, "food going down the wrong pipe" is used, it might be more correct to say, " the epiglottis wasn't functionally optimally".

SUBCLINICAL AND PATHOLOGICAL CONDITIONS OF THE EARS

EAR PROBLEMS

EAR INFECTIONS (Otitis Media)

Infection of the ear that is one of two types:

1) **Acute:** usually a bacterial infection (most commonly streptococcus pneumoniae) that follows an allergy or respiratory tract infection.

   Signs and Symptoms of Acute Ear Infections:

   - acute ear pain
   - fever/chills
   - irritability
   - red, swollen eardrum

2) **Chronic:** repeated swelling and pain of the middle ear.

   Signs and Symptoms of Chronic Ear Infections:

   - chronic ear pain and swelling
   - hearing loss

NOTE: Over one million children per year have tubes inserted into the middle ear due to ear infections.

Possible Causes of Ear Infections:

1) Infection (bacterial, viral or fungal) - especially due to trauma or exposure to chlorinated water
2) Poor functioning of the Eustachian tube, due to infection, allergy or obstruction
3) Allergies (food or environmental) - allergies trigger inflammation which blocks the Eustachian tube
4) Loud noises - continuous exposure to noise levels above 80 decibels
5) Medications - repeated antibiotic therapy for ear infections has been shown to increase the likelihood of the child getting another ear infection within a month. Antibiotics increase the risk of developing yeast and fungal infections.
6) Ear trauma
7) Air travel can increase risk due to pressure changes
8) Temperature extremes (cold weather) and high altitudes
9) Nutrient deficiencies
10) Poor immune functioning
11) Early bottle feeding - breastfeeding for a minimum of six months has protective effects against developing ear infections
12) Heavy metal toxicity
13) Iron deficiency

MENIERE'S DISEASE
Increased fluid pressure in the inner ear, which creates balance disturbances and can cause vertigo (dizziness), tinnitus (ringing in the ears) and hearing loss.

Signs and Symptoms of Meniere's Disease:

- dizziness
- loss of balance
- ringing in the ears
- hearing loss
- nausea/vomiting

Possible Causes of Meniere's Disease:

1) Metabolic problems - usually carbohydrate metabolism problems including hypoglycemia
2) Allergies (food and environmental)
3) Fluid retention prior to the menstrual cycle
4) Blood vessel spasm in the ear
5) Poor circulation
6) Poor dietary habits
7) High cholesterol levels
8) Obesity
9) Hypoadrenia

TINNITUS
Ringing in the ears

Signs and Symptoms of Tinnitus:

- ringing in the ears
- ear pain
- dizziness

Possible Causes of Tinnitus:

1) Excess ear wax
2) Blocked Eustachian tube
3) Meniere's disease
4) Decreased circulation in the ears
5) Continuous exposure to loud noises
6) Ear trauma
7) TMJ (Temporomandibular Joint) dysfunction
8) Hypertension
9) Atherosclerosis
10) Anemia
11) Drug use
12) Smoking
13) Tumor
14) Medications - may be a reaction to NSAIDs (aspirin, etc.); some people react to the salicylates in aspirin
15) Hypoglycemia
16) Poor diet - high fat/cholesterol diets decrease oxygen flow to the inner ear and could trigger tinnitus

Nutrient Applications:

1) Vitamin C - increases immune function.. Vitamin C is contraindicated in iron overload disease, gout and people prone to kidney stones.
2) Bioflavonoids - antioxidant and anti-inflammatory properties
3) Thymus extract - immune support and aids in decreasing food allergies (Burton Goldberg Group, Alternative Medicine: The Definitive Guide, Future Medicine Publishing, Inc. WA, p. 943).
4) Propolis - natural antibiotic
5) Beta-carotene - potent anti-oxidant and immune booster
6) Lactobacillus - essential if patient has been on repeated antibiotic therapy
7) Goldenseal and echinacea - potent herbal anti-bacterial agents
8) Ginkgo biloba - increases circulation in the ear; shown to be helpful in tinnitus (Giller, R., M.D., and Matthews, K., Natural Prescriptions, Ballantine Books, NY, p. 128).
9) Homeopathic ear drops may be beneficial
10) Manganese - deficiency has been linked to ear problems
11) N-acetyl cysteine - may thin mucus and help ears to drain (Giller, R., M.D., and Matthews, K., Natural Prescriptions, Ballantine Books, NY, p. 128).

Dietary and Lifestyle Applications:

1) Avoid allergies caused by food and the environment when possible. Follow an elimination/rotation diet.
2) Breastfeed infants for at least six months to provide increased protection.
3) Avoid antibiotics when possible to avoid both compromising the immune system and decreasing good bacterial flora. Use antibiotics as needed if the infection spreads to the mastoid bone (behind the ears) or the meninges (the membranes covering the brain and spinal cord). (Burton Goldberg Group, Alternative Medicine: The Definitive Guide, Future Medicine Publishing, Inc. WA, p. 702).
4) Avoid loud noises, smoking, alcohol and extreme temperature changes.
5) Eat a healthy diet, free of refined foods, saturated fats and cholesterol.
   NOTE: Increased fat levels in the blood have been directly correlated to hearing and ear problems.
6) Avoid public swimming pools when possible.
7) Clean ears carefully and thoroughly after bathing.
8) Heat applied locally to the ear may be helpful in decreasing pain and discomfort.
9) When sleeping, elevate the head or raise the crib to allow the Eustachian tubes to drain naturally.
10) Drink plenty of filtered water.
11) A vaporizer in the room during sleep may be helpful.
12) Check for iron-deficiency anemia.
13) Regular chiropractic adjustments are highly suggested.
14) For Meniere's disease, avoid alcohol, caffeine and smoking. Maintain blood sugar levels and check for hypoglycemic problems. Also check for food allergies.

THE PHYSIOLOGY OF THE ENDOCRINE SYSTEM

THE ADRENAL GLANDS

The adrenals are known as the "anti-stress glands" of the body. They are frequently depleted by stress including:

1) **Physical stress:** overwork and sleep deprivation.
2) **Chemical stress:** poor diet, environmental toxins, allergies, endocrine imbalances.
3) **Emotional/mental stress:** emotional upheavals, mental turmoil.
4) **Thermal stress:** extreme temperature changes.

Hans Selye, M.D. identified the effects that stress had on the body. He discovered that any of the above stressors would cause certain reactions in the body including:

1) Adrenal cortex enlargement
2) Thymus and lymph gland atrophy
3) Stomach and duodenal ulceration

Dr. Selye went on to highlight the series of events that happen due to prolonged stress. This series of events became known as the General Adaptive Syndrome which includes three stages:

1) **The Alarm Reaction:** fight or flight response: initial response to stress initiated by hypothalamic stimulation of the sympathetic nervous system and the adrenal medulla.
2) **The Resistance Stage:** after prolonged, continuous stress, the adrenals adapt and re-build themselves, increasing in size and function.
3) **The Exhaustion Stage:** at this point the person cannot deal with stress and has no reserves left. A person in the exhaustive stage will have a variety of complaints.

PHYSIOLOGY OF THE ADRENAL GLAND

ADRENALS: located above the kidneys and divided into two sections.

1) **Adrenal cortex** - bulk of the gland and it is divided into three zones:
   a) Zona glomerulosa - secretes hormones called mineralcorticoids
   b) Zona fasciculata - secretes glucocorticoids
   c) Zona reticularis - secretes gonaodocorticoids
2) **Adrenal medulla** - produces two principal hormones:
   a) **epinephrine** (adrenaline) - 80%
   b) **norepinephrine** (noradrenaline) - 20%

HORMONES PRODUCED BY THE ADRENAL GLANDS:

1) **Hormones produced by the adrenal cortex:** (all are produced from cholesterol)
   A) **Mineralcorticoids** - aldosterone is the mineralcorticoid hormone that is responsible for 95% of the mineralocorticoid activity; the other mineralcorticoids include corticosterone and desoxycorticosterone.

   FUNCTIONS OF THE MINERALCORTICOIDS:

   1) Control water and electrolyte homeostasis, especially sodium and potassium.
   2) Aldosterone acts on the kidneys by:

a) increasing retention of sodium, chlorides and water.
b) increasing excretion of potassium (thus large amounts are lost in the urine).

Aldosterone production is controlled by the renin-angiotensin pathway. Sodium deficiency, dehydration (decreased blood volume) or hemorrhaging cause the blood pressure to decrease. Decreased blood pressure causes the kidneys to secrete renin, which converts a precursor to angiotensin. Angiotensin ultimately stimulates the adrenal cortex to produce more aldosterone in hopes of increasing sodium and water reabsorption, and increasing blood pressure.

EFFECTS OF MINERALCORTICOID DEPLETION:

Fatigue, musculoskeletal problems, dehydration, excess perspiration, excess urination, heart palpitations and muscle twitches due to sodium-potassium imbalance, eyes sensitive to light, non-pitting edema (fluid retention that does not leave "pits" in the skin when pressed against)

CLINICAL TESTS FOR ADRENAL FUNCTION:

1) **Koenisburg's Test** - measures chlorides in the urine.
   NOTE: Excess sodium and chlorides in the urine indicates hypoadrenia.
2) **Ragland Test** - blood pressure test: systolic blood pressure drops 4 to 10 mmHg when standing up from a prone position.
3) **Pupillary Light Reflex** - pupil will dilate to light or constrict, but the pupil will be unable to hold constriction for a minimum of 30 seconds.
4) **Muscle Weakness** - sartorius, gracilis, posterior tibialis, gastrocnemius.

B) **Glucocorticoids** - the three glucocorticoid hormones include cortisol (most abundant), corticosterone, and cortisone.

FUNCTIONS OF THE GLUCOCORTICOIDS:

promote normal metabolism and increase resistance to stress; these hormones increase blood glucose levels and counteract inflammation.

A rapid increase in blood glucose - initiates the pancreas to produce insulin.

A rapid decrease in blood glucose - initiates the adrenals to produce glucocorticoids.

THUS, a diet high in refined carbohydrates is a big factor here in depleting the pancreas and adrenals.

Also, during the alarm reaction and resistance stage, glucocorticoid production is increased and this causes the thymus gland to atrophy. Therefore, in chronic stress, both the adrenal and thymus may need to be supported.

EFFECTS OF GLUCOCORTICOID DEPLETION:

Headaches, nervousness, allergies, blurred vision, erratic behavior, mood swings, anxiety

**The retina of the eye, epithelial tissue and nervous tissue do not store glucose, and thus are most affected by glucocorticoid depletion.

CLINICAL APPLICATIONS:

1) **Addison's Disease** - hyposecretion of glucocorticoids
   Symptoms: hypoglycemia, weight loss, muscle weakness, mental lethargy, low blood pressure, dehydration

2) **Cushing's Syndrome** - hypersecretion of glucocorticoids (mainly cortisol and cortisone)
Symptoms: fat redistribution as shown by tiny legs with a "moon face", a hump on the back, etc., skin flushing, stretch marks on the abdomen, poor wound healing, easily bruised

NOTE: Glucocorticoids are the anti-inflammatory hormones useful in joint inflammation and allergy reactions. If a patient has been on cortisone therapy for inflammation, as in arthritis or bursitis, adrenal function should be checked. Prolonged cortisone therapy will cause the adrenal glands to atrophy.

Also note that hypoadrenia can trigger brown patches of skin to develop on the body. This is due to the fact that chronically low adrenal function (exhaustion stage) will cause the pituitary to produce adrenocorticotropic hormone (ACTH) in excess amounts. ACTH is a hormone produced by the anterior lobe of the pituitary gland that influences the production and secretion of certain hormones of the adrenal cortex. The pituitary will continue to produce ACTH because the adrenals are not responding. This extra ACTH will stimulate the ovary to produce more estrogen and will also stimulate melanocyte stimulating hormone (MSH). MSH is a pituitary hormone that stimulates the skin to produce melanin, which may create a bronzing effect on the skin. (Schmitt, W. Common Glandular Dysfunction in Clinical Practice, North Carolina, 42).

C) **Gonadocorticoids** - sex hormones (estrogens and androgens) produced by the adrenal cortex. Estrogen is the female hormone concerned with the development of the female reproductive structures and sex characteristics. Androgen (ie. testosterone) is the male sex hormone that stimulates male characteristics. In men, the adrenal cortex produces the only source of estrogen. Women get an abundant supply of estrogen from their ovaries.

FUNCTIONS OF GONADOCORTICOIDS:
sexual characteristics and energy metabolism; very small amounts are produced, so effects are not significant.

EFFECTS OF GONADOCORTICOID HYPERSECRETION: (usually happens in the resistance stage of adrenal function)

Women - masculine characteristics such as excess body hair
Men - feminine characteristics

2) **Hormones Produced by the Adrenal Medulla:**
A) **Epinephrine** - 80% of hormonal secretion; vasoconstrictor
B) **Norepinephrine** - similar action to epinephrine

FUNCTIONS OF EPINEPHRINE AND NOREPINEPHRINE:

fight or flight response; aid the body to resist stress; mimic effects of sympathetic nervous system. During stress both hormones increase blood pressure and heartrate by constricting the blood vessels. They also relax the bronchials, triggering bronchodilation. Low blood sugar may stimulate epinephrine or norepinephrine secretion.

EFFECTS OF EPINEPHRINE/NOREPINEPHRINE DEPLETION:

decreased systolic blood pressure upon standing; no resistance to stress; altered fight or flight responses; bronchoconstriction.

NOTE: Always check asthmatics and bronchitis patients for hypoadrenia.

NOTE:
During pregnancy - when the baby's adrenal glands mature, they may take over if a mother's

adrenal glands are not functioning optimally, making the mother feel much better in the third trimester of pregnancy.

During menopause - estrogen output decreases from the ovaries; the adrenal glands will attempt to take up the slack; if a person complains of severe symptoms during menopause, check adrenal function.

THE THYROID GLAND

The thyroid gland regulates metabolism of every cell of the body. A poor functioning thyroid gland can cause a wide array of different symptoms since almost every cell of the body is affected by the thyroid gland. The brain, retina, thymus, spleen, lungs and gonads are the only organs whose metabolic rates are not controlled by the thyroid hormones.

PHYSIOLOGY OF THE THYROID GLAND

THYROID GLAND: located just below the larynx; the thyroid gland can store hormones for months until needed.

HORMONES PRODUCED BY THE THYROID GLAND:

1) **Thyroid Hormones**:
   A) **Thyroxine (T4)** - contains four iodine atoms; greater amount of T4 is produced than T3.
   B) **Triiodothyronine (T3)** - contains three iodine atoms; 3-4 times more potent than T4.

   FUNCTIONS OF THE THYROID HORMONES:
   1) **Regulate metabolism** - stimulate carbohydrate and lipid catabolism and increase the rate of protein synthesis; the overall effect is to increase the basal metabolic rate (BMR).
   2) **Regulate tissue growth and development** - work with growth hormone to increase body growth, especially nerve tissue growth.
   3) **Regulate nervous system reactivity** - the thyroid hormones can stimulate nervous system activity including increased blood pressure, heartrate, blood flow, nervousness and GI motility.

   THE THYROID HORMONES ARE REGULATED BY:
   1) Blood levels - if blood levels fall, the hypothalamus secretes thyrotropin releasing factor (TRF), which stimulates the pituitary to secrete thyroid-stimulating hormone (TSH). TSH stimulates the thyroid to release T3 and T4.

   NOTE: Pregnancy, cold weather and high altitudes also trigger the above reaction.

   Iodine combines with tyrosine to make T3 and T4. Hypothyroidism is rampant in the west due to low iodine content in the soils.

2) **Calcitonin (CT):** regulates blood calcium levels

   FUNCTIONS OF CALCITONIN:
   1) lowers blood calcium levels by increasing calcium absorption by bones and inhibiting the breakdown of bone.

   EFFECTS OF CALCITONIN:
   1) inhibits osteoclast activity (inhibits bone breakdown).
   2) inhibits parathyroid hormone (PTH); PTH increases calcium absorption in the gut, activates vitamin D, and increases osteoclast activity. PTH's main role is to increase blood calcium levels.

CLINICAL APPLICATIONS:

1) **Axillary Temperature Test**: best method.
   If body temperature is low, then metabolic rate is low and thyroid function is diminished. Low axillary temperature could also indicate hypoadrenia.

   TEST: Take axillary temperature first thing in the morning before arising. Shake down thermometer before going to bed, and upon waking place thermometer directly under armpit for 10 minutes. Do not move.
   Normal temperature = 97.8 to 98.2 F.
   Males - take temperature for one week.
   Females - monitor for full menstrual cycle, especially during menstruation.

ASSOCIATED DISEASES:

1) **Cretinism:** hyposecretion of thyroid hormones; dwarfism and mental retardation.
2) **Myxedema:** hypothyroidism in the adult; can produce facial swelling and droopy, swollen eyes.
3) **Goiter:** hypersecretion of thyroid hormones; enlarged thyroid, protruding eyes and high metabolic rate; can also be due to insufficient iodine in the diet.
4) **Hashimoto's disease:** can cause hypothyroidism; body becomes allergic to the thyroid hormone.

LAB TESTS:

1) **Primary hypothyroidism** = decreased thyroid hormone levels with increased TSH levels.
2) **Secondary hypothyroidism** = decreased thyroid hormone levels with decreased TSH levels (<2.0); pituitary is causing hypothyroidism due to lack of sufficient pituitary stimulation .

CONSIDERATIONS:

1) The thyroid gland is **important for the formation of progesterone.** Progesterone is needed for a healthy pregnancy, therefore, in the **case of a miscarriage,** thyroid function should be analyzed.
2) The thyroid gland influences the pituitary gland, parathyroid gland, adrenal glands and sex glands.
3) The **thyroid and adrenal gland balance** is very important. If adrenal function is low, the thyroid will not function properly and vice versa. If adrenal function is low, the thyroid will decrease the metabolic rate so as not to overtax the adrenals. Hypothyroidism in combination with hypoadrenia is not unusual, especially in highly motivated people (who keep "whipping the tired horse"). Treating the adrenals and thyroid together can be very important in this case. If you treat one without the other, the patient's symptoms can get progressively worse as the gap between the two widens. Going back and forth between thyroid and adrenal treatment protocols is classic in this case.
4) Both the adrenal hormones (epinephrine and norepinephrine) and thyroid hormones are derived from the **amino acid tyrosine.**

THE PITUITARY GLAND

The pituitary gland, also known as the hypophysis, is sometimes referred to as the "master gland" because it is the main endocrine gland and regulates many body functions. The pituitary gland is stimulated or inhibited by the hypothalamus, which is the principal intermediary between the endocrine system and the nervous system.

The pituitary gland is divided into two lobes:

A) **Anterior lobe** - responsible for secretion of seven hormones:
   1) **Growth hormone (GH)** - controls body growth.
   2) **Prolactin (PRL)** - initiates milk production by the mammary glands after birth.
   3) **Thyroid-Stimulating Hormone (TSH)** - stimulates synthesis and secretion of thyroid hormones.

4) **Follicle-stimulating hormone (FSH)** - stimulates egg and sperm production in the ovaries or testes, respectively.
5) **Luteinizing hormone (LH)** - stimulates ovaries to release egg, and prepares the body for fertilization.
6) **Adrenocorticotropic hormone (ACTH)** - stimulates adrenal cortex to release hormones.
7) **Melanocyte stimulating hormone (MSH)** - increases skin pigmentation through dispersion of melanin.

B) **Posterior lobe** - does not synthesize hormones. The hypothalamus produces two hormones, oxytocin and antidiuretic hormone, which are transported to the posterior pituitary, stored, and released when needed.

1) **Oxytocin** - stimulates smooth muscle cell contraction in the uterus during birth; stimulates contraction of mammary glands for milk ejection.
2) **Antidiuretic hormone (ADH)** - decreases urine volume by causing the kidneys to remove water from urine and return it to the blood; also increases blood pressure during hemorrhaging by constricting the arteries.

CLINICAL APPLICATIONS:

1) **Diabetes Insipidus** - dysfunction of the posterior lobe of the pituitary, in which ADH secretion is decreased due to hypothalamus damage.

Symptoms: large amounts of urine, excess thirst
Treatment: administer ADH

THE HYPOTHALAMUS

The hypothalamus coordinates activities of both the exocrine and endocrine glands. The **exocrine glands** have ducts or channels (i.e. salivary and mammary glands) and the **endocrine glands** are ductless glands that secrete hormones directly into the blood. The main endocrine glands include:

1) **Pineal** - not much is known about the pineal gland, but it is possibly an endocrine gland.
2) **Pituitary** - regulates all the endocrine glands with the above seven hormones.
3) **Thyroid** - regulates body metabolism.
4) **Thymus** - immune function regulator.
5) **Pancreas** - islets of Langerhans produce insulin.
6) **Gonads** - ovaries and testes, which are involved in sexual development.
7) **Adrenals** - help the body deal with stress.

The hypothalamus is thought to be the primary gland associated with aging. Light therapy is said to be extremely important for the pineal, pituitary and hypothalamus to increase longevity.

THE THYMUS GLAND

The thymus gland is known as the "center of the body's immune system". The thymus gland is a mass of lymphatic tissue that reaches maximum size in puberty (twice the size of an adult), and atrophies as we get older. The lymphatic tissue is eventually replaced by fat and connective tissue. The thymus gland is very vulnerable to free radical attack, thus antioxidants are necessary to increase immunity and prevent involution of the thymus gland.

The thymus gland produces four hormones:

1) Thymosin
2) Thymic humoral factor (THF)

3) Thymic factor (TF)
4) Thymopoietin

The thymus gland produces T-lymphocytes (T-cells), which are white blood cells responsible for cell-mediated immunity (immunity not controlled by antibodies). The thymus gland hormones circulate in the body fluids and increase T-cell activity in the T-cells that have already left the thymus and migrated to lymphoid tissue. In animals, if the thymus gland is removed before birth, cell-mediated immunity will not develop.

CLINICAL APPLICATIONS:
1) Associated muscle weakness: Infraspinatus

THE PINEAL GLAND

The pineal gland is also known as the "seat of the soul". It regulates endocrine function and is highly affected by sunlight and electromagnetic fields. Little is known about the pineal gland, but it is thought to be involved in important roles, including:

1) direct effect on the pituitary gland.
2) direct effect on the adrenals during stress.
3) inhibitory action on the thyroid.
4) regulation of the thymus gland.
5) aid in temperature regulation.

The pineal gland is extremely affected by light and may play a role in Seasonal Affective Disorder (SAD). Light therapy may be effective. Electromagnetic fields, such as those from computer screens, electric blankets, waterbeds and microwaves, also affect the pineal. The pineal gland is sensitive to stress. "Pineal gland extract given to animals has been shown to increase their life span" (Balch, Prescription For Nutritional Healing, Avery Publishing Group, Inc., N.Y., 189). Vitamin A deficiency can be degenerative to the pineal gland.

SUBCLINICAL AND PATHOLOGICAL CONDITIONS OF THE ENDOCRINE SYSTEM

ADRENAL PROBLEMS

HYPOADRENIA

Low adrenal function

Signs and Symptoms of Hypoadrenia:

- low energy
- allergies
- tired all the time
- environmental sensitivities
- symptoms begin after a stressful event
- headache when standing up
- dizziness or loss of vision when standing quickly
- low blood pressure or systolic blood pressure that drops when standing (Ragland Test)
- weak and shaky
- sensitive to bright light
- easily startled or frightened
- perfectionism
- Loud noises cause the heart to pound
- difficult time breathing
- "lump in throat" that hurts when upset
- pupillary light reflex test (can't hold pupil constriction to bright light - light sensitivity)
- chronically bad knees (sartorius and gracilus connection)
- weak ankles or aching calves (gastrocnemius, soleus and posterior tibialis connection)
- salt craving
- muscle twitches and arrhythmias from sodium/potassium imbalance

Possible Causes of Hypoadrenia:

1) Stress - continuous physical, chemical, emotional or thermal stress. During stress, ACTH (adrenocorticotropic hormone) is released by the pituitary gland. ACTH is responsible for increasing blood pressure by triggering sodium retention and potassium excretion. Under constant stress, this could result in water retention, which can lead to hypertension.
2) Nutrient deficiencies
3) Environmental pollutants or toxins
4) Heavy metal toxicity
5) Poor dietary habits - highly refined foods
6) Smoking marijuana for several months
7) Hypoglycemia - hypoadrenia is usually found in conjunction with sugar handling problems
8) Food allergies
9) Alcohol and/or drug abuse
10) Thyroid or pituitary imbalance
11) More often found in fair-skinned, blond, blue-eyed people
12) Excess use of cortisone therapy, for such conditions as asthma or arthritis, causes the adrenal glands to shrink in size.
13) Addison's disease - a rare disorder of the adrenal glands, in which the adrenal cortex is underactive. This creates a discoloration of the skin (bronzing), fatigue, decreased body hair, the inability to cope with stress, and constantly feeling cold.

Nutrient Applications:

1) Adrenal support - to offset adrenal hypertrophy and atrophy in later stages of adrenal stress; do not leave patient on high potency, long-term adrenal support due to the old concept of "beating a tired horse".
   NOTE: Adrenal glandular can increase blood pressure in hypertensive patients.
2) Thymus support - to offset thymus atrophy due to stress
3) Stomach support - to offset damage to the stomach lining due to stress
4) Parotid - helpful in detoxification of heavy metals
5) B-vitamins - pantothenic acid, pyridoxine (B-6), riboflavin (B-2) and niacin all are important co-factors for adrenal function
6) Vitamin C, B-6, zinc, magnesium and pantothenic acid are all needed for synthesis of adrenal gland hormones. Panthothenic acid is very important to prevent adrenal atrophy.
7) Potassium - needed to maintain potassium levels that fluctuate due to aldosterone changes during stress
8) Chromium - essential in glucose tolerance factor (GTF); needed to stabilize blood sugar fluctuations
9) Tyrosine - amino acid that is a precursor for epinephrine and norepinephrine
10) Bioflavonoids - anti-oxidant and anti-inflammatory properties
11) Potassium - **NOTE:** In some cases of adrenal hyperfunction (during resistance stage), aldosterone is increased and potassium may be needed to balance retained sodium.

Dietary and Lifestyle Applications:

1) Relaxation exercises and de-stressing activities are a must. Biofeedback, meditation, massage and yoga are suggested.
2) Eat a healthy diet, with no refined carbohydrates. Caffeine, the bromine in tea and chocolate all cause sodium excretion and interfere with the sodium/potassium balance, thus should be avoided. A diet rich in potassium foods (bananas, potatoes, dried fruit and asparagus) is suggested.
3) Moderate exercise is beneficial.
4) Avoid alcohol, smoking and environmental toxins when possible.
5) Check for thyroid and/or pituitary imbalances.
6) In any chronic inflammatory condition (any "itis"), hypoadrenia needs to be addressed.

THYROID PROBLEMS

HYPOTHYROIDISM

Low thyroid function

Clinical hypothyroidism: blood level abnormalities of the thyroid hormones (T3 and T4) that show up on standard diagnostic tests.

Subclinical or functional hypothyroidism: blood levels in normal ranges, but temperature tests and other indicators show a mild deficiency state, which can still cause dramatic symptoms.

Signs and Symptoms of Hypothyroidism:

- axillary temperature test below 97.5
- chronic constipation
- sensitive to cold weather
- slow heartrate
- chronic fatigue
- excess hair loss
- gain weight easily
- recurrent infections
- skin problems (dry, flaky skin)
- PMS
- Depression
- cold hands and feet
- cry easily (may need iodine)
- headaches/dizziness
- myxedema (facial swelling, droopy eyes)
- slow speech
- feel worse in the morning

- increased triglyceride and cholesterol levels due to increased fat utilization
- feel better after exercising due to increased metabolic rate
- cracking and peeling of skin on heels and hands (may need essential fatty acid support)
- symptoms worse at change of season (spring/fall)
- brittle fingernails
- short windedness (can't breathe deep enough)
- paranoia
- memory loss (may need RNA support)
- sudden change in personality
- loss of libido

Possible Causes:

1) Depressed immune function
2) Poor dietary habits
3) Food allergies/sensitivities
4) Nutrient deficiencies (mainly iodine, tyrosine, B-vitamins)
5) Hormone imbalances
6) Candida/parasites - a high amount of candida patients will not clear until thyroid function is addressed
7) Liver dysfunction - thyroid hormones are conjugated in the liver
8) Secondary hypothyroidism - due to anterior pituitary dysfunction (TSH<2.0 uU/ml)
9) Medications - estrogen compounds (i.e. the pill) will reduce T3 uptake

Nutrient Applications:

1) Thyroid glandular
2) Iodine (kelp) - needed for thyroid hormone synthesis; may have **metallic taste** in mouth with iodine deficiency or heavy mucus secretions

   NOTE: According to Walter Schmitt, D.C., a **bitter taste** in the mouth with thin mucous secretions indicates biliary dysfunction and a need for bile salts. Also note that iodine excess will cause thyroid suppression, thus iodine levels need to be regulated within very narrow limits (RDA = .1 mg). Iodine supplementation should never exceed 1 milligram for any length of time.
3) Tyrosine and copper - needed for thyroid hormone synthesis
4) Possible parotid, adrenal and thymus support if the patient has recurrence of symptoms and doesn't hold treatments

   NOTE: The salivary secretions from the parotid gland aid in separating iodine from foods in order to make the iodine available to the thyroid gland. Take parotid in combination with iodine support.
5) B vitamins - necessary for normal manufacturing of the thyroid hormones
6) Calcium and magnesium - calcium insufficiency may be a problem in thyroid imbalances, due to calcitonin (thyroid hormone) regulation of blood calcium levels.
7) Essential fatty acids - needed for proper functioning of the thyroid gland
8) Vitamins A and E, and zinc - aid in thyroid hormone production
9) If necessary, a prescription for natural thyroid extract may be necessary.
10) Manganese and vitamin B-12 - manganese is needed to activate enzymes which increase thyroid function. Manganese increases the body's need for B-12.

Dietary and Lifestyle Applications:

1) Eat a healthy diet. Avoid processed and refined foods. Consume foods high in iodine (fish, kelp, dulse, vegetables and potatoes), B vitamins (whole grains, nuts and seeds) and vitamin A (dark, green and yellow vegetables). Avoid foods that slow down thyroid function including broccoli, brussel sprouts, cabbage, spinach, kale, peaches and pears. (Burton Goldberg Group, Alternative Medicine: The Definitive Guide, Future Medicine Publishing, Inc. WA, p. 937). Avoid foods that prevent utilization of iodine (turnips, cabbage, mustard, soybean, peanuts, pine nuts and millet (when cooked these foods

are inactivated)). These foods contain goitrogens, which prevent the utilization of iodine. (Murray, M. and Pizzorno, J. Encyclopedia of Natural Medicine, Prima Publishing, CA, p. 389). Use iodized salt.

2) Estrogen-containing medications (the pill, tranquilizers) will decrease T-3 uptake. Avoid antihistamines and sulfa drugs which aggravate the problem.
3) Thyroid medication will increase bone loss significantly, thus a calcium supplement should be taken to counteract bone loss.
4) Mild exercise is important. It stimulates the thyroid gland.
5) Drink filtered water. Chlorine and fluoride will compete with iodine and block iodine receptor sites in the thyroid gland.

HYPERTHYROIDISM (Grave's Disease)

Hyperactive thyroid function; overproduction of thyroid hormones. Hyperthyroidism is very rare compared to hypothyroidism.

Signs and Symptoms of Hyperthyroidism:

- protruding eyes
- increased axillary temperature > 98.2F
- rapid heartbeat (>90 beats per minute)
- low heat tolerance
- moist skin and palms
- diarrhea
- increased appetite
- anxiety/difficult to relax
- difficult to gain weight
- Gastrointestinal distress
- goiter (enlarged thyroid)
- PMS
- Trembling
- fatigue
- excessive sweating
- increased appetite
- rash and swelling in front of lower leg
- malabsorption due to increased digestive processes

Possible Causes:

1) Depressed immune function
2) Poor dietary habits
3) Food allergies/sensitivities
4) Nutrient deficiencies (mainly iodine, tyrosine, B vitamins)
5) Hormone imbalances
6) Candida/parasites - a large percentage of candida patients will not clear until thyroid function is addressed
7) Liver dysfunction - thyroid hormones are conjugated in the liver

Nutrient Applications:

1) Thyroid glandular
2) High doses of iodine have been known to suppress thyroid function by a negative feedback system
3) Vitamin A - needed for increased metabolic rate
4) Thymus support
5) Amino acid support - to meet demands of increased metabolic rate
6) Multiple vitamin/mineral support for "hyper" metabolic demands
7) B vitamins

Dietary and Lifestyle Applications:

1) Eat a healthy diet. Avoid processed and refined foods. Avoid caffeine, nicotine and soft drinks, which stimulate the system. Avoid dairy products. Increase foods that slow down thyroid function including broccoli, brussel sprouts, cabbage, spinach, kale, peaches and pears.

2) Thyroid medication will increase bone loss significantly, thus a calcium supplement should be taken to counteract bone loss. "A study done at the University of Massachusetts revealed that levothyroxine, a drug commonly used to treat thyroid conditions, caused up to 13% bone loss. Over 19 million people take this drug for hyperthyroidism, enlarged thyroid, and thyroid cancer" (Balch, J., M.D., and Balch, P., CNC, Prescription for Nutritional Healing, Avery Publishing Group, Inc., NY, p. 214).
3) Drink filtered water. Chlorine and fluoride will compete with iodine and block iodine receptor sites in the thyroid gland.

PANCREAS PROBLEMS

HYPOGLYCEMIA

Low blood sugar due to oversecretion of insulin by the pancreas. Insulin clears glucose from the blood and increases cellular utilization.

Signs and Symptoms of Hypoglycemia:

- anxiety/nervousness
- rapid heartbeat
- fatigue/weakness/irritability if meals are missed
- double vision
- headaches relieved by sweets or alcohol
- extreme hunger
- weakness/shakes/jitters
- symptoms occur in afternoon, several hours after eating, or if waiting period between meals is too long
- dizziness
- digestive complaints
- memory problems

Possible Causes:

1) Insulin-dependent or non-insulin dependent diabetes mellitus
2) Poor adrenal function
3) Blood sugar imbalance problems
4) Poor dietary habits - excess sugars, refined foods and increased caffeine consumption or simply a lack of food
5) Nutrient deficiencies, especially chromium, zinc, B-6 and essential fatty acids
6) Hypothyroidism - approximately 50% of hypoglycemics have low thyroid function
7) Food allergies/sensitivities
8) Excess stress (physical, mental or emotional)
9) Excessive exercise
10) Alcohol or drug abuse
11) Smoking - alters blood sugar balance
12) Poor digestive function
13) Low pancreatic enzymes
14) Poor eating habits - skip meals
15) Hereditary factors
16) Candida/parasites

Nutrient Applications:

1) Chromium - essential in glucose metabolism, part of glucose tolerance factor (GTF)
2) B vitamins - important in carbohydrate metabolism
3) Adrenal and pancreas support
4) Vitamin C with bioflavonoids. Vitamin C is contraindicated in iron overload disease, gout and people prone to kidney stones.
5) Amino acid support
6) HCl and pancreatic enzymes - if needed for digestive support
7) Calcium and magnesium

8) Zinc

Dietary and Lifestyle Applications:

1) Eat smaller more frequent meals throughout the course of the day, which alleviates adrenal and pancreas stress by maintaining blood glucose levels. Do not skip breakfast.
2) Remove all refined sugars, processed foods, hydrogenated fats, caffeine and alcohol from the diet. Eat whole grains, seeds, nuts, nut butters, lean meats and fish. High fiber foods help stabilize blood sugar and should be combined with small protein snacks, especially during a blood sugar reaction.
3) Moderate exercise is beneficial.
4) Follow an elimination/rotation diet if food allergies are suspect.
5) Avoid stress. Practice relaxation exercises.

Considerations:

1) The brain needs a constant level of blood sugar in order to function correctly. Fluctuations in blood sugar can cause anxiety due to the effects on the brain.
2) The average American consumes more than 80 pounds of sugar per year, which is approximately 30 teaspoons per day.

DIABETES

Chronic degenerative disease marked by high amounts of glucose in the blood (>140 mg/dl). The disease is caused by a lack of, or resistance to, the hormone insulin. Insulin is secreted by the pancreas and regulates blood sugar levels by moving glucose from the blood into the cells. In the United States, diabetes is one of the leading causes of deaths and affects over six million people.

Types of Diabetes Mellitus:

1) **Type 1 - Insulin-dependent juvenile diabetes**
The body cannot manufacture the insulin necessary to get the glucose into the cells, and the glucose spills into the urine. The body is unable to use the glucose and basically starves to death.

Signs and Symptoms of Type 1 Diabetes:

- frequent urination
- fatigue
- excessive thirst
- weakness
- irritability
- unusual hunger
- nausea/vomiting
- weight loss

NOTE: Mostly found in children and can involve instant hypoglycemic reactions that are remedied immediately by eating a piece of candy or drinking fruit juice to bring the blood sugar levels back to normal. If the sugar administration does not work, it may be a problem of excess insulin administration, in which case the sugar will not hurt. Insulin injections are necessary in Type 1 diabetes to control the disease.

2) **Type 2 - Non-insulin-dependent adult-onset diabetes**
Insulin is still produced by the pancreas but the cells become resistant to insulin and glucose cannot move into the cells; usually seen in adults.

Signs and Symptoms of Type 2 Diabetes:

- family history of diabetes
- tingling/numbness in feet
- blurred vision
- obesity

- excessive thirst
- itching
- cuts that will not heal
- drowsiness

NOTE: Type 2 diabetes can usually be controlled by diet, weight management and exercise. These factors reduce insulin resistance. In most cases, insulin shots are not required unless blood sugar levels are out of control.

3) **Gestational diabetes** - temporary blood sugar problems brought on during pregnancy. Blood sugar levels need to be monitored so the fluctuations do not damage the fetus.

Signs and Symptoms of Gestational Diabetes:

- excessive thirst
- excessive hunger
- urgent need to urinate

Possible Causes:

1) **Type 1 -**
   1) Genetic predisposition
   2) Autoimmune problems - a high percentage of Type 1 diabetics have antibodies in their blood against their own pancreatic cells
   3) Food allergies
   4) Viral infections - may trigger an autoimmune response
   5) Free radical injury of pancreatic beta cells, which produce and secrete insulin.
   6) Nitrate compounds (smoked and cured meats) have been shown to destroy beta cells.
2) **Type 2 -**
   1) Genetic predisposition
   2) Obesity - it has been suggested that a person 30% or more overweight for over 30 years will develop diabetes
   3) Poor diet - refined, processed foods including sugar, saturated fats and refined carbohydrates, greatly contribute to diabetes
   4) Viral infections - may trigger an autoimmune response
   5) Food allergies
   6) Stress - increases adrenaline production, which increases blood sugar levels

Nutrient Applications:

1) Vanadyl Sulfate - maintains blood sugar balance; increases rate of glucose transport, relieving the insulin mechanism. It decreases insulin requirements and aids in synthesis and retention of muscle mass.
2) Chromium - necessary component of the glucose tolerance factor (GTF); aids in blood sugar regulation and cholesterol reduction. Chromium potentiates the action of insulin. (Murray, M. and Pizzorno, J. Encyclopedia of Natural Medicine, Prima Publishing, CA, p. 283).
3) B vitamins - (Werbach, M., M.D., Healing Through Nutrition, Harper Collins Publishers, NY, pp. 110-113).
   a) B-6 - shown to decrease insulin needs; found very effective in gestational diabetes
   b) Niacin - a necessary component of GTF; aids in insulin action
   c) Thiamine (B-1) - involved in carbohydrate metabolism and the Krebs Cycle. May help prevent diabetic neuropathy (nerve disease in diabetes).
   d) Biotin - aids in glucose utilization
   e) B-12 - involved in carbohydrate metabolism; helpful in diabetic retinopathy
   f) Folic Acid - involved in carbohydrate metabolism
4) Zinc - essential for insulin production (Burton Goldberg Group, Alternative Medicine: The Definitive Guide, Future Medicine Publishing, Inc. WA, p. 937).

5) Vitamin C - high amounts have been shown to decrease insulin needs and regulate blood sugar (Burton Goldberg Group, Alternative Medicine: The Definitive Guide, Future Medicine Publishing, Inc. WA, p. 652). Vitamin C is contraindicated in iron overload disease, gout and people prone to kidney stones.
6) Vitamin E - increased requirement is shown in diabetics; may help prevent complications of diabetes such as diabetic retinopathy and heart disease (Murray, M. and Pizzorno, J. Encyclopedia of Natural Medicine, Prima Publishing, CA, p. 283).
7) Magnesium - aids in insulin and blood sugar regulation; may help prevent diabetic retinopathy and heart disease (Werbach, M., M.D., Healing Through Nutrition, Harper Collins Publishers, NY, p. 117).
8) Manganese - needed for activating enzymes necessary in glucose metabolism (Werbach, M., M.D., Healing Through Nutrition, Harper Collins Publishers, NY, p. 117).
9) Copper - deficiency is associated with blood sugar problems (Werbach, M., M.D., Healing Through Nutrition, Harper Collins Publishers, NY, p. 116).
10) Selenium - may be a factor in glucose levels; potent antioxidant
11) Brewer's yeast - excellent source of chromium (GTF)
12) Omega-6 fatty acids - specifically black currant seed oil or evening primrose oil; aid in reversing nerve damage due to diabetic neuropathy (Jamal, G. et al. Treatment of diabetic neuropathy with gamma-linolenic acid (GLA) as evening primrose oil. JACN,6:86, 1987).
13) CoEnzyme Q10 - stimulates insulin production; shown to reduce fasting blood sugar levels and ketone bodies by 30%. (Werbach, M., M.D. Nutritional Influences on Illness, Keats Publishing, Inc. CT., p. 179).

Dietary and Lifestyle Applications:

1) A healthy diet is essential. Avoid refined, processed foods and increase complex carbohydrates and fiber. Soluble fiber, found in fruits and vegetables, should be emphasized. Two servings of beans per day may help control blood sugar levels (soak beans in several drops of iodine to alleviate gas-producing effects). Moderate amounts of lean meat, fish and unsaturated fats are helpful. Small, frequent meals are suggested. A vegetarian diet is helpful. Onions and garlic have blood sugar-lowering effects (Murray, M., N.D. Natural Alternatives to Over-the-Counter and Prescription Drugs, William Morrow and Company, Inc. NY, p. 179).
2) Regular, moderate exercise is essential.
3) Reduce weight if necessary.
4) Reduce stress. Practice relaxation exercises.
5) Eliminate alcohol, caffeine and smoking.
6) Follow an elimination/rotation diet to detect food allergies or sensitivities.

Considerations:

1) Diabetes can lead to many different complications including heart and kidney disease, neuropathy (nerve damage), eye problems (diabetic retinopathy and cataracts), atherosclerosis, gangrenous infections of the feet or legs, blindness and death. Another complication of diabetes is ketoacidosis, which is an accumulation of toxic acidic by-products that are produced by the body when the body starts burning fat and muscle for fuel, since it is unable to utilize glucose. The by-products of fat oxidation are responsible for the acetone breath of a diabetic in ketosis.

THYMUS PROBLEMS

DECREASED THYMUS FUNCTION

The thymus gland is the center of the body's immune function. It is of maximum size in puberty and atrophies as we get older. The thymus gland produces T-lymphocytes, which are white blood cells responsible for cell-mediated immunity (immunity that is not regulated or controlled by antibodies).

Signs and Symptoms of Decreased Thymus Function:

- repeated and prolonged infections
- infections lasting longer than seven days
- chronic swollen glands
- frequent flu-like symptoms
- neck soreness
- irregular heartbeat
- skin problems

Possible Causes:

1) Medications - Glucocorticoids cause the thymus gland to atrophy.
   NOTE: After organ transplants, glucocorticoids are given to decrease thymus function so that the immune system will not build antibodies to the foreign tissue. At the same time, the depressed immune system is not as able to fight infection. Also note that during chronic stress (adrenal alarm reaction or resistance stage), increased glucocorticoids are released from the adrenals, which inhibit thymus function and actually cause the thymus to atrophy.
2) Poor immune response
3) Nutrient deficiencies
4) Poor dietary habits
5) Candida/parasites
6) Heavy metal toxicity
7) Environmental pollutants and chemical toxins
8) Chronic stress
9) Toxic bowel - infectious agents fester in a toxic environment

Nutrient Applications:

1) Thymus extract - specific glandular support
2) Antioxidants to prevent thymic involution:
   a) Vitamin C - contraindicated in iron overload disease, gout and people prone to kidney stones.
   b) Vitamin E
   c) Bioflavonoids
   d) Zinc
   e) Selenium
   f) Beta-carotene
3) Vitamin A - epithelial repair and immune support
4) Vitamin B-6 - has been shown to increase thymic function and cell-mediated immunity
5) Echinacea/Goldenseal - increase immune function

Dietary and Lifestyle Applications:

1) Eat a healthy diet.
2) Practice relaxation exercises.
3) Avoid environmental pollutants whenever possible.
4) Keep the bowel clean and healthy.

Considerations:

1) In infectious mononucleosis, "patients usually require support of either the adrenal glands or the thyroid gland in addition to the thymus" (Schmitt, Common Glandular Dysfunction in the General Practice, Applied Kinesiology Study Program, NC, p. 54).
2) Thymus in combination with parotid, adrenal and spleen may be helpful for people under chronic stress. The thymus and parotid gland are thought to have a connection. According to Walter Schmitt, D.C. in his book Common Glandular Dysfunction in General Practice, obscure references

have been made to the idea that the thymus and parotid activate nutrient function, so that nutrients are sent to the areas they are needed most.

THE PHYSIOLOGY OF THE MALE REPRODUCTIVE SYSTEM

MALE REPRODUCTIVE ORGANS

THE ORGANS OF THE MALE REPRODUCTIVE SYSTEM INCLUDE:

Testes: male gonads which produce sperm in the seminiferous tubules.
Scrotum: outpouching that supports the testes; regulates temperature of the testes.
Sperm: gametes that initiate fertilization.
Epididymis: transports sperm out of the testes.
Ductus (Vas) Deferens: epididymis changes into the ductus deferens and carries sperm to the ejaculatory duct and on to the prostatic urethra. The ductus (vas) deferens is what is partially removed and tied in a vasectomy.
Prostate: secretes milky, white alkaline fluid into the prostatic urethra, which combines with sperm to form semen; this fluid makes close to 30% of semen volume.
Seminal Vessicles: secretes alkaline, viscous fluid, rich in fructose into the ejaculatory duct and combines with sperm and prostate fluid to form semen; this fluid from the seminal vessicles makes up 60% of semen volume.
Bulbourethral Gland: secretes mucus for lubrication; neutralizes urine.
Urethra: passageway for sperm during ejaculation and urination.
Semen: sperm plus fluid secretions from the prostate, seminal vesicles and bulbourethral glands; slightly alkaline pH of 7.35 - 7.50; also contains an antibiotic called seminal plasmin that destroys bacteria in semen and the vaginal tract.
NOTE: Average semen volume/ejaculation = 2.5 to 6 ml.
Average range of sperm ejaculated = 50-100 million/ml.
Considered sterile if ejaculated sperm falls below 20 million/ml.
Penis: organ used to introduce sperm into the vagina.

HORMONAL CONTROL

The hypothalamus releases **gonadotropin releasing factor (GnRF),** which triggers the anterior pituitary to release:

1) **FSH (Follicle Stimulating Hormone)** - initiates spermatogenesis in testes.
   Inhibin (a protein hormone) inhibits FSH secretion by the anterior pituitary once spermatogenesis required levels are achieved.

2) **LH (Luteinizing Hormone)** - stimulates testes to produce and secrete testosterone.
   Testosterone - synthesized from cholesterol or acetyl coenzyme A in the testes; principle male hormone.

   FUNCTIONS OF TESTOSTERONE:

   1) Controls growth and development of male sex hormones.
   2) Stimulates sexual behavior, final sperm maturation, male sex characteristics, bone growth and protein anabolism.
   3) Inhibits GnRF release when blood levels of testosterone reach a certain level.

SUBCLINICAL AND PATHOLOGICAL CONDITIONS OF THE MALE REPRODUCTIVE SYSTEM

MALE GENITOURINARY SYSTEM

Problems of the male genitourinary system include prostate enlargement, prostatitis, impotence and prostate cancer.

PROSTATE ENLARGEMENT (BENIGN PROSTATIC HYPERTROPHY (BPH) or HYPERPLASIA)

Enlargement of the prostate, which is the male sex gland located beneath the urinary bladder and surrounds the urethra (the duct where urine and semen pass in males). This problem can affect over 30% of males over 50 years of age.

PROSTATE FUNCTION: secretes a milky, white alkaline fluid into the prostatic urethra, which constitutes up to 33% of the volume of semen. This fluid enhances sperm motility and fertility during ejaculation. The prostate is also the first defense of the genitourinary system against infection.

Signs and Symptoms of Prostate Enlargement:

- increased urinary frequency
- need to urinate during the night
- decreased urine flow with increased strain
- difficulty in urinating or interruption of urine flow
- enlarged prostate
- painful urination

Possible Causes:

1) **Inflammation or abnormal tissue growth of the prostate**, which eventually blocks the urethra and interferes with normal urination. This can eventually affect the kidneys and bladder, producing such consequences as kidney infections, cystitis and uremia (retention of urine in the blood).
   NOTE: Testosterone is the culprit in the growth of prostate tissue. Testosterone is the principal male hormone and is synthesized from cholesterol or acetyl coenzyme A in the testes (the site of sperm production). As a man ages, **testosterone conversion to dihydrotestosterone (DHT)**, a very potent male hormone, **is increased, which enhances tissue growth of the prostate.** DHT is known to increase in the prostate cells mainly due to decreased rate of removal of DHT and increased uptake of testosterone by the prostate. **Prolactin,** another hormone, **is known to increase testosterone uptake and increase DHT synthesis. Beer and stress increase prolactin levels.** (Murray, M. and Pizzorno, J. Encyclopedia of Natural Medicine, Prima Publishing, CA, p. 283).
2) Chronic constipation - it does not cause BPH, but is a contributing factor that increases pain and discomfort when the gland is already enlarged.
3) Nutrient deficiencies - especially zinc and essential fatty acids
4) Heavy metal toxicity - especially cadmium
5) Environmental toxins and pollutants - pesticide toxicity has been shown to cause BPH
6) Excess beer consumption - increases prolactin production, which increases DHT
7) Excess stress - increases prolactin production, which increases DHT

8) High cholesterol levels - cholesterol metabolites (breakdown products of cholesterol) have been shown to enhance prostate hypertrophy, and are also carcinogenic
9) Food allergies and/or sensitivities

PROSTATITIS

Acute or chronic inflammation or infection of the prostate gland seen in men of all ages.

Signs and Symptoms of Prostatitis:

- difficulty upon urination
- increased frequency and urgency of urination
- pain during urination
- discharge from the penis after a bowel movement
- prostate tenderness and pain
- fever/chills
- blood or pus in the urine
- lower back pain

Possible Causes:

1) Infection - usually bacteria or chlamydia (an intracellular parasite transmitted during intercourse)
2) Nutrient deficiency
3) Immune depletion
4) Repeated sexual contact, especially with multiple partners. High sexual activity depletes the prostate of essential nutrients.
5) Injury
6) Heavy metal toxicity
7) Environmental pollutants

PROSTATE CANCER

Cancer of the prostate; it is the third most common cancer that afflicts men, following lung and colon cancer. It accounts for over 30,000 deaths per year in the United States.

Signs and Symptoms of Prostate Cancer:

- similar symptoms to benign prostatic hypertrophy plus:
- weight loss
- pain or swelling of the prostate
- blood in the urine

Possible Causes:

1) Hormonal imbalances
2) Genetic factors - black males have a higher risk
3) Chemical toxicity exposure
4) Cadmium toxicity
5) Vasectomy surgery will increase risk
6) Venereal disease
7) Repeated prostate infections

Nutrient Applications for Prostate Problems:

1) Zinc - BPH patients have low levels of zinc in the prostatic fluids. Zinc has been shown to decrease prostate size and symptomotology in BPH. (Murray, M. and Pizzorno, J. Encyclopedia of Natural Medicine, Prima Publishing, CA, p. 482).

   Zinc Functions:

   1) Inhibits prolactin secretion.
   2) Inhibits the enzyme that converts testosterone to DHT.
   3) Increases excretion of male hormones, thus decreases DHT production.

   NOTE: Zinc is required to metabolize male hormones. The prostate contains the highest amount of zinc of any body part.
2) Essential fatty acids - shown to reduce prostate size; theory is that prostaglandins prevent prostate enlargement and prostaglandin synthesis declines with age. EFA's provide prostaglandin support, which may decrease prostate enlargement. (Giller, R., M.D., and Matthews, K., Natural Prescriptions, Ballantine Books, NY, pp. 285-286).
3) Saw Palmetto - comes from the berries of the saw palmetto palm tree; known as "an aphrodisiac and sexual rejuvenator"; saw palmetto has been shown repeatedly to decrease urinary problems associated with BPH (Werbach, M., M.D., Healing Through Nutrition, Harper Collins Publishers, NY, p. 335).
4) Vitamins E and C - found in high amounts in prostate tissue; potent antioxidants (Burton Goldberg Group, Alternative Medicine: The Definitive Guide, Future Medicine Publishing, Inc. WA, p. 737). Vitamin C is contraindicated in iron overload disease, gout, and people prone to kidney stones.
5) Prostate and orchic (testicular) support
6) Cadmium homeopathic - if cadmium toxicity is suspect
7) Vitamin B-6 - enhances zinc absorption
8) Enzymes - aids in inflammation
9) Garlic - aids in preventing infection

Dietary and Lifestyle Applications:

1) Eat a healthy diet. Eat foods rich in zinc and essential fatty acids including nuts and seeds. An old folk remedy is that pumpkin seeds, taken daily, help in BPH, because they are very high in zinc and EFA's. Avoid spicy foods, caffeine, alcohol (especially beer), tobacco and high fat foods. One teaspoon daily of EFA's (linseed, flaxseed, soy, walnut, sunflower oils) may be helpful.
2) Avoid stress and practice relaxation exercises.
3) Avoid pesticides and environmental pollutants as much as possible. Eat organic foods.
4) Chronic constipation needs to be remedied, since it increases prostatic discomfort.
5) Mild exercise is suggested, but avoid bicycle riding due to increased pressure on the prostate.
6) Avoid exposure to very cold weather.
7) Hydrotherapy helps increase circulation to the prostate region. Sitz baths, in which the pelvic region is submerged in water and the feet are in a separate tub of hot water, are the recommended form of hydrotherapy.
8) Avoid sexual intimacy while infection is present.
9) Follow an elimination/rotation diet if food allergies are suspect.
10) Completely and immediately evacuate the bladder when you feel the need.

Considerations:

1) Finasteride (Proscar) is the only approved medication used for BPH.

   ACTION: Inhibits 5 alpha-reductase, the enzyme that converts testosterone to DHT. It is only 50% effective and if it is effective, the results are only noticeable after 6 months.

   SIDE EFFECTS: problems with ejaculation, decreased libido, impotence.

   NOTE: The extract of saw palmetto has been shown to be much more effective than Proscar in clinical trials, but is has been refused by the FDA as treatment for BPH (Murray, M., N.D. Natural Alternatives to Over-the-Counter and Prescription Drugs, William Morrow and Company, Inc. NY, p. 215).

IMPOTENCE

Inability to have or maintain an erection; 10 million men in the U.S. are suspected of having impotence problems

Signs and Symptoms of Impotence:

- inability to have or maintain an erection

Possible Causes:

1) Psychological factors - fear, guilt, anxiety, boredom, low self-esteem, immaturity; psychological factors are the cause of 75-80% of all impotency cases
2) Stress
3) Low male sex hormone levels
4) Infection and illness
5) Endocrine dysfunction - low thyroid or pituitary function
6) Injury
7) Vascular problems (i.e. arteriosclerosis) - affects the vessels in the penis, thus the penis does not engorge sufficiently
8) Medications - anti-depressives, hypertension medication
9) Mumps as an adult
10) High blood pressure or high cholesterol levels
11) Prostate and/or abdominal surgery
12) Diabetes - due to blood sugar fluctuations, which may trigger impotence
13) Food allergies/sensitivities
14) Alcohol or cigarette abuse - both decrease hormone levels of testosterone. Smoking also clogs the penile arteries.

Nutrient Applications:

1) Zinc - necessary for testosterone production
2) Yohimbe bark - dilates blood vessels and aids in norepinephrine release

   NOTE: Yohimbe can increase anxiety and heartrate if taken in large amounts. Check with a trained, licensed professional for amounts of yohimbe to use. It is best used in a synergistic formula where the effects of small amounts are optimized by supporting herbs and nutrients.
3) Damiana - aphrodisiac; enhances sexual activity
4) Ginseng - known for centuries as an aphrodisiac; anti-stress properties
5) Saw palmetto - often used in conjunction with damiana to promote sexual health
6) Gotu kola - excellent general tonic and helpful in impotence problems
7) Ginkgo biloba - dilates blood vessels to increase penile blood flow
8) Vitamins E and C - aid in sperm motility and prostate health

Dietary and Lifestyle Applications:

1) Eat a healthy diet with foods high in zinc and essential fatty acids (nuts, seeds and unsaturated oils). Avoid fried and spicy foods, caffeine and refined foods.
2) Avoid alcohol and tobacco.
3) Avoid stress and practice relaxation exercises.
4) Avoid pesticides and environmental pollutants as much as possible. Eat organic foods.
5) Avoid heavy metal exposure.
6) Strenuous exercise, saunas and hot tubs should all be avoided. All three decrease sperm count.
7) Medications, especially hypertensive drugs, tranquilizers and street drugs all can cause impotence. Ulcer medications (Tagamet and Zantac) may decrease sperm count.

Considerations:

1) Do not confuse natural age-related changes in men to impotence; as men age, erections may happen more slowly and/or be less engorged.

SEXUALLY TRANSMITTED DISEASES (STD)

Diseases that are transmitted by sexual intimacy (applies to both males and females). There are many types of STD's including:

1) **AIDS (Acquired ImmunoDeficiency Syndrome)** - AIDS is a severe breakdown of the immune system, which can manifest in a variety of complaints. It is a conglomeration of 28 known diseases combined with a positive HIV antibody test. Some of the diseases associated with an AIDS diagnosis include a conglomeration of candidiasis, pneumonia, Kaposis sarcoma (a form of cancer), cytomegalovirus, herpes, tuberculosis, and the list goes on.

   Signs and Symptoms of AIDS:

   - Symptoms associated with the 28 known diseases plus:
   - HIV positive
   - chronic swollen glands
   - rashes
   - night sweats
   - diarrhea
   - weight loss
   - fever

2) **Candidiasis** - yeast infection; much more common in females.

   Signs and Symptoms of Candidiasis:

   - thick vaginal discharge in females
   - itchy genitals
   - pain upon urination

3) **Chlamydia** - most common STD in the United States; infectious disease that causes genital lesions and lymph node inflammation in the genital area.

   Signs and Symptoms of Chlamydia:

   - usually no symptoms are present; if present, can include:

   Male:
   - clear, watery discharge from the penis
   - changes in urination
   - itchy genitals

   Female:
   - white, vaginal discharge and/or bleeding
   - changes in urination
   - pelvic pain
   - fever
   - pain during intercourse

4) **Genital Herpes** - caused by the herpes simplex virus type 2 (HSV2); HSV1 causes cold sores.

Signs and Symptoms of Genital Herpes:

- occurs within 7 days of sexual contact with an infected partner
- itching and burning in the genital area
- painful urination
- pimple-like bumps on the skin in the genital area, which eventually blister and burst, oozing pus

5) **Genital Warts** - caused by the Human Papilloma Virus (HPV) and can be transmitted by sexual contact or spread through unsanitary objects, such as tanning beds and underwear. Most warts are not visible. HPV is thought to be a cause of cervical dysplasia.

Signs and Symptoms of Genital Warts:

- cauliflower-type growths in the genital area
- burning and itching in the affected area

6) **Gonorrhea** - caused by bacteria (Bonococcus neisseria), which cause the mucous membranes of the genitals to become inflamed.

Signs and Symptoms of Gonorrhea:

- often no symptoms are present
- swelling and redness of the genitals
- painful and frequent urination
- vaginal or urethral discharge; yellow pus in males
- can spread to the joints and cause arthritis-type pains

7) **Syphilis** - caused by bacteria (Treponema pallidum), that cause lesions to an organ or tissue; syphilis is extremely dangerous and needs antibiotic treatment.

Signs and Symptoms of Syphilis:

- no symptoms present in early stages of disease
- sores or lesions on the genitals
- rash
- mouth sores
- sore throat
- fever

8) **Trichomonas** - caused by a protozoa (single-cell parasite).

Signs and Symptoms of Trichomonas:

- vaginal odorous discharge in females
- clear urethral discharge in males
- itching and burning of the genitals

Possible Causes of Sexually Transmitted Diseases:

1) Sexual activity, especially with multiple partners including kissing and intercourse
2) Infections - bacteria, virus, parasites, yeast
3) Blood transfusions
4) Intravenous drug injections (i.e. sharing needles)

5) Poor immune function

Nutrient Applications:

1) Immune support nutrients:
   a) Vitamin A - supports epithelial repair
   b) Vitamin C - potent immune enhancer and antiviral agent (magnesium and B-6 taken along with vitamin C will decrease the risk of developing kidney stones) (Werbach, M., M.D., Healing Through Nutrition, Harper Collins Publishers, NY, pp. 235-236). **NOTE:** Vitamin C is contraindicated in iron overload disease, gout, and people prone to kidney stones.
   c) Vitamin E - may decrease pain during herpes outbreak and help shorten the duration (Murray, M. and Pizzorno, J. Encyclopedia of Natural Medicine, Prima Publishing, CA, p. 283).
   d) Beta-carotene - increases number of T-cells
   e) Zinc - immune enhancer and antiviral agent
   f) B vitamins
   g) Goldenseal and echinacea - stimulate the immune system; echinacea has been shown to inhibit herpes virus proliferation (Zand, J. et al. Smart Medicine for a Healthier Child, Avery Publishing Group, NY, p.262). Berberine in goldenseal is an effective antifungal, antimicrobial and antiprotozoal agent.
2) Saw Palmetto - excellent support for men during any genital infection.
3) L-lysine and licorice root - helpful for herpes sufferers; lysine is suggested to inhibit herpes outbreaks, while arginine promotes it (Giller, R., M.D., and Matthews, K., Natural Prescriptions, Ballantine Books, NY, p. 184). Licorice root contains glycyrrhizic acid that prevents growth and inhibits the cell-damaging effects of the herpes virus (Murray, M. and Pizzorno, J. Encyclopedia of Natural Medicine, Prima Publishing, CA, p. 283).
4) Thuja - common homeopathic remedy used to treat warts
5) Folic acid - deficiency may increase the risk for cervical dysplasia (deficiency of vitamins A and C will do the same) (Giller, R., M.D., and Matthews, K., Natural Prescriptions, Ballantine Books, NY, pp. 79-78).
6) Hypericin – one of the active ingredients in St. John's Wort, is being tested with some success in AIDS patients

Dietary and Lifestyle Applications:

1) Eat a healthy diet. Remove refined foods, fatty foods, excess salt and coffee from the diet. Increase fresh fruits and vegetables. Vegetable juicing is beneficial. For herpes sufferers, increase lysine-rich foods including seafood, chicken, potatoes and brewer's yeast. Avoid chocolate, coconut, nuts and seeds, which are high in arginine and can aggravate herpes outbreaks.
2) Avoid alcohol and smoking.
3) Drink plenty of filtered water.
4) Reduce stress. This is especially important with herpes sufferers because stress intensifies the number and intensity of the outbreaks .
5) Avoid medication when possible due to immune suppressing effects.
6) During a herpes outbreak, cold compresses can be applied to the lesions to relieve the pain. Aloe vera can be applied topically as a salve. Do not touch the affected area and then touch your mouth, face, eyes, etc..
7) Be careful when receiving blood transfusions or when you have an open wound.
8) Practice safe sex and find out your partner's health and sexual history.
9) Pap smears are important for females to aid in early detection.
10) Make sure to get adequate sleep, and exercise moderately to reduce stress, promote healing, circulation and excretion.
11) Liver and bowel detoxification is suggested to enhance immune function.
12) Wear cotton underwear and non-restricting clothes and keep affected area dry and clean.

THE PHYSIOLOGY OF THE FEMALE REPRODUCTIVE SYSTEM

FEMALE REPRODUCTIVE ORGANS

THE ORGANS OF THE FEMALE REPRODUCTIVE SYSTEM INCLUDE:

Ovaries: female gonads which produce ova (eggs); promote ovulation (releasing of the egg); secrete progesterone, estrogen and relaxin (the female sex hormones).

Fallopian (uterine) tubes: transport egg from the ovaries to the uterus, usually the site of fertilization.

NOTE: Ectopic pregnancy results when the fertilized egg implants in the fallopian tubes or pelvic cavity, instead of the uterus. Ectopic pregnancies must be terminated before the tube ruptures.

Uterus: the womb; site of menstruation, implantation of the fertilized egg, fetus development and labor; ligaments hold the uterus in place.

A) **Fundus** - portion of the uterus above the tubes.
B) **Body** - central portion of the uterus.
C) **Cervix** - narrow portion of the uterus that opens into the vagina.

Vagina: passageway for menstrual flow, site of intercourse and birthing.

Vulva: external genitalia of the female.

Mammary Glands: located over the pectoralis major muscle; they secrete and eject milk (lactation); lactation is regulated by the hormones prolactin and oxytocin.

HORMONAL CONTROL

The hypothalamus releases gonadotropin releasing factor (GnRF), which stimulates the anterior pituitary to release:

1) **FSH (Follicle Stimulating Hormone)** - stimulates development of the ovarian follicle (egg and surrounding tissues); stimulates secretion of estrogen by the follicles for the first 14 days of the cycle.
2) **LH (Luteinizing Hormone)** - develops the ovarian follicle; production of LH increases right before ovulation, initiating ovulation; stimulates estrogen, progesterone and relaxin production by the ovarian cells, with progesterone production in higher amounts.

   THEREFORE:
   1) Higher amounts of estrogen are released the first 14 days of the cycle.
   2) Higher amounts of progesterone are released the second 14 days of the cycle. The progesterone levels drop suddenly 1-2 days prior to menstruation.

HORMONES

1) **Estrogen** - includes B-estradiol (principal estrogen), estrone and estriol, which are synthesized from cholesterol and acetyl coenzyme A in the ovaries; estrogens are the hormones of growth and sexual development.

FUNCTIONS OF ESTROGEN:

1) Development and maintenance of female reproductive system including the uterus, breasts and sex characteristics.
2) Controls fluid and electrolyte balance.

3) Increases protein anabolism.
4) Inhibits GnRF release when blood levels of estrogen reach a certain level.
NOTE: Some birth control pills work by inhibiting GnRF.

2) **Progesterone** - hormone of maturation.

FUNCTIONS OF PROGESTERONE:

1) Prepare the uterus for implantation of fertilized egg.
2) Prepare mammary glands for lactation.

3) **Relaxin** - functions during final stages of pregnancy; relaxes and dilates uterus to facilitate delivery.

THE MENSTRUAL CYCLE

The average cycle is every 28 days, but can vary from 24-35 days. The menstrual cycle is divided into four stages:

1) **MENSTRUATION (MENSES):** discharge of blood from the uterus, triggered by a sudden drop in estrogen and progesterone; lasts approximately five days. During menstruation approximately 20-25 ovarian follicles begin development (at birth each ovary contains approximately 200,000 follicles) and trigger GnRF secretion. This in turn stimulates FSH production. Only one follicle reaches maturity, the others die.

2) **PREOVULATORY PHASE:** time between menstruation and ovulation (release of the egg); lasts approximately 6-13 days in a 28 day cycle. Estrogen production increases and stimulates repair of the endometrial lining of the uterus that was shed during menstruation. Estrogen hormone and FSH secretion is dominant. Right before ovulation, LH is secreted in high quantities and FSH is inhibited.

3) **OVULATION:** the egg is released from the follicle into the fallopian tube (day 14). The follicular cells enlarge and form the corpus luteum (yellow body).

4) **POSTOVULATORY PHASE:** time between ovulation and the next menses; lasts approximately 15-28 days in a 28 day cycle. LH stimulates corpus luteum formation, which secretes estrogen and progesterone. Progesterone is the dominant hormone released. Progesterone prepares the uterus for implantation of the fertilized egg. FSH gradually increases and LH secretion gradually decreases. If fertilization does not occur, the corpus luteum degenerates and estrogen and progesterone levels decrease triggering menstruation. If fertilization does occur, the corpus luteum is maintained by the placenta (connection between mother and child).

SIGNS AND SYMPTOMS OF ESTROGEN/PROGESTERONE IMBALANCES

An imbalance in the estrogen/progesterone ratio can create many symptoms in the female patient. According to Walter Schmitt, D.C., in his book "Common Glandular Dysfunctions in the General Practice", imbalances in the estrogen/progesterone ratio can trigger the following symptoms:

1) **Excess Estrogen:** heavy flow, short cycles (21-25 days), breast tenderness, edema, large breasts, menstrual cramps.
2) **Low Estrogen:** short flow (1-2 days), scanty flow, long cycles, small breasted, possible cramping if accompanied by low progesterone.
3) **Excess Progesterone:** scanty flow, long cycles (32-35 days), small breasted, no cramps.

4) **Low Progesterone:** heavy flow, short cycles, definite menstrual cramps.
NOTE: Prostaglandins stimulate uterine contractions (menstrual cramps), but cannot do so with high levels of progesterone. Progesterone inhibits prostaglandins, but if pregnancy does not occur, progesterone levels fall quickly, while prostaglandin levels increase. This may be a cause for menstrual cramps.

CONSIDERATIONS:

1) Estrogen and progesterone require good liver function for complete breakdown.
2) Good thyroid function is necessary for proper progesterone production. Low thyroid function correlates with low progesterone production.

MENOPAUSE

Menopause refers to a women's last menses. Menopause usually occurs in a woman's late 40's to early 50's, but can vary widely between each individual. Menstrual cycles become less frequent. Physiologically, the ovaries, as they age, are unable to respond to FSH and LH stimulation. As a result, estrogen production decreases.

SUBCLINICAL AND PATHOLOGICAL CONDITIONS OF THE FEMALE REPRODUCTIVE SYSTEM

FEMALE PROBLEMS

DYSMENORRHEA

Menstrual cramps caused by forceful contraction of the uterine muscle; menstrual cramps are not "normal" and indicate that an imbalance is present.

Signs and Symptoms of Dysmenorrhea:

- intense cramps right before period
- backache
- lower abdominal pain
- bloating of abdomen
- pinching/pain sensations in inner thighs
- headache
- pain during period is getting worse
- light or heavy blood flow

Possible Causes:

1) Poor dietary habits
2) Hormonal or endocrine imbalances
3) Nutrient deficiencies
4) Endometriosis
5) Pelvic Inflammatory Disease
6) Obesity
7) Liver congestion - steroid hormones are broken down by the liver; B vitamins are needed for estrogen breakdown by the liver; the liver aids in detoxification of the bowel.
   NOTE: B vitamins may, in rare instances, be the nutrients needed to bring the entire endocrine system back into balance. Vitamin B deficiency symptoms include:
   1) symptoms worse during the second half of the cycle when estrogen degradation is highest and the liver needs extra B vitamins to breakdown the estrogen.
   2) edema and breast tenderness prior to menstruation.
   3) awakening in the middle of the night and difficult time getting back to sleep.
   4) headaches - tight band around the head.
   5) heart palpitations.
   6) shortness of breath.

   If B vitamin support is needed, increased dose two weeks prior to menstruation and smaller dose two weeks after menstruation is recommended. Note whether liver or bowel detoxification is needed.
8) Thyroid dysfunction or low pituitary function
9) Iron deficiency anemia
10) Spinal/pelvic subluxation - pelvic misalignment may need applied kinesiology technique called uterine lift
11) Ileocecal valve problems
12) Stress

13) Toxic bowel - puts extra load on the liver
14) Low progesterone levels - thyroid must function normally to produce adequate progesterone
15) Ovarian cysts
16) Overproduction of prostaglandins by the uterus - progesterone inhibits prostaglandins from producing uterine contractions

Nutrient Applications:

1) Calcium and magnesium - both relax the uterine muscle; magnesium inhibits inflammatory prostaglandin synthesis (Fontana-Klaiber, H., and Hogg, B. Therapeutic effects of magnesium in dysmenorrhea. Schweiz Rundsch Med Prax 79(16): 491-494, 1990).
2) Niacin or niacinamide - shown to relieve menstrual cramps (Werbach, M., M.D., Healing Through Nutrition, Harper Collins Publishers, NY, p. 251). Avoid high doses of niacin. Slow niacin release is suspected of causing liver damage.
3) Vitamin E - shown to regulate prostaglandins and aid in cramps (may use wheat germ oil source) (Werbach, M., M.D., Healing Through Nutrition, Harper Collins Publishers, NY, p. 252).
4) Proanthocyanidins - potent bioflavonoids shown to relax smooth muscle (Colombo, D., and Vescovini, R. Controlled Trial of Anthocyanosides from Vaccinium Myrtillus in Primary Dysmenorrhea. G Ital Obstet Ginecol 7:1033-1038, 1985).
5) Omega-6 fatty acids - containing gamma-linolenic acid (i.e. black currant seed oil and evening primrose oil) which is a PGE1 **anti-inflammatory** precursor. Some omega-6's, such as arachidonic acid, are PGE2 **inflammatory** precursors.
6) Potassium - smooth muscle relaxant
7) Vitamin B-6 - prostaglandin synthesis
8) Uterus and ovarian glandular support
9) Thyroid or pituitary support if necessary - the pituitary oversees the entire endocrine system and the thyroid oversees the ovaries
10) Herbs to aid in muscle relaxation including valerian, passion flower and skullcap

Dietary and Lifestyle Applications:

1) Eat a healthy diet containing whole grains, fresh fruits and vegetables, legumes, nuts and seeds. Avoid refined, processed foods, dairy products, salt, saturated fats, sugar, caffeine and chocolate. If avoiding dairy, substitute another calcium source, such as leafy green vegetables or broccoli. Decrease inorganic meat consumption. Increase intake of olive oil, fish, flaxseeds, and fiber.
2) Avoid alcohol and smoking.
3) Detoxify the bowel.
4) Decrease stress. Practice relaxation techniques.
5) Moderate exercise is beneficial.
6) Check for hypothyroidism (axillary temperature test). With consistently low axillary temperature, check pituitary function. Excess estrogen and poor adrenal function will also lower axillary temperature.
7) Check for food allergies, candida/parasites, heavy metals and hypochlorhydria.
8) A good multiple vitamin/mineral supplement is suggested.
9) A hot water bottle placed on the abdomen or a warm bath helps soothe cramps.
10) Drink plenty of filtered water each day.

AMENORRHEA

Absence of menstruation

Signs and Symptoms of Amenorrhea:

- lack of menstruation
- irregular periods

- regular strenuous exercise
- low caloric intake (anorexia)
- 5-10 pounds under ideal weight
- low sex drive
- vaginal itching or abnormal discharge

Possible Causes:

1) Hormonal imbalance
2) Poor diet
3) Nutrient deficiencies
4) Regular strenuous exercise
5) Anorexia
6) Biliary insufficiency
7) Emotional upsets
8) Thyroid or other endocrine imbalances
9) Zinc deficiency
10) Toxic bowel or congested liver
11) Iron deficiency anemia

Nutrient Applications:

1) B vitamins - B-1, B-2, niacin, B-6, B-12 and folic acid
2) Vitamin E - wheat germ oil is a good source
3) Ovary and uterus glandular support
4) Thyroid and/or pituitary support if needed
5) Essential fatty acids

Dietary and Lifestyle Applications:

1) Eat a healthy diet containing whole grains, fresh fruits and vegetables, legumes, nuts and seeds. Avoid refined, processed foods, dairy products, salt, saturated fats, sugar, caffeine and chocolate. Decrease meat consumption. Increase intake of olive oil and fiber. One to two teaspoons of high quality wheat germ oil or flaxseed oil is helpful.
2) Avoid alcohol and smoking.
3) Detoxify the bowel.
4) Decrease stress. Practice relaxation techniques.
5) Moderate exercise is beneficial.
6) Check for hypothyroidism (axillary temperature test). With consistently low axillary temperature, check pituitary function. Excess estrogen will also lower axillary temperature.
7) Check for food allergies, candida/parasites, heavy metals and hypochlorhydria.
8) A good multiple vitamin/mineral supplement is suggested.
9) Drink plenty of filtered water each day.

PREMENSTRUAL SYNDROME

Also known as PMS; a variety of symptoms triggered 7-14 days prior to menstruation.

Signs and Symptoms of Premenstrual Syndrome:

- mood swings
- cramps
- breast pain
- weight gain
- headaches
- crying for no apparent reason
- depression
- sugar cravings
- altered sex drive
- swelling in hands and feet

- abdominal bloating
- anxiety
- irritability

Possible Causes:

1) Hormonal and endocrine imbalances
2) Poor diet
3) Nutrient deficiencies
4) Psychological factors such as stress and anxiety
5) Liver/biliary congestion or toxic bowel
6) Lack of exercise
7) Alcohol abuse
8) Medications
9) Spinal/pelvic misalignment
10) Low thyroid or pituitary function
11) Obesity
12) High estrogen/low progesterone level right before menstruation, which may trigger premenstrual anxiety. Normally, progesterone is the dominant hormone released during the post-ovulatory phase, and drops off prior to menstruation.
13) Hypoglycemia
14) Heavy metal toxicity - lead interferes with estrogen's binding capacity
15) Salt retention
16) Increased aldosterone levels (adrenal hormones)
17) Increased levels of prolactin, which is the hormone that initiates and maintains lactation
18) Adrenal insufficiency

Nutrient Applications:

1) Calcium and magnesium - calcium supplementation has been shown to decrease PMS symptoms. Magnesium levels are decreased in red blood cells in PMS. Magnesium deficiency also alters the adrenal glands, which may be a factor in fluid retention (increased adrenal size and aldosterone production increases fluid retention) (Werbach, M., M.D., Healing Through Nutrition, Harper Collins Publishers, NY, pp. 328-329).
2) Gamma-linolenic fatty acids (i.e. black currant seed oil and evening primrose oil) - PGE1 anti-inflammatory precursors
3) Vitamin B-6 - aids in increasing intracellular magnesium levels; helpful in PMS; may help with acne. Also may help to decrease estrogen and increase progesterone levels.
4) Vitamin E - helpful in PMS symptoms; aids in breast tenderness by decreasing inflammatory prostaglandins and inhibiting prolactin
5) Beta-carotene and vitamin A - may decrease symptoms
6) Multi-vitamin/mineral support - good for comprehensive support
7) Vitamin B complex - B complex deficiency suppresses liver function
8) Bioflavonoids (especially proanthocyanadins) - potent antioxidants and smooth muscle relaxers
9) Milk thistle - potent liver detoxifier (Salmi, H,. and Sarna, S. Effect of silymarin on chemical, functional, and morphological alteration of the liver. A double-blind controlled study. Scand J Gastroenterol 17:417-421, 1982).
10) Zinc - antioxidant; helpful in PMS symptoms and acne
11) Vitamin C - potent antioxidant; aids in breast discomfort; regulates estrogen clearance from the body. Vitamin C is contraindicated in iron overload disease, gout, and people prone to kidney stones.
12) Herbs that help in PMS - dong quai, blessed thistle, cayenne, raspberry leaves, skullcap and squaw vine (contraindicated in pregnancy).
13) Chromium - to balance blood sugar levels

Dietary and Lifestyle Applications:

1) Eat a healthy diet. Refined foods such as sugar will promote hypoglycemia, magnesium excretion in the urine and fluid retention. Avoid saturated fats, dairy products, meat and chicken (eat only organic - free of hormones), processed foods, caffeine and chocolate. If avoiding dairy, substitute another calcium source, such as leafy green vegetables, or broccoli. Increase whole grains, fresh fruits and vegetables, legumes, seeds and nuts. Increase intake of olive oil, fish, flaxseeds and fiber. Fiber will bind and excrete excess estrogen.
2) Avoid alcohol salt, chocolate and tobacco.
3) Detoxify the bowel.
4) Decrease stress. Practice relaxation techniques.
5) Moderate exercise is beneficial.
6) Check for hypothyroidism (axillary temperature test). With consistently low axillary temperature, check pituitary function. Excess estrogen will also lower axillary temperature.
7) Check for food allergies, candida/parasites, heavy metals and hypochlorhydria.
8) A good multiple vitamin/mineral supplement is suggested.
9) A hot water bottle placed on the abdomen or a warm bath helps soothe cramps.
10) Drink plenty of filtered water each day.
11) Check for hypoglycemia and adrenal function.

Considerations:

1) Woman's immune systems peak prior to ovulation and decrease after ovulation. This may occur so that the egg and foreign sperm can unite and be accepted by the woman's body.

FIBROCYSTIC PROBLEMS

FIBROCYSTIC BREAST DISEASE (FBD)

Also known as cystic mastitis; uncomfortable to somewhat painful benign cystic swelling of the breasts, usually prior to menstruation. The cysts fill with fluid and fibrous tissue surrounds the cysts, creating pressure and pain.

Signs and Symptoms of Fibrocystic Breast Disease:

- small lumps in the breast
- breast pain and tenderness
- breasts tender to touch
- breast swelling

Possible Causes:

1) Increased estrogen levels both from natural sources and birth control pills.
2) Increased prolactin levels, a hormone secreted by the pituitary for lactation.
3) Poor diet - caffeine, tea and chocolate are all culprits. The theophylline in tea and the theobromine in chocolate aggravate the inflammation.
4) Bowel dysfunction - less than three bowel movements per week increase risk of fibrocystic breast disease (FBD) (Giller, R., M.D., and Matthews, K., Natural Prescriptions, Ballantine Books, NY, p. 139).
5) Poor liver function - the liver clears estrogen and needs B vitamins and the lipotropic factors (choline and inositol) in sufficient amounts to work efficiently.
6) Hypothyroidism and/or iodine deficiency. There is experimental evidence linking iodine deficiency in animals with cystic mastitis (Giller, R., M.D., and Matthews, K., Natural Prescriptions, Ballantine Books, NY, p. 140).
7) Asthma medications that contain caffeine could make the problem worse
8) Obesity
9) Antibiotics can upset intestinal flora and decrease proper elimination of estrogen

Nutrient Applications:

1) Essential fatty acids – e.g. gamma-linolenic acid and flaxseed oil have been used successfully for FBD
2) Vitamin E - has shown dramatic results in FBD
3) Thyroid and iodine (kelp or dulse) support
4) B complex - to aid in liver function
5) Beta-carotene - may aid in FBD
6) Vitamin B-6
7) Vitamin C - Vitamin C is contraindicated in iron overload disease, gout, and people prone to kidney stones.
8) Enzymes - to help reduce inflammation

Dietary and Lifestyle Applications:

1) Eat a healthy diet. Avoid caffeine, tea and chocolate. Avoid saturated fats, but increase intake of essential fatty acids (fish, walnuts, flaxseeds, etc.). Eat plenty of fiber. A vegetarian diet, which is low-fat (but balanced in essential fatty acids) -may be helpful, but organic meats should not present a problem. Be sure to consume adequate amounts of iodine (fish, kelp, dulse). Inorganic meat should be avoided due to high estrogen content.
2) Avoid alcohol and smoking.
3) Be careful of medications, especially birth control pills (estrogen) and asthma medications (caffeine).
4) Check for hypothyroidism.
5) Liver and bowel detoxification is suggested.

UTERINE AND OVARIAN PROBLEMS

UTERINE FIBROIDS

Noncancerous tumors in the uterus; much more prevalent in black women that white women.

Signs and Symptoms of Uterine Fibroids:

- usually no symptoms are present
- lower abdominal pain
- fullness/pressure in the lower abdomen
- menstrual cramps
- bleeding between periods
- increased urination
- heavy menstrual flow

Possible Causes:

1) Excess estrogen, from natural form, birth control pills or estrogen-replacement therapy given for menopausal symptoms
2) Hormone and/or endocrine imbalances
3) Poor diet
4) Nutrient deficiencies
5) Poor liver and/or bowel function
6) Past trauma or abuse

Nutrient Applications:

1) Vitamin C with bioflavonoids - flavonoids have anti-estrogenic substances. Vitamin C is contraindicated in iron overload disease, gout, and people prone to kidney stones.
2) Enzymes - to aid in inflammation and dissolve the fibroid
3) Essential fatty acids - precursors for anti-inflammatory prostaglandins
4) Beta-carotene
5) Selenium
6) Zinc
7) B vitamins

Dietary and Lifestyle Applications:

1) Eat a healthy diet. Avoid caffeine, tea and chocolate. Avoid saturated fats, but increase intake of essential fatty acids (fish, walnuts, flaxseeds, etc.). Eat plenty of fiber. A vegetarian diet, which is low-fat (but balanced in essential fatty acids) -may be helpful, but organic meats should not present a problem. Be sure to consume adequate amounts of iodine (fish, kelp, dulse). Inorganic meat should be avoided due to high estrogen content.
2) Avoid alcohol and smoking.
3) Be careful of medications, especially birth control pills (estrogen) and asthma medications (caffeine).
4) Check for hypothyroidism.
5) Liver and bowel detoxification is suggested.
6) Heal past abuse issues or trauma if necessary.

ENDOMETRIOSIS

Growth of endometrial cells (the cells lining the inside of the uterus) outside of the uterus anywhere in the pelvic cavity (ovaries, fallopian tubes, bladder, bowel, etc.). The cells still respond to hormonal fluctuations and fill with blood at each cycle, but have no place to shed or go at time of menstruation. Endometriosis usually affects women over thirty.

Signs and Symptoms of Endometriosis:

- menstrual cramps
- large clots during menstruation
- dull ache in the lower abdomen and pelvis
- excessive bleeding
- severe, incapacitating pain in the pelvis
- nausea/vomiting
- painful intercourse
- infertility
- pain intermittently throughout the menstrual cycle

Possible Causes:

1) Unknown. Possible theories include:
   A) Excess estrogen production.
   B) Early menstruation (early age of first menses), which means the woman has many more menstrual cycles before becoming pregnant.
   C) Reflux menstruation in which menstrual fluid backs up into the fallopian tubes and enters the pelvic cavity.
   D) Past trauma and/or abuse issues.

Nutrient Applications:

1) Vitamin C with bioflavonoids - flavonoids have weak estrogenic activity that may block the body's own production of estrogen. Vitamin C is contraindicated in iron overload disease, gout, and people prone to kidney stones.
2) Proteolytic enzymes - to aid inflammation and scarring

3) Essential fatty acids - precursor for anti-inflammatory prostaglandins
4) Vitamin E - aids hormone balance
5) B vitamins
6) Calcium and magnesium

Dietary and Lifestyle Applications:

1) Eat a healthy diet. Avoid caffeine, tea and chocolate. Avoid saturated fats, but increase intake of essential fatty acids (fish, walnuts, flaxseeds, etc.). Eat plenty of fiber. A vegetarian diet, which is low-fat (but balanced in essential fatty acids) -may be helpful, but organic meats should not present a problem. Be sure to consume adequate amounts of iodine (fish, kelp, dulse). Inorganic meat should be avoided due to high estrogen content.
2) Avoid alcohol and smoking.
3) Be careful of medications, especially birth control pills (estrogen) and asthma medications (caffeine).
4) Check for hypothyroidism.
5) Liver and bowel detoxification is suggested.
6) Moderate exercise each day is helpful.

CERVICAL DYSPLASIA

Abnormal cell development of the cervix, the tip of the uterus that connects the vagina. A diagnosis of cervical dysplasia, which is made by a gynecologist after a pap smear, is considered to be a precancerous lesion.

Signs and Symptoms of Cervical Dysplasia:

- a positive pap smear test, diagnosing cervical dysplasia

Class 1: normal cells

Class 2 - 4: "precancerous cells"; somewhere in between normal and cancerous cells. The higher the number the more abnormal the cell development

Class 5: cancerous cells

NOTE: The pap smear test is not that accurate. Repeated tests should be done to get consistent results.

Possible Causes:

1) Nutrient deficiencies, especially vitamins C, B-6, folic acid, and beta-carotene
2) Multiple sexual partners
3) Viral infections - especially Human Papiloma Virus and herpes
4) Oral contraceptive use - increases susceptibility to folic acid deficiency
5) Early age of intercourse
6) Poor diet
7) Past trauma and/or abuse
8) Smoking - depletes vitamin C stores
9) Environmental and/or chemical toxicities
10) Heavy metal toxicity

Nutrient Applications:

1) Folic acid - has been shown effective in treating cervical dysplasia (Giller, R., M.D., and Matthews, K., Natural Prescriptions, Ballantine Books, NY, p. 79).
2) Vitamin C - the lower the levels of vitamin C, the higher the risk of cervical dysplasia (Werbach, M., M.D. Nutritional Influences on Illness, Keats Publishing, Inc. CT., p. 135). Vitamin C is contraindicated in iron overload disease, gout, and people prone to kidney stones.

3) Vitamin A and beta-carotene - vitamin A and beta-carotene levels are both low in women with cervical dysplasia
4) Vitamin B-6 - also low in women with cervical dysplasia
5) Selenium - powerful antioxidant

Dietary and Lifestyle Applications:

1) Eat a healthy diet high in fresh fruits and vegetables and whole grains. Avoid saturated fats, hydrogenated oils, refined foods, caffeine or chocolate. Avoid inorganic animal meats and increase fiber intake.
2) Avoid smoking and alcohol.
3) Practice safe sex.
4) Avoid taking birth control pills.

OVARIAN CYSTS

Fluid-filled tumors of the ovary

Signs and Symptoms of Ovarian Cysts:

- no symptoms are usually present
- sudden onset of pain on one side of the abdomen that lasts several hours; usually occurs half way
- between menstrual cycles at time of ovulation
- bleeding

Possible Causes:

1) Hormone and/or endocrine imbalance
2) Liver toxicity
3) Toxic bowel
4) Poor diet
5) Nutrient deficiency
6) Past trauma and/or abuse

Nutrient Applications:

1) Vitamin C with bioflavonoids - flavonoids have weak estrogenic activity and may block the receptors of the body's own production of estrogen (Burton Goldberg Group, Alternative Medicine: The Definitive Guide, Future Medicine Publishing, Inc. WA, p. 665).
2) Proteolytic enzymes - to aid against inflammation and scarring
3) Essential fatty acids - especially Omega 3's and gamma-linolenic acid (i.e. black currant seed oil and evening primrose oil), precursors for anti-inflammatory prostaglandins
4) Vitamin E - aids hormone balance
5) B vitamins
6) Calcium and magnesium

Dietary and Lifestyle Applications:

1) Eat a healthy diet. Avoid caffeine, tea and chocolate. Avoid saturated fats, but increase intake of essential fatty acids. Eat plenty of fiber. A low-fat, dairy-free vegetarian diet is recommended. Be sure to consume adequate amounts of iodine (fish, kelp, dulse). Meat should be avoided due to high estrogen content.
2) Avoid alcohol and smoking.
3) Be careful of medications, especially birth control pills (estrogen) and asthma medications (caffeine).
4) Check for hypothyroidism.

5) Liver and bowel detoxification is suggested.
6) Nourish the liver with beets, carrots and lemons.
7) Avoid exposure to the cold, which may cause internal congestion.
8) Heal past abuse issues or trauma.
9) Avoid wearing high heels. Heels can cause pelvic problems and block pelvic circulation.

VAGINAL PROBLEMS

VAGINITIS (Vaginal Infections)

Inflammation of the vagina; very common in women.

Signs and Symptoms of Vaginitis:

- burning and itching of the vagina
- vaginal discharge, usually with an odor
- painful intercourse
- pain when urinating
- increased amount of vaginal discharges

Possible Causes:

1) Infectious agent - yeast (Candida), bacterial, viral (Herpes), parasites (Trichomoniasis)
2) Depressed immune function
3) Sexually transmitted diseases - herpes, gonorrhea, chlamydia, AIDS
4) Antibiotic use which destroys the "good bacteria" in the gut and increases susceptibility to infection
5) Birth control pills
6) Diabetes
7) Pregnancy - due to increased hormonal stimulation
8) Food allergies/sensitivities
9) Environmental or chemical toxicity
10) Recurrent urinary tract infections
11) Endometriosis
12) Medications - especially steroids and antibiotics
13) Increased sexual activity, especially with multiple partners. Avoid sexual activity during active infection. Be sure the partner is treated to prevent reinfection.
14) Tampons left in too long
15) Increased pH level of the vagina, which increases risk of infection
16) Tight fitting clothing (i.e. nylon tights)
17) Irritants - laundry detergents, latex condoms, physical trauma, etc.
18) Hormonal changes - especially in postmenopausal women or women who have had their ovaries removed
19) Personal hygiene products are potentially irritating

Nutrient Applications:

1) Vitamin C with bioflavonoids - immune enhancer. Vitamin C is contraindicated in iron overload disease, gout, and people prone to kidney stones.
2) Lactobacillus acidophilus and bifidus - to rebuild normal flora
3) B vitamins - needed for overall healing
4) Beta-carotene and vitamin A - aid in epithelial repair
5) Vitamin E - potent antioxidant and immune stimulant
6) Zinc - immune enhancer
7) Chlorophyll - may soothe inflamed membranes

8) Goldenseal/echinacea - immune stimulant; goldenseal is also a potent anti-bacterial agent
9) Iodine - may be used topically (with caution) as a douche; iodine has been shown to be effective in killing micro-organisms
   Source: Betadine (available at health food stores - does not sting or stain) (Murray, M. and Pizzorno, J. Encyclopedia of Natural Medicine, Prima Publishing, CA, pp. 533-535).

Dietary and Lifestyle Applications:

1) A healthy diet is suggested. Avoid saturated fats, refined, processed foods, especially sugar. Follow yeast diet if yeast infection is present.
2) Drink plenty of filtered water.
3) Avoid medications and birth control pills when possible.
4) Practice good personal hygiene.
5) Avoid nylons. Wear white, cotton underwear.
6) Avoid allergy-causing foods.
7) Pure apple cider vinegar (2-3 cups) in the bath water may be effective.

MENOPAUSAL PROBLEMS

MENOPAUSE

The time in a woman's life when ovulation stops (the ovaries stop producing estrogen) and menstruation ceases. Menopause usually occurs around 50 years of age and can last for up to five years. Prior to menopause, progesterone levels decrease and the excess estrogen can trigger a variety of symptoms. During menopause, estrogen levels gradually decline and eventually stabilize at a much lower level as the adrenals carry the load of making some estrogen . Not all women experience negative menopausal symptoms.

Signs and Symptoms of Menopause:

- irregular periods; eventual ceasing of menstruation
- low sex drive
- hot flashes
- heart palpitations
- memory loss
- night sweats
- irritability/mood swings
- nausea
- depression
- insomnia
- anxiety
- inability to concentrate
- vaginal dryness and pain
- incontinence
- water retention

Possible Causes:

1) Hormonal fluctuations - progesterone levels gradually decline, followed by estrogen levels decreasing
2) Stress - negatively affects the adrenals and decreases the amount of estrogen the adrenals produce that would normally compensate for the ovaries decreased production
3) Hypoglycemia - will enhance menopausal symptoms
4) Poor diet, lack of fat, and lack of exercise can bring on early menopause
5) Hypothyroidism
6) Physical trauma – traumas such as car accidents can bring on early menopause
7) Smoking - can bring on early menopause

Nutrient Applications:

1) Vitamin E - shown to provide symptomatic relief for vaginal dryness (both orally and topically) (Werbach, M., M.D. Healing Through Nutrition, Harper Collins Publishers, NY., p. 247).
2) Vitamin C with bioflavonoids - aids in menopausal symptoms. Vitamin C is contraindicated in iron overload disease, gout, and people prone to kidney stones.
3) Essential fatty acids - alleviates hot flashes, especially gamma linolenic acid (Balch, J., M.D., and Balch, P. CNC, Prescription for Nutritional Healing, Avery Publishing Group, Inc., NY, p. 241).
4) Boron - naturally elevates estradiol levels (Giller, R., M.D., and Matthews, K., Natural Prescriptions, Ballantine Books, NY, p. 245).
5) Calcium and magnesium - as a natural relaxant, and to prevent bone loss
6) Valerian, passion flower and chamomile - to relax, calm and relieve anxiety
7) Dong quai - helpful for the hot flashes and depression of menopause (Balch, J., M.D., and Balch, P. CNC, Prescription for Nutritional Healing, Avery Publishing Group, Inc., NY, p. 241). "Scientific investigation has shown that dong quai produces a balancing effect on estrogen activity and a tonic effect on the uterus" (Murray, M., N.D. Natural Alternatives to Over-the-Counter and Prescription Drugs, William Morrow and Company, Inc. NY, p. 294). Dong quai is contraindicated in pregnancy.
8) Vitamin B-6 - if taking hormone replacement therapy

Dietary and Lifestyle Applications:

1) A healthy, balanced diet is important. Foods high in phytoestrogens (weak estrogenic substances) are helpful for hot flashes including papayas, soybean foods, apples, carrots, potatoes, brown rice, whole wheat, rye and sesame seeds. Calcium rich foods, such as yogurt and green, leafy vegetables, are important to prevent osteoporosis. Legumes, seeds and nuts are a good source of minerals. Avoid dairy products, caffeine and alcohol. If avoiding dairy, choose an alternate calcium source, such as broccoli.
2) Avoid hypoglycemic symptoms by eating a balanced diet, eating regular meals throughout the day and incorporating protein and chromium into the diet.
3) Take a walk daily to relax the body and stimulate the energy system. Daily exercise also fights depression and alleviates anxiety.
4) Do not smoke. Smoking promotes early menopause.

Considerations:

1) At menopause, the risk of osteoporosis and heart disease increases due to the decrease in estrogen. Low estrogen levels promote increased bone loss. Also, estrogen plays a protective role against heart disease. Estrogen deficiency increases LDL levels and makes the blood vessels more prone to blood clots.
2) At menopause, many women face the choice of estrogen-replacement therapy. Natural, alternative means are always suggested due to the risks involved in taking estrogen therapy. The benefits versus the risks, are listed below:

ESTROGEN THERAPY:	
BENEFITS	**RISKS**
May prevent osteoporosis, but new bone may be more brittle	Increases risk of breast and endometrial cancer
Reduces risk of heart disease	Gallstones
Prevents hot flashes and insomnia	PMS symptoms
	Hypertension
	Liver problems
	Fluid retention/weight gain

Many women are trying natural progesterone replacement therapy. Progesterone stimulates osteoblast activity (bone formation) and is thought to be helpful in preventing osteoporosis. It is also used to aid in the symptoms associated with PMS and menopause. Do not use the synthetic, chemically derived progesterone, which has numerous side effects (fluid retention, nausea, insomnia, allergies, masculine characteristics, etc.). Natural progesterone, as of yet, has not been reported to cause serious side effects.

SUBCLINICAL AND PATHOLOGICAL CONDITIONS FOR MISCELLANEOUS CONDITIONS

EDEMA

Abnormal fluid accumulation in the body

Signs and Symptoms of Edema:

- bloating and swelling usually in the feet and ankles, but can occur anywhere in the body
- if pitted edema (pressure into the skin creates "pits"), a doctor should be consulted immediately

Possible Causes:

1) Food allergies/sensitivities
2) Environmental allergies
3) Kidney/bladder problems
4) Liver problems
5) Heart problems
6) Vitamin B deficiency
7) Protein absorption/assimilation problems

Nutrient Applications:

1) Dandelion root - effective diuretic herb that contains potassium; also potent liver support (Hoffmann, D., The New Holistic Herbal, Element, MA, p. 196).
2) Potassium - to restore electrolyte balance, especially if taking a diuretic
3) Kidney and liver support
4) Vitamin B-6 - to aid in reducing water retention (Balch, J., M.D., and Balch, P. CNC, Prescription for Nutritional Healing, Avery Publishing Group, Inc., NY, p. 164).
5) Alfalfa - beneficial herb for edema
6) Celery seed - diuretic and blood cleanser
7) Uva ursi - contains phenolic glycosides that have "diuretic and urinary antiseptic action"
8) B-complex
9) Free form amino acids - for edema caused by poor protein assimilation (Balch, J., M.D., and Balch, P. CNC, Prescription for Nutritional Healing, Avery Publishing Group, Inc., NY, p. 164).

Dietary and Lifestyle Applications:

1) Eat a healthy diet. Avoid caffeine, salt, alcohol, fried foods, dairy products and refined foods. If avoiding dairy, substitute another calcium source, such as leafy green vegetables. Focus on whole grains and watery fruits and vegetables (cucumbers, potatoes, beets, onions, apples and cabbage). Increase fiber intake.
2) Moderate exercise is suggested.
3) Sauna, steamrooms and hot baths are beneficial.
4) Drink plenty of filtered water.

INSOMNIA

Inability to get to sleep or stay asleep during the night

Signs and Symptoms of Insomnia:

- inability to fall asleep at night
- waking up several times during the night; hard to fall back to sleep

Possible Causes:

1) Stress and emotional factors - anxiety, depression, etc.
2) Poor diet
3) Drug and/or alcohol abuse
4) Poor adrenal function - increased cortisone levels
5) Illness - GI problems, nerve problems, bladder infections, asthma
6) Electromagnetic disturbances - electric blankets, waterbeds, power lines, clocks, etc.
7) Environmental sensitivities
8) Food allergies/sensitivities - histamine release alters brain chemistry and can alter sleep patterns
9) Hypoglycemia
10) Chronic pain
11) Nutrient deficiencies, especially calcium and magnesium
12) Hypothyroidism and other endocrine problems
13) Medications

Nutrient Applications:

1) Calcium and magnesium - sedative effect on the body
2) B vitamins - niacinamide (a form of vitamin B-3) at bedtime (1 gram) has been shown to be helpful (Werbach, M., M.D. Healing Through Nutrition, Harper Collins Publishers, NY., p. 225).
3) Chlorella - sedates the nerves; source of natural tryptophan
4) Herbs - passion flower, skullcap, valerian, chamomile, kava kava
5) Amino acids - may help insomnia if person has amino acid deficiencies

Dietary and Lifestyle Applications:

1) Eat a healthy diet. Avoid caffeine and allergy foods.
2) Avoid alcohol and drugs when possible.
3) Practice relaxation exercises - massage, yoga, deep breathing, meditation.
4) Follow an elimination/rotation diet to identify food allergies.
5) Check for hypothyroidism and other endocrine imbalances.
6) Avoid electromagnetic stress, including waterbeds, electric blankets, power lines, etc.. Move electrical appliances away from the bed.
7) Regular exercise in the afternoon or evening may help induce sleep.
8) Sunlight exposure (in moderation), is helpful to balance circadian rhythms ("the biological clock").
9) Herbal teas, including chamomile and passion flower, before bed are excellent.
10) A warm bath with baking soda before bedtime may be helpful.

NUTRIENT APPLICATIONS

GENERAL DISCLAIMER

The nutritional suggestions and research reported in this book are not offered to treat, mitigate or cure disease, and should not be used as a substitute for sound medical advice. This book is designed to be used in conjunction with the services provided by a trained, licensed healthcare practitioner.

CAUTION

Caution should be used in all conditions, especially concerning pregnancy and children, when taking herbal supplements or high potency nutrients. A physician knowledgeable in natural and preventative medicine should be consulted.

It is the reader's responsibility to be aware of certain contraindications, toxicology and drug-nutrient interactions which may occur. A concise table of drug-nutrient interactions has been provided for information, however, competent resources, such as "Shils and Young, Modern Nutrition in Health and Disease", Lea & Febiger, Phil, Pa 1988, should be consulted for the RDA's and upper limits of vitamins and minerals (Contraindications and Toxicology). As an example, vitamin C supplementation to people with iron overload disease (2% of the population) can be harmful and even fatal. Less information is available on herbs and other supplements, and several resources are recommended, such as the "Lawrence Review of Natural Products", Facts and Comparisons, St. Louis, Missouri. 1996, and the German monographs.

ALFALFA

Alfalfa is from the legume family and contains vitamins A, B-1, B-6, B-12, C, E, niacin, pantothenic acid, biotin and folic acid, along with essential and nonessential amino acids. Additionally, it contains chlorophyll, along with major minerals and trace elements, such as calcium, magnesium, phosphorus, potassium, manganese, iron, zinc and copper (Heinerman, John. Heinerman's Encyclopedia of Fruits, Vegetables and Herbs. 1988; Parker Publishing, West Nyack, NY p. 3). Alfalfa also contains high amounts of vitamin K, which is necessary for the formation of prothrombin in the blood-clotting process.

Research recently has shown that alfalfa might have **cholesterol lowering** and **anti-atherosclerotic** effects. The saponins found in alfalfa are thought to help bind cholesterol and bile salts in the gut. Alfalfa seeds lower low density lipoprotein cholesterol and apolipoprotein B concentrations in patients with type II hyperlipoproteinemia (Atherosclerosis May 1987; 65(1-2):173-79).

Alfalfa is an **infection fighter**; the high chlorophyll content in alfalfa was used by doctors in the 40's for treating infections from surgical incisions, bed sores and inner ear problems (Heinerman, J. Heinerman's Encyclopedia of Fruits, Vegetables and Herbs. 1988; Parker Publishing, West Nyack, NY. p. 2). Alfalfa extracts containing a high manganese content reportedly **improved the condition of a diabetic** who failed to respond to insulin, as reported in the Journal of Nutrition (J of Nutr August, 1984, and as cited in Heinerman, J. Heinerman's Encyclopedia of Fruits, Vegetables and Herbs. 1988 Parker Publishing, West Nyack, NY. p. 3).

Alfalfa is a tonic and diuretic and is helpful in bowel and urinary complaints. "Alfalfa is a **tonic, stimulant, appetizer and diuretic**, and also r**elieves urinary disorders and edema**" (Sharon, Dr. M. Complete Nutrition. 1994. Prion Publ., London, England. p. 135). It is important to note that some people may have a sensitivity to alfalfa. Alfalfa contains L-canavanine, which can cause reactions in susceptible people.

ALOE VERA

"All is well, aloe is on board" - Christopher Columbus.

The pulp of the aloe vera leaf contains mostly **water**, in a **mucilaginous gel** that can provide water to injured tissue without sealing off the air needed for tissue repair (Heinerman, J. Heinerman's Encyclopedia of Fruits, Vegetables and Herbs. 1988; Parker Publishing, West Nyack, NY. p. 5). In addition to water, the gel is packed with **complex carbohydrates, enzymes, amino acids, vitamins and minerals** (Heinerman, J. Heinerman's Encyclopedia of Fruits, Vegetables and Herbs. 1988; Parker Publishing, West Nyack, NY. p. 5). Known for its healing properties, it is used for many conditions, including topically for **cuts** and **burns**. Aloe is known as an **intestinal purgative** that **stimulates colon activity** and is **helpful in constipation**. Aloe vera contains **acemannan**, which is the polysaccharide component of aloe thought to have **antiviral and immune-enhancing activity**. Among aloe's other virtues, it is known to help in **insect bites and stings, edema (swelling), periodontal surgery, cold sores and candidal dermatitis** (caused by infection of Candida Albicans) (Heinerman, J. Heinerman's Encyclopedia of Fruits, Vegetables and Herbs. 1988; Parker Publishing, West Nyack, NY. p. 4).

Aloe vera aids in the **healing of stomach disorders and ulcers**, by providing tissue protection to the gastro-intestinal mucosa. (Balch JF Presc for Nutr Healing 1990, Garden City Park, NY). "Aloe vera **improves wound healing and inhibits inflammation**" (Davis RH. J Am Podiatr Med Assoc 1994;84(2)77-81). Aloe vera extracts have been shown to **decrease wound diameters** by almost 50% (J Am Podiatr Med Assoc 1991;81(9):473-8). A research study showed that aloe vera **reduced inflammation, regenerated epithelial cells, and increased overall wound healing** by 72 hours - "This acceleration in wound healing is important to reduce bacterial contamination" (J Dermatol Surg Oncol 1990;16(5):460-7). Aloe vera is also **helpful in food allergies,** which is suspected in association with ulcers. In fact, Delazzari et al propose that their data on IgE levels and gastric bacteria, "lend support to the hypothesis of an underlying immuno-allergic reaction in some forms of gastric or duodenal ulcer" (Scand J Gastroenterol 1994 (Suppl) 201:11). And so, in addition to the soothing effect of aloe vera on the mucosa, it may be helpful also by way of influencing food allergies.

AMINO ACIDS

"Amino acids will always be an integral part of nutritional support in all patients. The use of specific amino acids in pharmacologic doses may be beneficial to critically ill patients, indicating that such compounds are conditionally essential" (Surg Clin North Am 1991;71(3):459-76). The amino acid **histidine** is found in **parsley,** and has been found to be a strong **inhibitor of tumor development** (Mutation Research 77:245-50, as cited in (Heinerman, J. p. 260).

"Arginine, glutamine, the long chain polyunsaturated omega-3 and omega-6 fatty acids, and, to a lesser extent, ribonucleic acid and the vitamins E, C, and A have pharmacological effects when given in amounts in excess of what is needed to prevent nutritional deficiency. These effects are exerted primarily via the immune system, and immunoenhancing diets that embody the recently developed principles of nutritional pharmacology have been shown to reduce infectious complications by approximately 75% in surgical patients and hospital stay by more than 20% in surgical patients and patients in the intensive care unit in three independent, prospective, randomized studies, two of which were double-blinded. These findings suggest that specialized diets can be designed that will be of benefit to patients with cancer, atherosclerosis, intestinal diseases, autoimmune diseases, infections, and trauma" (Arch Surg 1993;128(11):1242-5).

ANISE STAR SEED

Anise is an aromatic plant, which smells a lot like licorice. "As an infusion, anise **helps the digestion, relieves flatulence, improves appetite, and alleviates cramps, nausea and colic** in children" (Sharon, Dr. M. Complete Nutrition, 1994. Prion Publ., London, England. p. 135).

ANTIOXIDANTS

<u>Good sources for antioxidants are</u> fresh fruits and vegetables; especially cruciferous vegetables such as broccoli, and the dark-colored fruits and vegetables. Antioxidants function to reduce the reactivity of

molecules called free radicals. **Free radicals** carry a single electron in their outer shell, making them **highly reactive.** Unfortunately, sometimes they react with various cellular components and **destroy** them in the process. The double bond, present in the fatty acid of the cell membrane, is in a vulnerable position for the free radical to steal an electron. The **loss of the electron** converts the fatty acid into a **radical,** which in turn converts the next fatty acid into a radical, and so on, known as the "**chain reaction**" of lipid peroxidation. With the change to a radical, the composition of the fatty acid is drastically affected. Since every cell membrane is composed of a phospholipid bilayer which includes these fatty acids, the disruption eventually ends in **membrane rupture and cell death** when the chain is not interrupted.

Antioxidants, which **stabilize radicals** and **halt the chain reaction**, can **prevent** that **damage** and **maintain** the **integrity of cell membranes.** The antioxidant vitamins work in different capacities to fight against cellular damage. For instance, vitamin C is an important aqueous radical quencher, which means that it works against the beginning radical formation in the watery portion of intracellular and extracellular components. Vitamin E is known as the major lipid antioxidant, and it works mainly against the lipid peroxidation of lipid cell membranes. Vitamin E is known as the "chain-breaker", because it stops the chain reaction of damage. Beta-carotene, which is a precursor to vitamin A, is also a lipid antioxidant, however it functions mainly in areas of low oxygen concentration.

The antioxidant vitamins decrease cellular damage related to many diseases, and therefore have been reported to be associated with the decreased incidence of many diseases, including gastric cancer. For instance, supplements of vitamin C, vitamin E and beta-carotene were reported in Nutrition Reviews to decrease risk of gastric cancer Rev. (Nutr Rev. 1994; 52(3):75-83).

"Vitamins A, E, C and carotenoids are able to protect cells and **enhance humoral and cellular immune responses** in disease" (Nockels, C.F. The role of vitamins in modulating disease resistance. 1988. Vet Clin North Am Food Anim Pract 4(3):531-42). In a clinical trial, 300 women who had developed precancerous cells in the cervix entered a study where half of them received treatment consisting of vaginal sponges which released a synthetic relative of **vitamin A**. In the moderate cases, the **precancerous spots disappeared** in the treated women (Science News. 1994;143(22):341). Numerous studies point to the beneficial effects of the **antioxidant vitamins** in cancer protection (Dietary carotenes, vitamin C and vitamin E as protective antioxidants in human cancers. Annu Rev Nutr 1992;12:139-59). **Beta carotene** seems to have a protective antioxidant effect on DNA, as Japanese researcher Keizo Umegaki of the National Institute of Health and Nutrition in Tokyo just reported last February that **beta-carotene, "significantly reduces chromosome damage**" (Science News. 1994; 145:126).

Antioxidants help **protect** against oxidative damage to the sensitive cells of the **digestive tract**, especially the mucosal cells, which contain the villi responsible for food breakdown and absorption. Additionally, the efficacy of natural plant medicinal products was enhanced in patients who were able to degrade them into compounds with antioxidant activity; in other words, **the ability to increase free radical scavengers dramatically increased the positive response to herbal therapy.** In patients responding the best, their gastric juice produced the most compounds with antioxidant activity, including **beta-carotene and vitamin E.** This led researchers to report that, " These findings suggest that one of the factors determining the **clinical response to natural herbal medicinal products** is the ability of the patient's digestive system to degrade the product to **liberate bioactive compounds (with antioxidant activity)"** (Planta Med 1991;57(4):299-304).

UV light can be a source of free radicals, and since the eye has a high phospholipid content, the eye is quite susceptible to free radical attack. For instance, macular degeneration was one of five retinal disorders studied in the massive **Eye Disease Case-Control Study**, which obtained data from 421 patients with macular degeneration and 615 controls. Serum levels of **carotenoids, vitamins C and E, and selenium** were evaluated, and subjects were classified by level of the micronutrient (low, medium, and high). Persons in the **medium and high carotenoid** groups had, **"markedly reduced risks"** of macular degeneration. Risk in the "high" group was reduced to one half, and risk in the "medium" group was reduced to one third, demonstrating a dose-dependent result. **"An antioxidant index which combined all four micronutrient measurements showed statistically significant reductions of risk with increasing levels of the index... these results suggest that higher blood levels of micronutrients with antioxidant potential, in**

particular, carotenoids, may be associated with a decreased risk of the most visually disabling form of age-related macular degeneration " (Arch. Ophthalmol. 1993, 111:104-9).

Authors of "Antioxidant protection of the ageing macula" report epidemiological evidence that suggests **patients with macular degeneration have a lower intake of carotenoids**, and, "moreover, a preliminary therapeutic trial in patients with AMD (Age-related macular degeneration) or diabetic retinopathy showed that **supplementation with beta-carotene, vitamin C, vitamin E and selenium halted the progression of degenerative changes and in some cases even brought improvement"** (Age and ageing 1991, 20:60-69). The clinical trial they refer to involved over 500 patients who received 500 mg vitamin C, 400 IU vitamin E, 9 mg beta carotene and 250 ug selenium daily for 7 to 12 years. The authors note that even though the retina contains higher concentrations of carotenoids, vitamin E and vitamin C than many other tissues, "the fact that the development of AMD still occurs indicates that in these cases **the balance between lifelong exposure to light and antioxidant protection has been disturbed in favor of light damage.** A higher intake of these antioxidant nutrients may thus be required to counteract the influence of light" (Ibid, p. 66).

The radicals formed from UV light can alter proteins, and the accumulation of damaged proteins sometimes occludes the eye in **cataracts**. Jacque and Chylack, authors of, "Epidemiologic evidence of a role for the antioxidant vitamins and carotenoids in cataract prevention", classified their subjects into three levels of vitamin C and beta-carotene status: low, intermediate, and high. **Persons with the lowest vitamin C intake had 11 times the risk of developing cataracts** as persons with the highest intake (Am J Clin Nutr. 1991, 53:3520S-25S). In the same study, **low plasma carotenoid levels corresponded to a seven-fold risk** over those with high levels.

In a review of the research on cataracts and antioxidants, The Annals of the NY Acad Sci. notes that, "Epidemiological and laboratory studies indicate that **cataractogenesis is causally related to photooxidative stress...** It appears possible to increase eye levels of some antioxidants... **several studies noted a correlation between enhanced dietary antioxidant intake or elevated plasma antioxidant levels and diminished risk of developing cataracts.** Inasmuch as age-related degeneration of the macula may be related to nutrition in similar ways as cataracts, these observations regarding benefits of antioxidant status may have extra value" (Annals NY Acad Sci, Beyond Def, 1992; 669: p. 118).

Vitamin E comes to the rescue after free radical damage. When free radical damage has already disrupted the lipids in the cell membrane, it is up to vitamin E to "stop the chain reaction". It donates a hydrogen to the radical, and neutralizes its activity. This is why vitamin E is called the major lipid antioxidant in the body.

When the red blood cell membrane is peroxidized, it loses its ability to change shape and squeeze through the vessels, and leads to a rupturing of the membrane, or hemolysis. Vitamin E has demonstrated a protective effect against this hemolysis in blood diseases, including sickle cell anemia. "In these diseases, there is extra oxidant stress, or a decrease in other protective mechanisms, so that the effects of vitamin E are more readily seen" (Halliwell and Gutteridge, Free Radicals in Biology and Medicine, 1990. New York, Oxford University Press, p. 173).

Two MD's were prompted to recommend antioxidant supplementation in The New England Journal of Medicine in Nov. of 1993. They cited the studies of Rimm, et al., who examined thousands of people, and determined that vitamin E reduced the risk for heart disease (New Eng J Med, 1993; 328:1444-56). In a letter to the editor, they pointed out that, "A substantial number of physicians in the United States are sufficiently convinced of the potential benefits of vitamin E to supplement their own diets with it. If vitamin E is good enough for physicians, should it not be good enough for our patients?" (James H. O'Keefe, Jr., MD, Mid America Heart Institute, Kansas City, Mo., and Carl J. Lavie, MD, Ochsner Heart and Vascular Institute, New Orleans, La. p. 1424).

When the lipid membrane of the cell is disrupted, along with the lipid membranes of intracellular structures, it's no wonder that so many disruptions of homeostasis result. It is also no surprise that there are so many strong associations between vitamin E and related diseases. Perhaps Isadore Rosenfels, MD had this in mind when he stated that, "Vitamin E is an antioxidant whose time has come".

Due to the accumulated scientific research that points to the protective qualities of antioxidant vitamins, more and more researchers and physicians are admitting that supplementation may be necessary to achieve this protection. Russian researchers have been prompted to advise, "It is probable that an increased intake of antioxidants (**ascorbic acid, carotenes, tocopherols, bioflavonoids, selenium,** etc.) would, along with other corrective provisions, **suppress** the steep increase of **cardiovascular disease"** (Vnitr Lek 1992; 38:1096-1104).

Besides these antioxidant vitamins, there are other substance which possesses antioxidant activity (see also bioflavonoids, or vitamin P). The minerals zinc and selenium, for instance, are reported to have this activity. Zinc is an essential element in **superoxide dismutase (SOD),** a potent radical scavenging enzyme. Research demonstrates that high levels of **SOD** , "protect mitochondria from oxidative damage that probably occurs with ageing in the retinal pigment epithelium (Invest. Ophthalmol. Vis. Sci. 1992, 33:1909-18). Selenium is an essential element in another radical scavenging enzyme, glutathione peroxidase.

Turmerin, which forms 0.1% of the weight of the spice **turmeric**, contains three residues of methionine that are partly responsible for its antioxidant activity. **Free Radicals in Biology and Medicine** (1991, 11:277-83), found **turmeric** to be **the most effective protectant** against DNA oxidative damage in human lymphocytes, amongst the ingredients they tested.. **Turmeric used widely as a spice would probably mitigate the effects of several dietary carcinogens**" (Plant Foods Hum. Nutr 1993, 44:87-92). Curcumin is a component of turmeric that has potent antioxidant activity. Other spices of nature, in the limelight for their antioxidant properties, are: **cloves, cumin, red chilies, ginger, coriander, and black pepper** (Mol Cell Biochem 1992, 111:117-24; Indian J Biochem Biophys. 1993, 30:130-4).

Other substances with antioxidant activity are coenzyme Q 10, quercetin (a bioflavonoid), and proanthocyanidins, which are powerful bioflavonoids found in the dark-colored fruits and vegetables, pine bark extract, and grape seed extract. Ginkgo biloba is an herb possessing antioxidant activity.

APPLE PECTIN

Apple pectin is a form of **fiber** found in the cell walls of plants. Pectin has a high ability to bind water, which **aids in digestion and elimination.** Besides absorbing water, pectin can **decrease the amount of fat absorbed.** Pectin may be helpful for diabetics because it slows down food absorption after meals. It also helps bind unwanted metals and toxins, and lowers cholesterol levels by binding the cholesterol and bile acids in the gut, aiding in excretion.

Pectin, "may **protect gastric mucosa** by strengthening the mucus-phospholipid layer" (Scand J Gastroenterol 1993;28(10):894-8). "...the formation of indomethacin-induced ulcers is related to...decreased synthesis of intestinal mucus glycoprotein. When pectin, a soluble fiber was given together with solid stock food, ulcer formation was significantly inhibited" (Nippon Shokakibyo Gakkai Zasshi 1991;88(10):2636-43). Pectin has also demonstrated an ability to **increase bile acids and decrease cholesterol, mainly by increasing cholesterol excretion** (Vopr Pitan. 1992(2):47-50). Fibers such as pectins remove candida toxins by binding to them and promoting excretion.

A fiber product containing apple pectin was given for 9 weeks to type II diabetics exhibiting hypercholesterolemia; **cholesterol and triglyceride concentrations were significantly reduced** (Leber-Magen-Darm. 1993;23(5):204-9). In Germany, there is a soft drink containing apple pectin called "anticholest", which reduced cholesterol up to 30% in a clinical trial and also **increased the good cholesterol (high density lipoprotein cholesterol, or HDL-C)**. The trial noted that the lack of side effects and ease of administration are important in long term compliance, essential to management of a progressive disease such as atherosclerosis (Wien-Klin-Wochenschr 1992;104(11):314-6).

ARTICHOKE

Artichoke is a **diuretic**, and **stimulates bile evacuation.** Extracts of the leaves and roots were once used to treat **arteriosclerosis, jaundice and post-operative anemia** (Sharon, Dr. M. Complete Nutrition. 1994. Prion Publ., London, England. p. 136). The main ingredient of artichoke is cynarin, which is known for **protecting and regenerating the liver.** It aids in liver congestion by stimulating bile elimination from the liver. Jerusalem artichoke is high in inulin, which contains fructooligosaccharides (FOS). These FOS attract good bacteria to the gut which counteracts populations of bad bacteria.

BARBERRY (Berberis vulgaris)

Barberry has a high alkaloid content of berberine, with **antibacterial and antimicrobial** properties, and is reported to be one of the herbs used to treat Candida. It is speculated that berberine enhances immune function by **increasing blood flow to the spleen and by activating macrophages.**

Barberry **promotes secretion of bile**, and is therefore considered to be **beneficial in liver disorders**; it also **dilates blood vessels and lowers blood pressure** (Sharon, Dr. M. Complete Nutrition. 1994. Prion Publ., London, England. p. 136). Barberry root bark preparations are toxic in large quantities or for long periods of time, and should not be used by children under two or pregnant women (Mayell M. The Natural Health First Aid Guide; p. 422).

BASIL

Basil leaves, which stimulate the appetite, are generally used as a culinary herb, however, "infusions of the leaves can also be used to **relieve flatulence, stomach cramps, constipation and enteritis**" Basil is also used to treat Candida albicans (Heinerman, John. Heinerman's Encyclopedia of Fruits, Vegetables and Herbs. 1988. Parker Publishing, West Nyack, NY p. 20).

BAYBERRY

Bayberry bark has medicinal properties similar to barberry; it **relieves, cures and prevents varicose veins** (Heinerman, John. Heinerman's Encyclopedia of Fruits, Vegetables and Herbs. 1988. Parker Publishing, West Nyack, NY p. 22). It **reduces fevers and intestinal parasites, and alleviates liver and kidney problems.** It's of value in **stopping bleeding of the lungs, bowels and uterus,** and also in **treating excessive menstruation and vaginal discharge** (ibid, p. 23). Bayberry (Myrica cerifera) is a **stimulant and astringent** that promotes sweating (Ody, The Complete Medicinal Herbal).

BEETS

(See also Betaine)

Beets, being a richly colored vegetable, have a high concentration of proanthocyanidins, which are powerful plant bioflavonoids. Beets have long had a reputation for being good liver cleansers. Beets may be good for **hypoglycemia** (Heinerman, John. Heinerman's Encyclopedia of Fruits, Vegetables and Herbs. 1988 Parker Publishing, West Nyack, NY p. 31). **Betaine** accounts for the red color in beets (Heinerman, John. Heinerman's Encyclopedia of Fruits, Vegetables and Herbs. Parker Publishing, West Nyack, NY p29-31), and helps to **convert cholesterol into bile acids,** important in **fat metabolism.**

BERBERINE

Berberine is a hydrophilic alkaloid isolated from goldenseal (hydrastis canadensis). It dissolves slowly in water with alkaline reaction and forms salts by replacement of a hydroxyl group. In addition to being **antibacterial, antipyretic, and antimalarial,** it is used as **bitters for the stomach** (Merck Index, 11th ed. Merck & Co. Inc., Rahway, N.J. 1989). Caution should be used when berberine is used as an extract apart from the whole goldenseal herb; it is the berberine in goldenseal that is responsible for the contraindication during pregnancy.

BETA-CAROTENE

(See also Antioxidants)

The antioxidant effect of beta-carotene **helps to combat free radical damage** to the cells of the body, especially the intestinal mucosal cells and cells of the eye, which are highly susceptible to oxidative damage. Beta-carotene **protects** the body from the irritating effects of **smoke and other pollutants**, promotes **tissue healing**, and may be helpful in **preventing ulcers.**

Beta-carotene **stimulates digestive rumen bacteria, improves digestion and, "increases the utilization of fatty acids**" (vitamin E has an additive effect) (J Dairy Sci 1993;76(2):600-5). Supplements of beta-carotene, vitamin E and vitamin C are believed to **decrease risk of gastric cancer** (Nutr Rev 1994;52(3):75-83).

BETA-GLUCANS

Beta-glucans are polysaccharides which make up some of the **insoluble fiber** in oat bran, for instance, that help it to its claim to fame for lowering cholesterol. The beta attachment is less easily broken down in the intestine than the alpha bond, hence it is less absorbable. It is interesting to note that **beta-glucans** have been heralded as, "agents that rapidly **enhance host resistance to a variety of biologic insults** through mechanisms involving **macrophage activation**" (Int J Immunopharmacol. 1992, 14:1363).

BETAINE

Betaine is the carboxylic acid derived by oxidation of choline; "the hydrochloride salt is used as a **gastric acidifier**" (Dorland's Pocket Medical Dictionary, 24th ed. WB Saunders Co., Phil, Pa. 1989). Betaine is listed in the Merck index as a **hepatoprotectant (liver-protecting)** (p. 1202) , and the compound **betaine** hydrochloric acid (**HCL**) is used in supplementation form to **aid in digestion**, and may even **reduce food sensitivities** by improving digestion (Murray MT & Pizzorno JE. Encyclopedia of Natural Medicine. 1991; Prima Publ., Rocklin, Ca., p. 496). In a 17 year old boy who developed severe **gastrointestinal distress** manifested by **chronic diarrhea,** "The diarrhea was **successfully treated with betaine**" (J Gastroenterol Hepatol 1993;8(1):60-2).

BILBERRY

Bilberry's actions include: astringent, tonic, antiseptic, urinary antiseptic, prevents vomiting, and lowers blood sugar (Ody p. 109). "Anthocyanidins in bilberry act to prevent capillary fragility and inhibit platelet aggregation. Bilberry is therefore demonstrated to be an anti-inflammatory herb" (Weiner, M.A. Herbs that Heal. 1994. Quantum Books, Mill Valley, Ca. p. 84). Promising test results on animals and in the laboratory suggest that bilberry has antiviral properties against herpes simplex virus II, influenza, and other viruses, antihistamine activity, anti-ulcer activity, anti-cancer activity, and may prevent atherosclerosis (Weiner, M.A. Herbs that Heal. 1994. Quantum Books, Mill Valley, Ca. p. 84). "Many clinical tests have shown that bilberry anthocyanosides given orally to humans **improve vision** in healthy people and also help treat people with eye diseases such as pigmentary **retinitis..**. Bilberry extracts administered in controlled experiments, conducted with persons suffering from diabetes, exhibited **normalization of capillary collagen thickness** and **reduced blood sugar levels** in humans and animals" (Weiner, M.A. Herbs that Heal. 1994. Quantum Books, Mill Valley, Ca. p. 84)

BLACK CHERRY

The Mohegans used to allow the ripe, wild black cherry to ferment in a jar for a year, and then they would drink the juice to **cure dysentery**. "The most widespread popular use of wild cherry bark is as a **cough sedative.** It acts as a **tonic** and calms irritation, **diminishing nervous excitability**. It has been employed in the treatment of **bronchitis**, and because it slows heart action, has been used in **heart disease** characterized by frequent, irregular, or feeble pulse. It has also been considered a **good remedy for weakness of the stomach** or of the system coupled with general or local irritation" (Weiner, M.A. Herbs that Heal. 1994. Quantum Books, Mill Valley, Ca. p. 115-16). Black cherries remove toxins from tissues, which is important in gout, and helpful for the glandular system; they also aid in gall bladder and liver function (Balch, P.A. Prescription for Cooking 1987. PAB Books, Tx).

BLACK COHOSH

Black Cohosh **reduces hypertension** and has a **sedative action on the nerves** (Heinerman, John. Heinerman's Encyclopedia of Fruits, Vegetables and Herbs. p. 41). Black Cohosh (Cimicfuga racemosa) is a **diuretic, antirheumatic, anti-inflammatory, antitussive (inhibits cough reflex), sedative, and uterine stimulant**, which should be avoided in early pregnancy (Ody, The Complete Medicinal Herbal). It is indicated in **colds, flu, fever, headache and sore throat, nervous conditions, cramps, rheumatism, arthritis, and it "raises the energy of the body"** (Tierra, L. The Herbs of Life. 1992. The Crossing Press, Freedom, Ca. p. 50).

Black cohosh contains phytoestrogens, which are plant substances believed to balance the female system. The popular Remifemin is actually a trade name of an extract of black cohosh, which is "the most widely used and thoroughly studied natural alternative to hormone replacement therapy in menopause" (Murray, M & Pizzorno, J. Enc of Nat Med. 1998. Prima Publ., Rocklin, Ca.). Clinical trials show that this extract has relieved hot flashes, depression, and vaginal atrophy (Gyne. 1982;3:14-16; Med Welt 1985;36:871-874; Therapeuticum 1987;1:23-31; Arch Gynecol Obstet 1993;254:817-18). In a large trial of over 600 women, the extract relieved both psychological and physical symptoms in more than 80% of the patients Since phytoestrogens exhibit weak estrogenic activity, the extract was tested for its effect on breast cancer cells. Growth of the cells usually depends on the presence of estrogens in vitro (cell culture), however. experiments showed inhibitory effects of the extract on breast cancer cells instead of stimulatory effects (Arch Gynecol Obstet 1993;254:817-18). In addition, the inhibitory effects of the anti-estrogen drug tamoxifen are potentiated with black cohosh extract (Murray & Pizzorno, ibid).

BLACK CURRANT SEED OIL

(See Essential Fatty Acids)

BLACK RADISH ROOT

Black radish root is reported to support the gallbladder and the gastrointestinal tract valves. It is used as a detoxifying herb for the bowel and lymphatics.

BLACK WALNUT

Black walnut is an **effective remedy for fungal infection** and **eradication of intestinal parasites** (Heinerman, John. Heinerman's Encyclopedia of Fruits, Vegetables and Herbs. Parker Publishing, West Nyack, NY p236). Black walnut has been utilized to eliminate kidney and gallstones, and remove excess phlegm in bronchitis and asthma (ibid, p. 237). It contains a crystalline compound which therapeutically treats hypertension, skin cancer, and muscular paralysis due to electrical shock (ibid, p. 238).

BLESSED THISTLE

Blessed Thistle was used by the Zuni to treat venereal disease and lower fever. Among the thistle's reported characteristics are that of appetite stimulant, indigestion and flatulence reliever, antibacterial/ anti-yeast/anti-tumor activity (Weiner, M.A. Herbs that Heal. 1994. Quantum Books, Mill Valley, Ca. p. 87).

BLUE COHOSH

Blue Cohosh was used by the Indians to promote rapid delivery during childbirth. It has also been employed to purge the intestinal tract of worms, as a diuretic, and to produce sweating. Listed in the U.S. Pharmacopoeia as an antispasmodic, diuretic and emmenagogue, "Scientific investigations... include anti-inflammatory activity, antihypertensive activity, and usefulness in the treatment of cirrhosis of the liver" (Weiner, M.A. Herbs that heal. 1994. Quantum Books, Mill Valley, Ca. p. 128).

BLUE VERVAIN

Blue Vervain has **analgesic**, **anti-inflammatory** and **antidiarrheal** properties, **relieves pain, sleeplessness, and tiredness, and helps in fevers and infections** (David B. Mowry, PhD. The Scientific Validation of Herbal Medicine. 1986. Keats Publishing, New Canaan, Conn. p. 117-206).

BUCKTHORN BARK

Buckthorn is such a **powerful laxative** that it should be used with caution (Wild, R., ed. The Complete Book of Natural and Medicinal Cures. 1994. Rodale Press, Emmaus, Pa. p. 250). Buckthorn berries contain anthraquinone glycosides, which are responsible for their **cathartic effect,** and which are similar to Cascara Sagrada, with buckthorn being the milder of the two. Buckthorn has shown **activity against Candida, staphylococcus, herpes, and influenza.** (Weiner, M.A. Herbs that Heal. 1994. Quantum Books, Mill Valley, Ca. p. 97).

BUCKWHEAT

Buckwheat has a **favorable effect on satiety,** thereby decreasing food cravings. In an informal study at the Anthropological Research Center in Salt Lake City, 11 overweight people ate buckwheat pancakes for 2 weeks (2-3 each time) every other morning and every other evening, and were permitted to eat anything else, no matter how sweet or fattening, for lunch (oatmeal was given at alternate dinners and breakfasts). All 11 noted a substantial decrease in frequency of snacks, as well as volume of food. Seven people lost an average of 15.75 lbs, with 4 losing in excess of 22 lbs. (Heinerman, John. Heinerman's Encyclopedia of Fruits, Vegetables and Herbs. p. 167).

BUCKWHEAT GRASS JUICE

Buckwheat is high in rutin (a bioflavonoid), which is excellent for capillary strengthening and decreases the likelihood of hemorrhages. It is also high in vitamins K, E and the B-complex, phosphorus, potassium, calcium and some iron and manganese. Buckwheat neutralizes acidic wastes and is good for the blood and kidneys (Balch, P.A. Prescription for Cooking 1987. PAB Books, Tx. p. 123).

BURDOCK ROOT

Burdock root has a reputation as an antibiotic, antifungal, anti-inflammatory and anti tumor substance. It is helpful as a detoxifying blood purifier, a diuretic, and pain killer, and is advantageous in weight loss for strengthening and purifying the blood (David B. Mowry, PhD. The Scientific Validation of Herbal Medicine. 1986. Keats Publishing, New Canaan, Conn. p. 279).

BUTTERNUT BARK

Butternut bark is useful as a **laxative, in liver disorders, in fever and infection, and in treating parasites/worms** (David B. Mowry, PhD. The Scientific Validation of Herbal Medicine. 1986. Keats Publishing, New Canaan, Conn. p. 117-229).

BUTYRIC ACID (formed from fiber)

The American Journal of Clinical Nutrition this year reported that butyric acid, "may have an **essential function in maintaining the health of the colonic mucosa**, particularly against **inflammatory conditions** and those conditions associated with **abnormal cell proliferation**" (Am J Clin Nutr 1995;61:75-81). **Butyrate**, one of the short chain fatty acids, could be significant, as it has anti-neoplastic **(prevents malignant growth)** properties" (Scand J Gastroenterol Suppl 1993;200:80-6). **Butyric acid/ butyrate**, produced during fermentation, **reduces colonic pH** and **inhibits** secondary bile acids that are **carcinogenic** (Ibid, p. 80).

Short chain fatty acids and glutamine are known to **suppress pouchitis**, which is an **inflammation of the ileal reservoir** (Ann Chiro 1993;47:1039-42).

CABBAGE

The Merck Index reports that cabbage contains **vitamin U,** the anti-ulcer vitamin, used in "**treatment of gastric disorders**" (Merck Index, Merck & Co., Rahway, NJ. 1989, p. 1581). Cabbage juice has been shown to be very beneficial in the **treatment of ulcers and constipation**. Cabbage contains high amounts of **glutamine**, which is the **principle fuel for the gastro-intestinal tract,** and is an essential ingredient of **intestinal mucus secretion.** Cabbage has a relatively high sulphur, chlorine and iodine content, which aids in **cleansing the mucus membrane** of the stomach and intestinal tract. Cabbage has been shown in a study to **speed the healing of ulcers** by 92%, compared to 32% in non-treated ulcer patients. (Werbach, M. Healing Through Nutrition. 1993. Harper Collins Publ., NY, NY. p. 318).

Cabbage, "contains several agents, including dithiolethiones, which appear to **inhibit carcinogenesis**.....studies have demonstrated that oltipraz (one of these compounds) is a potent **inducer of detoxification enzymes"** (including those involved in GI toxicity), and has also proven effective against **acetaminophen damage**. (J Cell Biochem Suppl 1993;17F:278-91). Cabbage juice **suppresses Candida yeast infection**, and **alleviates symptoms of PMS** (Heinerman, John. Heinerman's Encyclopedia of Fruits, Vegetables and Herbs. p. 56). Cabbage has been reported to exhibit some inhibitory activity against Helicobacter pylori, the bacteria suspected of causing most ulcers to form. It is believed that the active ingredient s-methyl-cysteine sulfoxide may be the compound in cabbage that the body transforms into a potent antibacterial agent (Journal of Food Science 1994;59).

CALENDULA

Calendula, "removes blood stagnation, aids blood and skin, liver, heart and lungs... promotes the rapid healing of wounds and aids persistent ulcers, burns, bruises, injuries, varicose veins and bleeding" (Tierra, L. The Herbs of Life. 1992. The Crossing Press, Freedom, Ca. p. 53). Reported therapeutic properties include that of astringent, antiseptic, antifungal (effective in vaginal yeast infections), anti-inflammatory, wound-healing, menstrual regulator, and bile stimulator (Ody, The Complete Medicinal Herbal).

CAPRYLIC ACID

Caprylic acid is effective in the treatment of **Candida**, and is described as, "a short chain, saturated **fatty acid** found to have **anti-fungal activity**, whose efficacy approaches that of nystatin" (Crook, W. MD. The Yeast Connection. 1983. Professional Books, Jackson, Tenn. pp. 352-53). Both injection and under skin implants of caprylic acid, "**cause lysis of tumor cells with little damage to normal tissue**" (AJCN 1991;53(4supp):1082S-1086S). Hepatic **tumors** in mice treated once daily were **totally obliterated after four days**, leaving normal liver cells unaffected. Because of this action of caprylic acid, the American Journal of Clinical Nutrition notes that it represents, "**a novel mode of antitumor action**" (AJCN 1991;53(4supp):1082S-1086S).

CARNITINE

Carnitine is a **"vitamin-like" molecule** that **transports fatty acids across the mitochondrial membrane** for oxidation, a process that is vital to **energy production**; its involvement in mitochondrial transport is believed to play an integral role in **branched chain amino acid metabolism** (Shils M & Young V, eds. Modern Nutrition in Health and Disease., 7th ed. 1988. Lea & Febiger, Philadelphia, Pa. p. 453). Vitamin C is needed for carnitine synthesis, and, "Muscle carnitine may therefore be a highly sensitive indicator of ascorbate status. Furthermore, **symptoms such as fatigue and lassitude** seen in vitamin C-depleted human volunteers **may be the result of poor energy production due to decreased carnitine biosynthesis**" (ibid, p. 422).

L-carnitine has been shown to have a **protective effect against ammonium acetate** (Biochem Pharmacol 1991;41(12): 1957-61) and **fully protected mice** at a dose that kills 100% of untreated controls (FEBS Lett 1984; 166:331-334).

CARROTS

Carrots are an excellent source of **beta-carotene, fiber** and many other **important nutrients.** Carrot juice or soup is helpful in **diarrhea, intestinal infection** and **intestinal disorders** (Balch P.A. Prescription for Cooking 1987. PAB Books, Tx. p. 62). When a trial was conducted on a diet high in carrot content, **microbial fermentation efficiency was increased** 2.6 times over a sweet potato diet, the carrot diet improved digestibility and, "played an important role in the nutritional physiology... and **enabled maximum utilization of the food substrates**" (Br J Nutr 1991;65(2):249-58).

CASCARA SAGRADA

Cascara sagrada is an herb that has long been used for its **laxative** properties. It contains anthraglycosides that **increase peristalsis** in the large intestine. It also has **bitter properties** that **aid in digestion**. "Cascara sagrada's **purgative power** has earned it a reputation as the world's most widely used laxative and made it the main ingredient in several over-the-counter laxatives" (Wild, R., ed. The Complete Book of Natural and Medicinal Cures. 1994. Rodale Press, Emmaus, Pa. p. 273). Cascara sagrada is fast acting, with most results showing up within 8 hours. However, on a long term basis, the colon needs fiber to keep the muscles of the colon exercised, and, "a **bulk laxative,** such as psyllium, is a better choice for **long-term chronic constipation**" (Wild, R. ibid, p. 274). Cascara sagrada should be used with caution, as the correct aging of the bark is necessary to avoid toxic chemicals. "Your best bet for taking cascara sagrada safely is to purchase a product that contains this herb as its active ingredient and to follow the product directions for use... **avoid** using cascara **if you are pregnant or have ulcers, ulcerative colitis, irritable bowel syndrome, hemorrhoids or other gastrointestinal conditions**" (Wild, R., ed. The Complete Book of Natural and Medicinal Cures. 1994. Rodale Press, Emmaus, Pa. p. 274).

CATNIP

Catnip leaves, "make an **effective** and aromatic infusion for an **upset stomach, colic and flatulence**" (Sharon, Dr. M. Complete Nutrition. 1994. Prion Publ., London, England. p. 137). Catnip has also been utilized as an antibiotic and appetite stimulant, and aids in bronchial infections, colds, and digestion (Mowry, Scientific Validation of Herbal Medicine, pp. 73-76).

CAT'S CLAW

Cat's claw (Uncaria tomentosa) has emerged from the tropical rainforests in Peru as a plant which is so high in phytochemicals that it possesses remarkable abilities as an adaptogen, immune stimulant, and digestive tonic. Although cat's claw has many polyphenols, glycosides, triterpenes and plant sterols which contribute to its activity (J Nat Products 1991;54:453-59), the most immunologically active alkaloid, according to pending patents, is isopteropodine (U.S. patents No. 4,844,901 (July 1989) and No. 4,940,725 (July 1990)). Laboratory testing has shown this alkaloid to have a pronounced effect on phagocytosis (ability of the white blood cells to engulf bacteria and debris) (Planta Medica 1985;51:419-23).

CAYENNE

Cayenne, also known as capsicum, has been shown to have a soothing effect on ulcers and has been used to treat digestive disorders including nausea, gas and indigestion. Cayenne stimulates gastric secretions and soothes the intestinal mucosa (Wild, R., ed. The Complete Book of Natural and Medicinal Cures. 1994. Rodale Press, Emmaus, Pa. p. 275). Cayenne contains a naturally occurring, photosynthetic bacterial carotenoid, capsorbin, which is a highly effective scavenger of singlet oxygen (reactive oxygen species) (Lipids 1994;29(2):149-50).

CELERY

Celery stems are rich in **iron, magnesium and carotene**; celery leaves **stimulate appetite, are diuretic, and bring on menstruation.** The seeds and stalks of celery contain a **sedative** compound called, "phthalide". and are also reported to **relieve flatulence** (Sharon, Dr. M. Complete Nutrition. 1994. Prion Publ., London, England. p. 137). In mainland China, celery juice **reduced hypertension** in 14 of 16 patients. Juice was mixed with equal amounts honey and about 8 tsp was taken orally three times each day for up to a week (Heinerman, John. Heinerman's Encyclopedia of Fruits, Vegetables and Herbs. p. 77). Celery **seed** is also reported by William Keller, PhD, professor and head of the Division of Medicinal Chemistry and Pharmaceutics at the Northeast Louisiana University School of Pharmacy in Monroe, to reduce blood pressure (Wild, R., ed. The Complete Book of Natural and Medicinal Cures. 1994. Rodale Press, Emmaus, Pa. p. 277). Lab animals given a daily dose of the phthalide compound experienced a 12% **reduction in their systolic blood pressure** over a four week time period; additionally, the compound may **lower cholesterol** (Wild, R., ed. The Complete Book of Natural and Medicinal Cures. 1994. Rodale Press, Emmaus, Pa. p. 278). Another compound in celery seed, sedanolide, along with butyl phthalide, **reduced the incidence of tumors** in laboratory animals from 38-57 %. (Heinerman, John. Heinerman's Encyclopedia of Fruits, Vegetables and Herbs. p. 77).

CHAMOMILE

One of the compounds in chamomile is **azulene.** It has been shown to be helpful in **prevention of allergic seizures, relieves asthmatic attacks in children, and has a beneficial effect on hayfever** (Heinerman, John. Heinerman's Encyclopedia of Fruits, Vegetables and Herbs. Parker Publishing, West Nyack, NY p. 81). **Chamomile** is the major ingredient we find in **relaxing, sleep-inducing** herbal teas. While it has had long reputed fame as a **soothing relaxant,** chamomile also has effective **anti-inflammatory** activity, which has proven effectiveness in treating patients (Eur J Clin Pharmacol. 1993;44:315-8). Chamomile also has **antiviral** activity, which makes it effective against the infections resulting from trauma/inflammation (Vopr Virusol. 1991;36:18-21). In addition to all the many therapeutic qualities chamomile possesses, researchers have recently discovered that chamomile has the ability to **increase positive images, shifting all mood ratings and frequency judgments in a more positive direction** (Br J Med Psychol. 1992;65:197-9).

CHICKWEED

Chickweed **relieves flatulence and constipation,** and can also be used to **soothe bruises and skin irritations**; the high potassium content of chickweed **reduces food cravings** (Sharon, Dr. M. Complete Nutrition. 1994. Prion Publ., London, England. p. 137).

CHINESE HERBS

In a controlled study of over 60 patients with chronic gastritis, **Chinese herbal treatment improved the cure rate of the gastric mucosa** atrophy due to HbP infection**,** and **increased antibacterial action** up to 96.7% over controls taking Sucrafati and Doperidone (Chung Kuo Chung Hsi... 1992;12(10): 598-601). In a study of over 485 chronic atrophic gastritis patients and over 53 Chinese medicinal herbs, **Corydalis and Coptis were found to be among the most sensitive to HbP bacteria** (Chung Kuo... 1992;12(9):521-3).

The Chinese herbs Oldenlandia diffusa and Scutellaria barbata (skullcap) are used in traditional Chinese medicine for **treating liver, lung, and rectal tumors**", and "these Chinese medicinal herbs **possess cancer chemopreventive properties**" (Mutat Res 1992;Jun 1;279(3):p. 209).

Dong-quai (Angelica sinensis, has been used for several thousand years to treat female problems. It relieves PMS, anemia and weak glands, regulates monthly periods, corrects hot flashes and vaginal spasms, and alleviates menopause (Heinerman, John. Heinerman's Encyclopedia of Fruits, Vegetables and Herbs. p. 7). Dong-quai is an herb that possesses, "both proven estrogenic activity and a long historical use in treating various female complaints" (Murray M. Enc Nat Med, p. 462). Dong quai contains phytoestrogens, which are believed to balance female hormonal problems.

Du Huo (**Angelica** pubescens) is an **analgesic, anti-inflammatory, and antirheumatic** (Ody, P. The complete Medicinal Herbal. Dorling Kindersley Ltd, London. 1993).

Chai Hu (**Bupleurum** chinense) is a **liver stimulant, antibacterial, anti-inflammatory, and analgesic, which stimulates bile flow and reduces cholesterol** (Ody, P. The Complete Medicinal Herbal. 1993. Dorling Kindersley Ltd, London). When fractions of the Japanese root bupleurum were tested for inhibition of gastric lesion formation, "The most potent anti-ulcer activity was observed in the pectin-like polysaccharide (bupleurum extract)" (Planta Med 1991;57(6):555-9).

Chuan Xiong (**Ligusticum** wallicbii) is a **circulatory stimulant, reduces blood pressure**, and it is a **natural sedative** (Ody, P. The Complete Medicinal Herbal).

Di Gu Pi (**Lycium** chinense) **lowers blood cholesterol** (Ody, P. The complete Medicinal Herbal. Dorling Kindersley Ltd, London. 1993).

Ze Xie (Alisma **plantago**) is a **diuretic, antibacterial, liver cleanser,** and **reduces blood pressure** (Ody, P. The complete Medicinal Herbal. Dorling Kindersley Ltd, London. 1993).

CHLORELLA

Chlorella is green, fresh-water algae that is high in all the amino acids, low in fat and contains substantial amounts of vitamins, minerals and plant chlorophyll. It has an abundance of beta-carotene, iron, iodine, zinc and vitamin B-12 and is also the richest natural source of DNA. Chlorella is also very effective in removing toxins from the body and provides relief for intestinal gas and chronic constipation.

Chlorella has unique health-promoting characteristics, including **antitumor resistance, bacterial resistance and viral resistance**. It has demonstrated the ability to **restore leukocyte, natural killer cell and interferon activity** (Nat Immun Cell Growth Regul 1990;9(2):121-8; Int J Immunopharmacol 1990;12(8):883-91). This has led to the announcement in Critical Reviews in Food Science and Nutrition that the microalgae Chlorella, "are being used as **nutrient dense foods**. They have significant amounts of **lipid, protein, chlorophyll, carotenoids, vitamins, minerals and unique pigments.** They may also have **potent probiotic compounds that enhance health**" (Crit Rev Food Sci Nutr 1991;30(6):555-73). Chlorella demonstrated **metal-removing properties** when used as a treatment for polluted stream samples (Biomed Environ Sci 1992;5(2):99-108).

CHLOROPHYLL

Chlorophyll is the main component of the plant's blood, just as hemoglobin is the main component in human blood. Magnesium is the center of the chlorophyll molecule, just as iron is the core of the hemoglobin molecule, thus chlorophyll is **high in magnesium**. Chlorophyll **provides intestinal nourishment** and has a **soothing effect on the lining of the mucosa**. It is an **intestinal detoxifier** due to its neutralizing effects on guanidine, an intense alkaline substance found in the intestines caused by constipation or cell trauma.

"Silkworm excreta containing **chlorophyll metabolites** have long been used for their **medicinal activities** in the Far East" (J Nat Prod 1992;55(9):1241-44). In 27 patients who had, "demonstrated a functional imbalance of the peripheral **blood phagocytizing (bacteria-scavenging) cells...chlorophyll administration corrected the metabolic shifts", and increased neutrophil activity** (Vestn-Dermatol-Venerol 1990;(8):67-9).

CHOLINE

Choline is a lipotropic factor (hastens fat removal/decreases deposits in the liver), and a major constituent of phosphatidylcholine, essential to the lipid layer of cell membranes. Choline as phosphatidylcholine is a basic component of soy lecithin. "Supplementation with choline restored the amount of phosphatidylcholine in cells..." previously depleted in choline (Biochem J 1993;291(Pt 2):419-27). "...phosphatidylcholine may **protect gastric mucosa** by **strengthening the mucus-phospholipid layer**" (Scand J Gastroenterol 1993;28(10):894-8).

Choline **decongests the liver of excess fats**, and it is also an integral part of the **neurotransmitter acetylcholine**. Choline helps the liver and gallbladder function correctly and is vital to brain chemistry.

CHONDROITIN SULFATE A (trachea)

Chondroitin sulfate consists of **high viscosity mucopolysaccharides** (glycosaminoglycans). These substances act as the **flexible connecting matrix** between the tough protein filaments in cartilage to form a system, "similar to reinforced rubber" (Merck Index, p. 2217). They are the most abundant mucopolysaccharides in the body, occurring in skeletal and soft connective tissue. Chondroitin sulfate is listed as an **antihyperlipoproteinemic** (Merck Index, p. 2217), and in the amount of 1-3 grams daily, "can **help lower cholesterol**" (Int Med Res 1978;6:217, as cited in: (Wright, Jonathan V. M.D. Healing with Nutrition. 1990. Keats Publishing, Inc. New Canaan, Conn. p. 569).

CHROMIUM

Chromium is a **blood sugar regulator**. Chromium is part of the glucose tolerance factor **(GTF)**, which is thought to **potentiate the action of insulin at the cellular level.** "Chromium may help restore some of the body's sensitivity to insulin and thus make better use of glucose... a recent study yielded results suggesting that many Americans, of all ages, get amounts of chromium in their daily diets that are **below the minimum safe and adequate allowance... chromium supplementation is expected to assume an important place in preventive medicine**" (Hendler, S.S., M.D. The Doctor's Vitamin and Mineral Encyclopedia. 1990. Simon & Schuster, NY, NY p. 124).

CINNAMON

Cinnamon is a **disinfectant, stimulant, and anti-flatulent**, and is also **helpful for nausea** (Sharon, Dr. M. Complete Nutrition. 1994. Prion Publ., London, England. p. 137). In addition, cinnamon may help **soothe indigestion, control blood sugar, prevent stomach ulcers, ward off urinary tract infections, and fight tooth decay and gum disease** (Wild, R., ed. The Complete Book of Natural and Medicinal Cures. 1994. Rodale Press, Emmaus, Pa. p. 282).

Cinnamon has been used in the **prevention and treatment of candidiasis** (ChungHua Hu Li Tsa Chih 1993;28(12):711-2). In the Journal of Food Science 1974, (as cited in Duke, JA. Handbook of Medicinal Herbs. CRC Press, Boca Raton, Fl. 1985), 20 mg of cinnamon spice per yeast extract inhibited up to 99% of molds.

CITRUS FRUITS

Citrus fruits contain limonene, which increases the enzymes that **decrease carcinogens**, and **enhance the ability of immune cell function** (Weiner, M.A. Herbs that Heal. 1994. Quantum Books, Mill Valley, Ca. p. 113). They also contain glucamase, which inactivates carcinogens and eliminates them. Citrus fruits include oranges, lemons, limes, and grapefruit. Juices of **lemon, grapefruit and orange** have been recommended by Airola for **glaucoma** (Airola, P. Handbook of Natural Healing. 1993. Health Plus Publishers, Sherwood, Oregon). .

CITRUS SEED EXTRACT

Citrus seed extract is reportedly helpful against **yeast, viruses, bacteria and protozoa**. William G. Crook M.D. (Chronic Fatigue Syndrome and the Yeast Connection. Professional Books, Jackson, Tenn. 1992 p. 37) recommends that for Candida, "...nonprescription antifungal medications including Lactobacillus acidophilus, caprylic acid, **citrus seed extracts**, garlic products and/or other substances that **curb the growth of Candida albicans in the digestive tract.**

CLEAVERS

Cleavers is an **antibiotic, a diuretic, a hypotensive, and helps in kidney/urinary problems** (David B. Mowry, PhD. The Scientific Validation of Herbal Medicine. 1986. Keats Publishing, New Canaan, Conn. p. 81-83). Other attributed properties of cleavers include **mild astringent**, and **lymphatic cleanser** for a range of conditions, including **glandular fever, tonsillitis, and prostate disorders** (Ody, The Complete Medicinal Herbal).

CLOVES

Cloves, a sweet smelling spice, possesses **antioxidant activity** (Mol Cell Biochem 1992;111:117-24; Indian J Biochem Biophys1993; 30: 130-4). This spice is a **powerful, penetrating antiseptic**, which is also known to **curb alcoholic cravings** (Heinerman, John. Heinerman's Encyclopedia of Fruits, Vegetables and Herbs. p. 108). Cloves are known to aid in **parasitic infestations, hernia, hiccuping,, and abdominal pain** (Balch, P.A. Prescription for Cooking. 1987. PAB Books, Tx. p. 173). Cloves help to: **relieve traveler's diarrhea, calm indigestion, soothe minor wounds, and ease toothache** (Wild, R., ed. The Complete Book of Natural and Medicinal Cures. 1994. Rodale Press, Emmaus, Pa. p. 284). In fact, its reputation for relieving tooth pain for hours was demonstrated with a flair in the movie, "Marathon Man", when Dustin Hoffman applies oil of cloves to his drilled teeth to eliminate the pain.

COENZYME Q10

This **vitamin-like nutrient** is one of the **electron carriers in the electron transport system** (ATP generation), and may **help cells utilize oxygen** (Mayell, M. The Natural Health First Aid Guide; p. 298). Oxygen supply is necessary for **tissue repair and immune function**; this could be why coenzyme Q purportedly **increases antibody count** and is helpful in **treating candidiasis.** In a test for oxidative performance in patients with myopathies, **treated patients experienced higher oxygen consumption and threshold to higher workload,** indicating, "**improvement of mitochondrial function**" (Neurology 1992;42(6):1203-8).

Coenzyme Q concentration in the mitochondrial membrane is not believed to be saturated for NADH (another important energy enzyme) oxidation, and, "This provides a rationale for the **reported therapeutic effects of coenzyme Q** under conditions when its concentration is decreased" (Clin Investig 1993;71(8 Suppl):S66-70). Perfusion of Coenzyme Q into rat livers **prevented oxidative stress and mitochondrial damage** (Clin Investig 1993;71(8 Suppl):S66-70).

Lieberman notes that coenzyme Q10, "has demonstrated excellent results in clinical trials on periodontal disease" (Mayell p. 298). "The studies have been positive in showing a speedup of healing time, reduced pockets, and improvements in other factors associated with gum disease" (ibid, p. 298). The therapeutic potential of this antioxidant is discussed in, "Antioxidant systems - physiology and pharmacotherapy trends" by P. Grieb (Mater Med Pol 1992 24(4):217-222).

Two patients with mitochondrial encephalomyopathy received 150 mg/d of coenzyme Q10 during ten months of treatment. After treatment, the bicycle ergometer exercise test indicated a **significant improvement with a decrease in resting blood lactate level, an increase in oxygen consumption during exercise, and an increase in the kinetics of lactate disappearance during the recovery period.** A shift of the ventilatory threshold to **higher workload** was present...These observations indicate an **improvement of mitochondrial function** and a shift from **high to low glycolytic activity** in both patients consequent to Coenzyme Q treatment" (Neurology 1992;42(6):1203). This is because the mitochondria make energy (ATP) during aerobic, or oxygen-dependent activity, while glycolytic activity is anaerobic, or not dependent on oxygen.

COLLINSONIA

Collinsonia stimulates, tones and cleanses the mucus membranes of the gastrointestinal tract. It assists in hemorrhoid and varicose vein problems. It is referred to in herbal literature as a "vascular astringent". In most patients with hemorrhoids or varicose vein problems, the patient has a congested liver. Bile salts should be combined with collinsonia because bile salts alone may be irritating.

A tincture of the roots is used as a **diuretic, and as a tonic for indigestion** (J Nat Products Oct 1992;55(10):1468-76). Sometimes called, "knobroot", it acts as a **saponin** (forms a stable foam in water), and as a **protective mucilage** (Merck Index, 11th ed. Merck & Co. Inc., Rahway, N.J. 1989 p. 2477).

CORN SILK

Corn silk has **effective diuretic properties** which have been used to **treat diabetes and hypertension** (David B. Mowry, PhD. The Scientific Validation of Herbal Medicine. 1986. Keats Publishing, New Canaan, Conn. p. 82). Corn silk has also been used in the treatment of **cystitis, edema, hepatitis, and prostate problems** (ibid, p. 233-235). "An **estrogenic and ovulation induction effect** was observed in animal studies. Preliminary animal experiments with an aqueous extract have found **immunostimulant activity,** as well as the **stimulation of interferon induction and macrophage migration**" (Weiner, M.A. Herbs that Heal. 1994. Quantum Books, Mill Valley, Ca. p. 132).

CRANBERRY

Cranberry's constituents are anthocyanidins, catechin, and triterpenoids. It has a high acid content, which acidifies the urine and **kills the bacteria which cause urinary infections**. Hence, its reputation for clearing urinary tract infections - "Cranberry also **prevents the bacteria from adhering to cells,** allowing the bacteria to be flushed from the system" (Weiner, M.A. Herbs that Heal. 1994. Quantum Books, Mill Valley, Ca. p. 136).

CRANESBILL

Early American Indians relied upon cranesbill root, otherwise called geranium maculatum, to treat **diarrhea, dysentery, leukorrhea and hemorrhoids.** "These people passed this knowledge on to the early settlers, and thus into the black bag of many early physicians, who discovered it would also **reduce chronic menorrhagia**" (Mowry, D. Scientific Validation, p. 186).

CREATINE

Creatine has become a popular supplement for weight lifters to enhance performance. Some evidence shows that improvements in muscle growth may result from creatine supplementation, although this is still debated by many. A 1996 study reported that creatine decreased the performance of sprint swimmers, but it was hypothesized that it may have been because of an increase in body mass and drag forces. Creatine can have some side effects, including nausea. Creatine is not a steroid precursor, such as the "androstenedione" that is being taken by some baseball players (including Mark McGuire, who broke the record for home runs). Creatine is a substrate for creatine phosphate, which is an energy source in the body for ATP, which is the body's exchange for energy. Creatine phosphate is a substrate for anaerobic energy, however, which means "without oxygen". Activities like weight-lifting are anaerobic; aerobic activity becomes anaerobic at very high intensity. There is no indication that creatine would make any difference in mild aerobic activity.

DAMIANA

Damiana is used in the **treatment of constipation, coughs, and kidney stones** (Mowry, Scientific Validation p. 152). It is rumored to be a **sexual stimulant and aphrodisiac**, and has been utilized in problems of infertility (ibid p.152). "Damiana is **one of the most popular and safest of all plants claimed to have an aphrodisiac effect**" (Weiner, M p. 137).

DANDELION

Dandelion is an excellent liver remedy and has a high carotenoid content (even higher than carrots). It aids in liver congestion, hepatitis, jaundice, gallstones, inflammation of the bile duct and enhances bile flow (Tierra, the Herbs of Life p. 59; David B. Mowry, PhD. The Scientific Validation of Herbal Medicine. 1986. Keats Publishing, New Canaan, Conn. p. 17, 18, 177-179). "The plant was noted to have an almost specific affinity for the liver, modifying and increasing its secretions... Dandelion has also been found effective in relieving arthritis" (Weiner, M. Herbs that Heal p. 139). "Dandelion is commonly administered as a home remedy for mild constipation and stomach ache. Dandelion leaf tea, drunk often, is recommended as an aid for promoting digestive regularity" (Weiner, M. Herbs that Heal, p. 139). Kiowa women used to boil the dandelion blossoms and drink the tea to relieve menstrual symptoms (ibid p. 138). Dandelion and fennel seed are natural herbal cleansers, and good sources of calcium, phosphorus, and potassium.

DEGLYCYRRHIZINATED LICORICE POWDER (DGL)

Most traditional ulcer medications decrease acid production without building up protective intestinal cells (H_2 receptor antagonists actually cause further deterioration of these cells). To increase the integrity of the mucus\bicarbonate producing cells, a natural licorice extract, "deglycyrrhizinated licorice (DGL)", has been utilized. DGL increases the life span of these intestinal cells, improves the quality of protective substances, and improves blood supply of nutrients (Glick L. Lancet ii:817, 1982).

DGL has been effective in treating both gastric and duodenal ulcers, and **can reduce the gastric bleeding** caused by aspirin (Rees WDW et al. Scand J Gastroenterol 14:605-7.1979). When DGL was compared to antacids and H_2 receptor antagonists in over 800 patients, all had a high healing rate. DGL, however, had a **significantly lower relapse rate** (Kassir ZA Irish Med J 78:153-56, 1985). When 33 gastric ulcer patients were treated with DGL or a placebo, the ulcer size was significantly reduced in the DGL group (by 78%) compared to the placebo group (34%) (Murray, M. Enc. Nat. Med.; p. 523).

DGL also cleanses the colon. It has been shown to be beneficial for colitis, diverticulosis, gastritis, stress and nausea. Glycyrrhizin decreases a form of testosterone by-product that encourages growth of prostate cancer; it also protects DNA from damage (Health Mar-Apr 1995; p. 60). DGL has exhibited some activity in inhibiting the bacteria considered to be responsible for most ulcer development (helicobacter pylori) (Am J Nat Med 1995;2:16).

DEVIL'S CLAW

Devil's claw reportedly has **anti-inflammatory and analgesic properties**, and is used in **rheumatoid arthritis and osteoarthritis.** "Harpagide and other extracts of Devil's Claw have been evaluated in recent times in clinical trials involving human subjects with arthritis and have shown a beneficial effect...In many excellent animal studies, Devil's claw has shown **analgesic activity, anti-inflammatory activity, smooth muscle relaxant activity, and antihypertensive activity"** (Weiner, M.A. Herbs that Heal. 1994. Quantum Books, Mill Valley, Ca. p. 140).

DONG-QUAI

(See Chinese herbs - Angelica sinensis)

DULSE

Dulse is a seaweed that is high in **iodine, protein, iron and calcium**. Seaweed extracts have, "**demonstrated therapeutic efficacy**" as an **antiviral** agent (Cancer Lett 1991;56(3):197-205), and can be effective **stimulators of immunity** (Radiats Biol Radioecol 1994;34(2):236-9). Seaweed structures have been known to influence the **chemotactic activity of macrophages, and possess antitumor properties**

(Carbohydr Res 1993;243(1):211-16). In diets containing a seaweed extract, "...a more-intense **positive reaction in the hepatic cells**" for antioxidant activity was evident, compared to controls (Nutr Cancer 1991;15(3-4):221-8).

ECHINACEA

Echinacea is a natural herb that has been used in many scientific studies for its ability to **enhance the immune system.** It is known to **stimulate macrophages and antibodies**. By increasing the number and enhancing the activity of bacteria scavenging cells, echinacea, **"mediates protection against systemic infections"** (Int. J. Immunophar. 13:27-37). Also used for **fevers** and **wound healing**, echinacea **boosts the power of vitamin C** to **combat infection**. "Current pharmacology indicates Echinacea is **antitumor, antiviral, and an immunostimulant.** It is also effective against **herpes and influenza,** is used for **wound healing,** has been proven to **activate reticulo-endothelial layer to increase alpha, beta, and gamma globulin** (which is the formation of antibodies), and to **increase the rate of phagocytosis** (Weiner, M. Herbs That Heal. p. 141). Echinacea has compounds which have demonstrated **potent inhibition of hyaluronidase,** a component in snake venom that destroys the ground substance of bone and connective tissue. This is why it is reputed to heal snakebites (Mayell. The Natural Health First Aid Guide. Pocket Books, NY, NY. 1994. p. 422).

In fact, hyaluronic acid (HA) is the substance that occurs in the tissues between cells to "cement" them together, forming a very effective barrier against infection. There is now a theory that destruction of this protective barrier is one of the precursors to **rheumatoid arthritis.** "There is an enzyme that attacks HA in a way not fully understood. When it does, the HA quickly loses viscosity, like jello tuning to water. This is the weak link in the system. If the enzyme is allowed to destroy the integrity of the HA barrier, pathogenic bacteria such as staph and strep penetrate the tissues and make you sick. A similar mechanism is thought to be involved in rheumatism and tumor formation and at the beginnings of malignancy. Echinacea has been shown to **prevent the enzyme from dissolving HA**. It's that simple. The herb acts to effectively close down one of the major routes of bug-invasion. It **inhibits the spread of infection** that may have already occurred. A possible mode of action is that echinacea and HA combine together to form a complex that is resistant to enzyme invasion and that **facilitates fibrous connective tissue regeneration. Cortisone-like activity** has also been discovered in echinacea that could help account for some of its **anti-inflammatory activity**. In addition, echinacea **accelerates the production of granulomatous tissue (necessary for healing) and has a stimulating effect on the lymph system, increasing its ability to carry waste tissue away from areas of infection.** Echinacin, the active constituent of echinacea, exhibits **interferon activity.** It protects cells against virus related diseases, such as **herpes, influenza, canker sores, etc. ... and stimulates T-cell activity"** (David B. Mowry, PhD. The Scientific Validation of Herbal Medicine. 1986. Keats Publishing, New Canaan, Conn. p. 119).

Since the body can develop resistance to the polysaccharides (sugars) in the cell wall of echinacea, it is recommended to avoid constant stimulation of the immune system with echinacea. Typical advice is to take the herb for 8 weeks and then refrain from taking it for at least a week.

ELUTHERO (Siberian Ginseng)

Siberian ginseng is widely used by Russians to **improve stamina and resist stress** (Wild, R., ed. The Complete Book of Natural and Medicinal Cures. 1994. Rodale Press, Emmaus, Pa. p. 303). It is utilized to combat fatigue, and normalize blood sugar levels, whether high or low (Mowry, D Scientific Validation, p. 27). "Ginseng species **stimulate the central nervous system in small amounts and depress the central nervous system in large doses**; they **protect** the body and nervous system **from stress**; they **stimulate and increase metabolic function**; **increase physical and mental efficiency; lower blood pressure and glucose levels when high, and raise them when low; increase gastrointestinal movement and tone; increase iron metabolism; and cause changes in nucleic acid (RNA) biosynthesis" (ibid, p. 288).**

Most of the activity of Siberian ginseng is attributed to the eleutheroside content, which has demonstrated adaptogenic abilities, defined by Brekhman as having normalizing action, irrespective of the direction of the pathological state (Farnsworth NR et al., Econ Med Plant Res 1985;1:156-215). It is believed that this adaptogenic capability may act through the pituitary-adrenocortical system (Filaretov AA et al. Effect of adaptogens on the activity of the Pituitary-Adrenocortical System in Rats. (Russian). Bull Eksper Bio Med 1986;101:573). One of the components in Siberian ginseng has demonstrated antiplatelet activity, which means it may help prevent blood clotting (J Nat Prod 1987;50:1059). Recommended dosage can be up to 600 mg/day of the solid extract.

Even though Siberian ginseng is not considered a "true" ginseng by some (it is in the same family, but not the same genus), all the ginsengs should be used with caution in combination with drugs associated with the treatment of conditions related to symptoms of excess ginseng supplementation, i.e. blood pressure drugs, heart medication, and particularly digitalis-like drugs. A physician should be consulted about combinations. Possible antiplatelet activity means that Coumadin and other blood-thinning drugs should be used with cauthion when combined with herbs possessing this activity.

ENZYMATIC AIDS

Pancreatic enzymes: Pancreatic enzymes are necessary for the complete breakdown of food particles. Incomplete breakdown can result in digestive problems, nutrient deficiencies, and activation of the immune system. Hydrochloric acid (HCL) decreases as we age, and the low pH thatHCL creates in the stomach is necessary to start the body's signals for the food to move on. Without the proper signals, the pancreatic enzymes can't be released into the small intestine to finish digesting food. Pancreatic extracts **stimulate pancreatic enzyme secretion** (Digestion 1993;54(Suppl 2):35-9). "Pancreatic enzymes have an **influence on the release of some gastrointestinal hormones** (i.e. cholecystokinin, motilin and gastric inhibitory peptide)" (Digestion 1993;54(Suppl 2):p.15). Oral pancreatic enzymes can be of great benefit to patients with chronic **pancreatitis** (Digestion 1993;54(Suppl 2):p. 30). Pancreatic extracts, which contain these enzymes, have effectively corrected the malabsorption resulting from pancreatic insufficiency.

Bromelain: Extracted from pineapple, bromelain is a **protein-digesting enzyme**. It is an **excellent anti-inflammatory** enzyme (Merck Index, 11th ed. 1989. Merck & Co. Inc., Rahway, NJ, p. 1382) used for post-traumatic injury and swelling. It is helpful in cardiovascular disease by **decreasing platelet aggregation** and clot formation. Bromelain therapy has become quite popular for use in **rheumatoid arthritis** to decrease joint inflammation.

Bromelain is an **effective wound healing agent** (Mayell M. The Natural Health First Aid Guide; p. 291). "Bromelain is quite effective as a substitute for pancreatic enzymes in the treatment of pancreatic insufficiency, but best results are obtained if it is used in combination with pancreatin and ox bile. Bromelain has also been shown in many studies to aid the body's response to **inflammation and swelling**" (Murray M and Pizzorno J Encyclopedia of Natural Medicine. Prima Publishing, Rocklin, Ca. 1991, p. 54). "Immunomodulation and the release of cytokines may contribute to the **therapeutic effect** of these preparations" (Oncology 1990;47(6):475-7). "In some patients...pancreatic insufficiency is severe enough to cause malabsorption, which can be effectively **corrected by oral pancreatic extracts**" (Digestion 1993;54(Suppl 2):43-7). Bromelain reduces bruising, especially the bruising due to tooth extractions, and can prevent the side effects from causing pain (Mayell p. 291).

Bromelain, "...has **therapeutic effects in the treatment of inflammation and soft tissue injuries**" (Med Sci Sports Exerc 1992;24(1):20). In the study published in Medicine and Science in Sports and Exercise, bromelain **reduced skeletal muscle injury** in the treated groups. (Med Sci Sports Exerc 1992;24(1):20-25). Following injury, an application of bromelain twice daily **significantly increased the maximum muscle force** in the treated group, indicating that bromelain can be helpful for a quick recovery from injury.

The **smooth muscle relaxant** properties of bromelain contribute to the documentation for **relieving menstrual cramps**. It is believed that bromelain works by **correcting the inflammatory prostaglandin imbalance** (premenstrual tension is also relieved with a balance) (Murray M. Enc Nat Med p. 478).

Pancreatin: Pancreatin refers to preparations of enzymes secreted by the pancreas; pancreatin has one of the greatest potentials in medicine; pancreatic enzyme deficiency is said to be at the root of many degenerative diseases. Pancreatin is often used in treatment of indigestion, malabsorption and inflammatory conditions.

Pancreatin contains the enzymes amylopsin, trypsin and steapsin. "**It converts not less than 25 times its weight of starch into soluble carbohydrates and not less than 25 times it weight of casein into**

proteoses (hydrolyzed protein) within 5 minutes. Its greatest activity is exhibited in neutral or faintly alkaline media; mineral acids or excess alkali hydroxides or carbonates render it inactive" (Merck Index, 11th ed. Merck & Co. Inc., Rahway, N.J. 1989 p. 6953). Good mixing of pancreatin with the B-12 intrinsic factor - R protein complex and with the protein containing meal seems to be **important for digestion of protein as well as fat** (Orv Hetil 1990;131(5):241-4. "Pancreatin is most often employed in the treatment of pancreatic insufficiency characterized by impaired digestion, malabsorption, nutrient deficiencies and abdominal discomfort... It is best to use a full-strength undiluted pancreatic extract (8-10X USP) with additional enzymes added (see bromelain)" (Murray M and Pizzorno J Encyclopedia of natural Medicine. Prima Publishing, Rocklin, Ca. 1991, p. 53).

<u>**Papain:**</u> Extracted from papayas, papain soothes the stomach and aids in protein digestion. Papain has been shown "to be effective in celiac disease patients by digesting the wheat gluten and rendering it harmless." (Murray M. Enc. Nat. Med. p. 226). Bezoars, (obstructions in the GI tract) can cause ulceration, bleeding and perforation, with symptoms of discomfort, nausea and vomiting, however, "Dissolution of the undigested bolus by ingestion of proteolytic enzymes such as papain may be tried" (Kinderarztl Prax 1990 58(10):531-4).

<u>**Pancreatic Lipase**</u>: A new high lipase preparation was tested in a **randomized, double-blind crossover study in children (18) with cystic fibrosis**. "There were **fewer gastrointestinal symptoms** when pancreatic enzyme was supplied as the high lipase preparation. There was also a **significant improvement in fat absorption**", with **reduction in fat output and energy loss** (Arch Dis Child 1993 68(2):227-30).

ESSENTIAL FATTY ACIDS (EFA'S)

Essential fatty acids (EFA's) are important in the diet because EFA's are a main component of phospholipids, the main constituent of cell membranes. Phospholipids help determine the fluidity and integrity of the cell membranes, and the type of fat ingested will play a major role in determining the health of the cell membranes. Saturated fats (i.e. butter or lard), trans-fatty acids (i.e. margarine or deep fried foods), or excess arachidonic acid (i.e. processed meats and dairy) all decrease cell membrane fluidity and function, while "good" essential fatty acids (i.e. fish oils) enhance cell membrane fluidity and function. Arachidonic acid is an essential fatty acid which is vital to development and maintenance of life, however, the average diet provides an excess. Essential fatty acids also play an important role in inflammation, hormone synthesis, nerve transmission and many other body system functions. Black currant seed oil (BCSO), for instance, can be made into arachidonic acid if it is lacking, but prevents against the symptoms of excess. This is because BCSO will force a pathway of antiinflammatory substances to be produced, whereas arachidonic acid excess leads to production of substances which can be inflammatory, clotting, and vasoconstrictive (tightens blood vessels and raises blood pressure).

The essential fatty acids are sometimes collectively referred to as vitamin F. EFA's are **essential for normal growth.** They are the **major component in cell membranes and function in energy production, steroid synthesis** and **keep the skin and tissues youthful** due to their lubricating quality.

A **balance of the fatty acids is essential. Allergic eczema** is believed by some to be caused by an **imbalance of fatty acids** in the body (Heinerman, John. Heinerman's Encyclopedia of Fruits, Vegetables and Herbs. Parker Publishing, West Nyack, NY p. 134). Heinerman proposes that allergy relief can be experienced after taking fatty acid supplements a month before season (ibid, p. 184). In fact, Heinerman believes that a **host of diseases**, including coronary artery disease, hypertension, hypercholesterolemia, allergic eczema, cancer, premature aging, chronic inflammation and autoimmune disorders are **related to an imbalance of fatty acids in the body** (ibid, p. 134).

Arachidonic acid:

Arachidonic acid can be synthesized from linoleic acid (omega 6). While **linoleic acid (unsaturated vegetable oils)** is needed for **normal immune response** (J Am Coll Nutr 1991;10:406-28), an imbalance of the series 2 products (prostaglandins) that linoleic makes when it is converted to arachidonic acid can have unfavorable results. Some linoleic acid can be made into gamma linolenic acid (eg. BCSO), which has a favorable prostaglandin pathway, while arachidonic acid sources, like processed red meat, will go directly to series 2 products. A balance of the other fatty acids is necessary, and in fact, "**In a number of diseases, plasma levels of linoleic acid are normal or elevated while those of gamma linolenic and further metabolites are below normal**" (Pgs, Lts & EFAs 1991;42:245-9). An example of an oil high in **linoleic acid** (omega 6) is **sesame seed oil.** Sesame seeds are rich in protein, zinc, calcium, copper, magnesium, phosphorus and potassium. Sesame also contains some vitamin A, E and most of the B vitamins.

Fish oil:

An example of oil high in omega 3unsaturated fatty acids is **fish oil**. Fish oils are comprised mostly of **docosahexaenoic acid (DHA) and eicosapentaenoic acid (EPA)**. These are highly unsaturated fatty acids; some examples are shark liver oil, halibut liver oil, and skip jack oil. Salmon, red trout, and herring are fish which are relatively high in omega 3 fatty acids. The omega 3 fatty acids make prostaglandins of the 3 series, which are antiinflammatory and vasodilating (relax blood vessels), as opposed to the 2 series from arachidonic acid, which can be inflammatory, pain-producing, and vaso-constrictive when they are in excess.

Fish oil seems to have many **beneficial effects on the cardiovascular system.** In fact, "The mechanisms by which dietary n-3 fatty acids might **modulate the morbidity and mortality from coronary heart disease** have been related to their effects on plasma lipids and lipoproteins, eicosanoid metabolism, and platelet-endothelial cell interactions. In addition, more recent studies have shown **positive effects on myocardial function and blood pressure**" (AJCN 1993;57:634).

Omega-3 fish oils, combined with black currant seed oil, resulted in the **smallest mammary tumors** when compared to a 23% corn oil diet that enhanced tumor growth in a study of rats (Pgs, LTs & EFA 1993;48:309-14). In addition, the effect of fish oil on **ulcerative colitis** was investigated in 87 patients. Treatment with fish oil resulted in, "**measurable clinical benefit**" - there was a trend toward achieving remission (being taken off corticosteroids) faster in the patients taking 4.5 grams fish oil daily for a year (Gut 1992;33(7):922-8).

Artificial formulas, unlike human milk, do not contain any **long-chain** polyunsaturated fatty acids (PUFA's). The PUFA's found in **fish oil**, such as **docosahexaenoic acid (DHA)** and **eicosapentaenoic acid (EPA),** are an example of **very long chain PUFA's.** Their high degree of unsaturation is needed for **membrane fluidity**. In the 1960's, **clinical signs of essential fatty acid (EFA) deficiency** became apparent in infants fed skim-milk based **formulas** (Am J Clin Nutr 1993;57:807S-12S). "The demand of the fetal and neonatal brain for docosahexaenoic acid (DHA)... increases substantially during the last trimester of pregnancy and the first months of postnatal life. Consequently, the use of these artificial formulas could lead to a considerable deterioration of the EFA status after birth, especially in children who are born prematurely" (Am J Clin Nutr 1993;57:829S). Arachidonic acid is a crucial element also needed for brain development; remember that linoleic acid sources can be made into arachidonic acid. Some nutritionists caution against early introduction of fish oil because of allergy-development. Flax seed oil, which is an alpha-linolenic acid, can be elongated in the body to the longer chain EPA and DHA fatty acids.

In a study on infants performed 57 weeks after birth, a **fish oil supplemented formula** was compared to human milk and a corn oil based formula. The corn oil based diet, which lacked the long chain **DHA** present in the fish oil formula and human milk, caused **impaired visual acuity** at both 36 and 57 weeks. **"The study supports a role for omega-3 long chain PUFA's as required nutrients for the optimal maturation of visual and cortical function in preterm infants"** (Am J Clin Nutr 1993;57:807S-12S).

DHA was found to be associated with **psychomotor and mental development** indexes in preterm infants, when it was measured in 211 diabetics for four years (AJCN 1993;57:801S-6S). Another study concluded that, "the **early dietary fat** regimen can influence the **development of brain** and visual function" (AJCN 1993;57: 807S-12). Subtle **clinical symptoms, including peripheral neuropathy,** "may occur in response to an **insufficiency** of the specific metabolic derivative of alpha linolenic acid, namely **DHA** (AJCN 1993;57: 807S-12).

It appears that a balance of long chain polyunsaturated oils (omega 6) with the longer chain omega 3 fatty acids, such as EPA & DHA, or flax seed oil (which is converted in the body to the longer chain fatty acids) is necessary for optimal growth and development.

Flax seed oil:

The conversion of flax seed oil, or alpha-linolenic acid, in the body to the longer chain fatty acids is challenged by Shils and Young (Modern Nutrition in Health and Disease), who say that the conversion process is slow, however, clinical results indicate that flax seed oil does have antiinflammatory effects, suggesting that the oil is made into prostaglandins of the 3 series by conversion to the longer chain omega 3's (EPA & DHA). Michael Murray, for instance, cites good results which have been obtained in studies involving people with high blood pressure, high cholesterol, rheumatoid arthritis, and impaired immune systems (Murray, M Enc. Nutr Supplements. Prima Publ, Rocklin, Ca. 1996).

Black currant seed oil:

Black currant seed oil is a balanced oil which contains some linoleic acid, but is also one of the few oils containing gamma linolenic acid (makes prostaglandins of the one series). It has strong **antiseptic** properties, and is used in the **treatment of Candida yeast infection, whooping cough, hypertension, and various skin diseases, including arthritic inflammations** (Heinerman, John. Heinerman's Encyclopedia of Fruits, Vegetables and Herbs. Parker Publishing, West Nyack, NY p. 36). A study on **rheumatoid arthritis** patients showed, "A **significant improvement** in morning stiffness was noted in the rheumatoid arthritis **patients receiving black currant seed oil**" (British J Rheumatology 1993;32:1055-8). Black currant seed oil also has a **profound effect on the immune system**, and, "A correlation was found between the degree of **developing resistance to infection, virus accumulation in the brain, blood, spleen and thymus...**" (Vopr Virusol 1993;38:170-3).

Vessel wall thrombus formation was decreased when a diet rich in black currant seed oil was fed. "This latter effect was better obtained when gamma linoleic acid was present suggesting a secondary effect of this fatty acid". Platelet adhesion was significantly decreased on the fish oil diet. "We conclude that **both fish oil and black currant seed oil rich diets inhibit platelet/vessel wall adhesion**" (Thromb Res 1990;59(5):819-30).

Evening primrose oil (EPO):

In two Canadian studies, both the main constituent in evening primrose oil (EPO), gamma-linolenic acid (GLA) and the plant oil (EPO) itself, **significantly reduced blood pressure -** (Heinerman J. p. 134). The blank currant seed also contains gamma linolenic oil, which reduces both hypertension and arthritic inflammations (Heinerman, John. Heinerman's Encyclopedia of Fruits, Vegetables and Herbs. Parker Publishing, West Nyack, NY p.36).

Kenneth Vaddadi, a psychiatrist at the University of Leeds in England, has achieved successful results using evening primrose oil in clinical trials. It appears that seven 500 mg capsules daily in conjunction with vitamins B-3, B-6, C and zinc achieve better results (Heinerman J. Heinerman's Encyclopedia; p. 134). Thirty women with severe PMS took 3 gms of primrose oil from the 15th cycle day to menses during 2 cycles, and placebo for 2 cycles. Symptoms, especially depression, were alleviated. Up to 6 capsules a day gave therapeutic benefits (ibid, p. 134). In two Canadian studies, both the main constituent in evening primrose oil (EPO), gamma-linolenic acid (GLA) and the plant oil (EPO) itself, significantly reduced blood pressure (Ibid, p. 134).

Supplementation of **evening primrose oil** (10% gamma linolenic acid) was tested on **dermatitis,** and **anti-inflammatory** substances were increased. The abnormal fatty acid pattern seen in dermatitis is believed to be involved in the pathogenesis of the disease, "and should therefore be the target for future **therapeutic approaches with fatty acid supplements**" (Lipids 1991;26:557-60). In another study of 12 volunteers, gamma linolenic acid-enriched oil not only **inhibited** the **inflammatory** substance LTB4, but the larger dose (1.5g) had a greater inhibition than the .5 g dose (AJCN 1992;55:39-45).

Borage oil:

Borage oil is a source for gamma linolenic acid, also, however it is controversial as to whether or not chemical structures in it are carcinogenic. A preferred source would be black currant seed oil.

EUCALYPTUS

Eucalyptus leaf oil contains a chemical, eucalyptol, that has **decongestant and antiseptic action;** researchers at the University of California at Irvine discovered that an ointment containing eucalyptus

increased blood flow to the muscle tissue and may be a **treatment for muscle soreness** (Wild, R., ed. The Complete Book of Natural and Medicinal Cures. 1994. Rodale Press, Emmaus, Pa. p. 293).

EVENING PRIMROSE OIL

(See Essential Fatty Acids)

EYEBRIGHT

Eyebright is an anti-inflammatory medicinal herb (Mayell p. 363). It contains vitamins A, B-3 (niacin), B-5 (pantothenic acid), B-12, C, D, and E; its properties lead to the recommendation that it is, "**good for all eye disorders**" (Balch, Presc for Nutr Healing, 1990, Avery Publ., NY, p. 52).

FENNEL SEED

Fennel has a reputation for **relieving gas and colic**, and therefore may be helpful for new parents! (Wild, R., ed. The Complete Book of Natural and Medicinal Cures. 1994. Rodale Press, Emmaus, Pa. p. 277). Fennel seed and dandelion are natural **herbal cleansers**, and good **sources of calcium, phosphorus, and potassium.**

FENUGREEK SEED

Fenugreek seeds contain mucilage, a gummy substance that coats and soothes irritated mucus membranes. Fenugreek has a reputation for: relieving constipation, reducing cholesterol soothing sore throat and cough, easing minor indigestion, relieving diarrhea, minimizing symptoms of menopause, and helping to control diabetes (Mowry, D. pp. 37-41, 110, 255, 260).

FEVERFEW

Feverfew contains a compound called parthenolide, which helps to **control the expansion and contraction of blood vessels in the brain.** Since migraine headaches are caused by abnormal contraction and expansion of brain blood vessels, feverfew is helpful, but only as a preventive over a long period of time (will not relieve a migraine in progress) (Wild, R., ed. The Complete Book of Natural and Medicinal Cures. 1994. Rodale Press, Emmaus, Pa. p. 295). Other less supported claims for feverfew are that it **relieves menstrual cramps and arthritic inflammation** (Wild, R., ed. The Complete Book of Natural and Medicinal Cures. 1994. Rodale Press, Emmaus, Pa. p. 295). Avoid taking feverfew if an allergy to any plant members of the daisy family exists, if a clotting disorder exists, or in pregnancy (Wild, R., ed. The Complete Book of Natural and Medicinal Cures. 1994. Rodale Press, Emmaus, Pa. p. 298).

FIBER

Fiber consists of polysaccharides such as **cellulose, hemicellulose, pectin, gums, waxes and lignins**. Fiber produces **butyric acid, a short chain fatty acid** which is manufactured by the intestines through bacterial fermentation of fiber. Butyric acid is the **main energy source for the intestinal epithelial cells** and helps **repair and regenerate damaged cells.** Many fibers can absorb 7-8 times their weight in water, which softens stools and decreases transit time. Fiber may **decrease size of hemorrhoids and prevent hemorrhoidal bleeding.** It also is said to "**lower cholesterol levels and slow the absorption of sugar in diabetics**, which may decrease the need for insulin in some people with diabetes." (Larson, D. Mayo Clinic Family Health Book, 1990. William Morrow & Co. Inc. NY, NY. p. 635).

Consumption of fiber **stimulates fermentation**, and, "fermentation is probably the key factor in the protective effect of fiber on colon carcinogenesis...**Butyrate,** one of the short chain fatty acids, could be significant, as it has **anti-neoplastic properties**..." (Scand J Gastroenterol Suppl 1993;200:80-6). These short chain fatty acids (butyric acid), produced during fermentation, **reduce colonic pH and inhibit secondary bile**

acids that are carcinogenic (Ibid p. 80). Additionally, the delayed passage rate induced by fiber results in **greater absorption of some of the amino acids** (J Nutr 1994;124(6):833-41). Braaten, JT, Wood PJ, and Scott FW et al. published a study on the effect of **oat fiber**, and found that, "**Oat gum lowers glucose and insulin after an oral glucose load**" (AJCN 1991; 53:1425-30).

FISH OIL

(See Essential Fatty Acids)

FO-TI

Fo-Ti is a Chinese herb, utilized for abscesses, fever, toxins, arthritis, atherosclerosis, cancer, hypertension, colic, constipation, enteritis, gout, pain and ulcerations, among other things (David B. Mowry, PhD. The Scientific Validation of Herbal Medicine. 1986. Keats Publishing, New Canaan, Conn. pp. 288-89).

FRUIT

Fruit contains essential plant enzymes which help us digest our food. One of the reasons for decreasd pancreatic enzyme activity is the result of decreased quantities of these enzymes in our food. They also contain vitamins and bioflavonoids (health-giving plant substances); citrus fruit is especially high in vitamin C. The dark colored fruits and vegetables have high concentrations of proanthocyanidins, which are powerful bioflavonoids.

Grapes have ellagic acid, which **blocks the production of particular enzymes needed for cancer cells**. They also possess phenols, antioxidants, and resveratrol. Kumquats **satisfy sweet and sour cravings** at the same time, having sweet rinds and tart pulps (Heinerman, John. Heinerman's Encyclopedia of Fruits, Vegetables and Herbs. p. 101), making them an excellent choice for **diabetics** or those interested in **weight control.** Kumquats seem to **lower blood pressure** (Heinerman, J Heinerman's Encyclopedia of Fruits, Vegetables and Herbs).

Chinese rhubarb juice and tea are used in mainland China to **treat cancer** (Heinerman, John. Heinerman's Encyclopedia of Fruits, Vegetables and Herbs. p. 298). Vol 20 of Pharmacology (1st supplement) noted that two of the **laxative** compounds in rhubarb, rhein and emodin **blocked** Erlich and mammary **tumors** in mice by 75% at the relatively high dose of 50 mg/kg/day. The 1984 issue of J. of Ethnopharm. also reported **decrease of malignant melanoma** at same dosage (Heinerman, J p. 298). The anthraquinones in rhubarb have **laxative** action, and **relieve itching** and **pain of psoriasis and arthritis**, and also **relieve constipation** (ibid, p. 299). 890 cases of upper GI bleeding) were treated with a 97% success rate. Rhubarb contains tannic acid, which **constricts blood vessels**. 100 cases of **pancreatitis** and 10 cases of **inflammation of the bladder** were **successfully treated** with full recovery noted in most (ibid, p. 300). **Total cholesterol, low density lipoprotein cholesterol, and triglycerides all decreased** from elevated levels in rabbits (ibid, p. 300).

The semi-dried leaves of the **mango** are used for **hypertension**. This **sedative** action to the leaves may be due, in part, to eremophilene, which also occurs in the herbal tranquilizer, valerian The seed contains gamma linolenic oil, which **reduces hypertension and arthritic inflammations** (Heinerman, John. Heinerman's Encyclopedia of Fruits, Vegetables and Herbs. p. 36). Persimmon juice is used to treat Candida (Heinerman J, p. 274)

GARLIC (Allium sativum)

Allicin is the molecule responsible for the odor of garlic, and also for many of the purported benefits it offers as an herb. Allicin, "has been known for very many years as an antimicrobial compound. Its inhibitory spectrum includes Candida species" (Odds, FC. Candida and Candidosis.1988. Bailliere Tindall, Philadelphia, Pa. p. 312). Several studies demonstrate the **power of garlic to combat Candida** (Prasad G & Sharma VD. Efficacy of garlic treatment against experimental candidiasis in chicks. Br. Vet. J. 1980; 136:448-51; Sandhu DK et al. Sensitivity of yeasts isolated from cases of vaginitis to aqueous extracts of garlic. Mykosen. 1980; 23:691-98; Tynecka et al. Inhibitory action of garlic on growth and respiration of some microorganisms. Acta Microbiol. Pol. (ser. B) 1973; 5:51-62).

F.C. Odds points out that, "Various plant metabolites have been purified and adopted widely as pharmaceuticals in medical practice and there is no reason why a compound such as allicin should not be studied and derivatives prepared for preclinical evaluation (for Candida)... However, the human intuitive psyche seems eternally destined to lag centuries behind the tangible achievements of human intellect (ibid, p. 312). "Neither Nystatin, nor amphotericin B... displayed such a high activity as garlic juice (against Candida)" (Crook, W. MD. The Yeast Connection. Professional Books, Tenn. pp. 355-356). With garlic having so many claims to fame, it's not surprising that in ancient times, the Egyptians would trade a healthy male slave for 15 pounds of garlic (Chalmers, I. The Great Food Almanac. 1994. Collins Publ., San Francisco, Ca. p. 184).

Garlic has a **significant antiarrhythmic effect on the heart**, suppressing premature ventricular contractions and tachycardia (fast heart rate) (J Ethnopharmacol 1994;43(1):1-8). Garlic's **antibacterial** characteristics have been tested even against drug-resistant varieties, and shown to have therapeutic activity (Indian J Med Res 1991;93:33-6). Garlic's properties include: **cancer inhibition** (Carcinogenesis 1994; 15(9):1881-5; J Cell Biochem Suppl 1993;17F:91-4; Pharm Res 1992;9(12):1668-70); **radiation protection** (Photochem Photobiol 1993;58(6):813-7), **sinusitis relief** (Vestn Otorinolaringol 1991;(2):62-3), and **cholesterol/triglyceride reduction** (Arzneim. 1993;43(9):978-81; J Postgrad Med 1991;37(3):132-5). Dietary intake of garlic is related to **reduced incidence of gastric cancer** (Prev Med 1993;22(5):712-22). A garlic derivative demonstrated **specific inhibition of esophageal cancer** (J Cell Biochem Suppl 1993; 17F:91-4).

The Journal of Clinical Gastroenterology recently reported the case of a patient with severe hepatopulmonary syndrome who failed conventional somatostatin therapy, and declined liver transplantation. This syndrome is believed to arise from **disordered gut peptide metabolism.** On her own, she took **large doses of powdered garlic, and experienced improvement** (J Clin Gastroenterol. 1992;15(3):248-50).

A garlic preparation **significantly lowered blood pressure** in nine patients with severe hypertension (Pharmacotherapy 1993; 13(4):406-7). The preparation contained 1.3% allicin at a dose of 2400 mg. Blood pressure fell an average of 7 mmHg systolic and 16 mmHg diastolic as soon as 5 hours after treatment, with no side effects. One of the amino acids of garlic has demonstrated **antidiabetic** effects, significantly decreasing serum lipids and glucose (Indian J Exp Biol 1992;30(6):523-6). A double-blinded controlled study in 1987 used 18 mg garlic oil to 20 healthy volunteers over a four week period. Cholesterol dropped 16% in the treated group, but not at all in the controls. HDL levels rose 23%, and **blood pressure dropped** from 94 to 88 mmHg. (Barrie S et al. Effects of garlic oil on platelets, serum lipids and blood pressure in humans; J Orthomolec Med 1987;2:15-21). It is thought that one of the mechanisms involved in lowering cholesterol is the ingredient nicotinic acid, which plays a major role in inhibiting HMG-CoA reductase activity (rate limiting enzyme in cholesterol synthesis) (Lipids 1993;28(7):613-19).

In one study using a combination garlic-ginkgo biloba product, the Christmas season was chosen to test the effectiveness of garlic's reputation for **lowering cholesterol**, since it is the period of the year with the most cholesterol-rich meals. 43 patients with elevated cholesterol levels were tested, with a significant difference after two months of treatment. It was followed by a two week wash-out period, in which no garlic-ginkgo was given, and, "During this period the total cholesterol value returned to 293.5 +/- 90 mg/dl, showing the **effectiveness of garlic treatment**" (Arnneimittelforschung 1993;43(9):978-81).

Garlic extracts have been found to be **safe and effective in treating parasites.** Thirty six children were administered two capsules, 2x day for three days, and their parasites were eliminated; garlic, "was found to be efficient, safe and **shortens the duration of treatment**" (J Egypt Soc Parasitol 1991; 21(2):497-502). The sulfides in garlic may also work in a way similar to that of penicillin and sulfa drugs, to **counter the growth of bacteria** . Garlic has even been shown to have, **"significant antidiabetic effects"** in diabetic rats. Administration of it, **"decreased significantly the concentration of serum lipids, blood glucose and activities of serum enzymes like alkaline phosphatase, acid phosphatase, lactate dehydrogenase and liver glucose-6-phosphatase.** It increased significantly liver and intestinal HMG CoA reductase activity and liver hexokinase activity" (the net overall effect on enzyme activity was to **decrease the enzymes which favor high blood glucose and cholesterol, and to increase the enzymes which favor the opposite**) (Indian J Exp Biol 1992;30(6):p. 523).

GENTIAN

Gentian stimulates the natural production of HCl, aids digestion, dispels liver heat and regulates the gallbladder. Gentian violet has antimicrobial activity (Int J Dermatol 1992;31(3):210-3), and scientists, "have recently demonstrated that gentian violet possesses a bactericidal effect" that was effective in 14 hospital patients when antibiotics had failed to eradicate the infection (Nippon Ronen Igakkai Zasshi 1993;30(9):795-801). In 92 cases of chronic obstructive parotitis (the parotid glands secrete saliva), gentian violet was used as an effective treatment to increase saliva flow (Chung Hua Kou Chiang Hsueh Tsa Chih 1992;27(4):200-2).

GINGER ROOT

In herbal literature, ginger has been touted as a **digestive stimulant** and has been used to **improve weak digestion** (Wild, R., ed. The Complete Book of Natural and Medicinal Cures. 1994. Rodale Press, Emmaus, Pa. p. 298). Ginger tea taken 30 minutes before meals has been known to be **helpful as a digestive aid**. Ginger has been used for **colitis, diverticulosis, gas, indigestion, vomiting, colon cleansing, morning sickness and nausea** (Mowry, D. Scientific Validation; pp. 48, 218, 197-200). Ginger is an excellent **carminative** (a substance that promotes elimination of intestinal gas) and as an **intestinal spasmolytic** (relaxes and soothes the intestinal tract). Ginger contains some of the **most powerful candida substances available** (Duke, JA. Handbook of Medicinal Herbs. 1985. CRC Press, Boca Raton, Fl.).

GINKGO BILOBA

Ginkgo Biloba is a potent free radical scavenger which is known to prevent alterations of vessels/capillaries (EXS 1992; 62:299-307). It is a, "specific and potent antagonist of PAF, a potent inflammatory autocoid (hormone)" (J Ethnopharmacol. 1991;32(1-3):135-9). The influence of ginkgo biloba on improving microcirculation (Fortschr Med 1990;108 (29):557-60; Arzneim. 1990 40(5):589-93) has important implications for delivery of nutrients to the liver/tissues via the blood.

Test results published in **Drugs Exp Clin Res** (1991, 17:571-4), "confirm that the **antioxidant properties** of **Ginkgo biloba** can **protect the retina against lipoperoxidation**". In a randomized, open clinical trial involving 42 patients with pathophysiological visco-elasticity values (the elasticity of their blood vessels had already been compromised), the effect of a single intravenous injection of 50, 100, 150, or 200 mg of **Ginkgo biloba** extract was investigated. A **significant increase in microcirculation and visco-elasticity** was noted. The response was dose dependent, with effects increasing as the dose increased. "**The present study thus confirms the positive effect of Ginkgo biloba extract on the microcirculation and whole-blood visco-elasticity values, already found in earlier studies, and shows it to be dependent on the dose employed**" (Fortschr Med. 1993, 111:170-2).

A German study was conducted on 24 patients with retinal insufficiency. Utilizing a randomized, double-blind study, **Ginkgo biloba** was used as a treatment, with a **significant increase in retinal sensitivity** seen within four weeks. Results in the lower dose group (80 mg/day) were not seen until the dose was increased to 160 mg/day. "**The results presented here show that damage to the visual field by chronic lack of blood flow are significantly reversible"** (Klin Monatsbl Augenheilkd. 1991, 199:432-8).

Free radicals are responsible for much of the damage induced by ischemia (lack of adequate blood flow) and reperfusion (dilation of blood vessels and return of oxygen). This leads to **damaging ion shifts in the eye,** which were **prevented** by administration of 100 mg/kg/day **Ginkgo biloba** for 10 days in a rat model. It is interesting to note that the drug allopurinol, which was also tested, failed to correct the retinal shifts. In diabetic retinopathy, the basal membrane of the retinal capillaries thicken, and the permeability of the retinal vessels is compromised. The authors in, "Oxidative stress in the diabetic retina" discuss the role of free radicals and the, "utilization of a **free radical scavenger**, such as **Ginkgo biloba**, in the **prevention of the retinal impairment in diabetes"** (EXS 1992, 62:299-307).

Since ginkgo can increase circulation and decrease clotting, it ahould be used with caution in combination with blood-thinning drugs such as Coumadin. High amounts should be avoided.

GINSENG

Ginseng is touted as being a, "regulator of basic body functions, a restorer of memory and sexual drive, and a general remedy for the ailments and incapacities of aging" (Chalmers, I. The Great Food Almanac. 1994. Collins Publishers, San Francisco, Ca. p. 185). There are several different varieties of ginsengs. There is Panax ginseng, American ginseng, and Siberian ginseng, among others. Siberian ginseng is in the same family of other ginsengs, but is not the same genus. The Siberian ginseng is tolerated better than the other "true" ginsengs as far as the upper limits causing side effects. It appears to be one of those herbs that seems to fascinate because of its association with the exotic East and all of its accompanying mystery. "North America exports well over 90% of all the ginseng it grows, while importing more than 90% of the ginseng it uses" (Chalmers, I. The Great Food Almanac. 1994. Collins Publishers, San Francisco, Ca. p. 186). Ginseng not only has powerful antioxidant properties, it has been found to be effective against ischemia and anoxia (absence of oxygen supply to the tissues) (Nippon Yakurigaku Zasshi 1991, 98:435-42), proving it to be of value in treating the reduced blood supply of macular degeneration . In September of last year, Chinese scientists reported calcium channel blockade action with ginseng (Chung Kuo Yao Li Hsueh Pao 1993, 13:403-6). Since calcium channels are responsible for the contraction of the smooth muscle surrounding blood vessels, this action could be beneficial for improving circulation in macular degeneration.

Tinctures of ginseng extracts had a tendency to **inhibit carcinogenesis** of the uterus cervix and vagina when administered orally, and when applied locally, "effectively inhibited carcinogenesis of uterus cervix and vagina" (Biull Eksp Biol Med 1993;116(11):534-36).

All the ginsengs should be used with caution in combination with drugs associated with the treatment of conditions related to symptoms of excess ginseng supplementation, i.e. blood pressure drugs, heart medication, and particularly digitalis-like drugs. A physician should be consulted about combinations. Possible antiplatelet activity means that Coumadin and other blood-thinning drugs should be used with caution when combined with herbs possessing this activity.

GLANDULARS

Glandulars are thought to **provide precursor substances that the body can use to support and enhance the function of a specific gland.** They may provide the potential "life force" the body needs to enhance function of a specific organ or gland. Glandulars are tissue concentrates, usually of a bovine source, which stimulate the glands of the immune system, such as thymus, spleen, and adrenal. Glandular therapy began in the late 19th century when doctors suggested to their patients that eating the glandular parts from a cow that corresponds to the weaknesses in their own bodies may help them to heal. The Egyptians and Greeks used glandular therapy many years ago because they believed in the concept that "like heals like" (Haas, E. MD. Staying Healthy with Nutrition. 1992; Celestial Arts, Berkeley, Ca. p. 283).

In the late 1800's, desiccated thyroid glandular was used for patients with hypothyroidism or goiter. Once thyroxine (T4) was isolated, it replaced the use of the thyroid glandular. Many doctors felt that the whole glandular was superior, due to better utilization and absorption. The same phenomenon occurred when insulin was isolated in the early 1920's. Insulin replaced the use of the whole pancreas gland and became therapy for treating diabetes.

Glandular therapy has been a source of conflict in the allopathic community. Currently, there is not much research being done in this field. One example of work done in this field was by Dr. Bates at Minnesota Metropolitan Medical Center, in which he showed that beef derived thymus gland, when fed orally to animals, was capable of **enhancing the T-lymphocyte function.** In another study, **thymus extract was shown to normalize altered T-cell ratios in EBV patients. Spleen extracts have been shown to increase WBC counts in extreme leucopenia and helped patients with typhoid fever or malaria.** (Murray M. Enc. Nat. Med p. 217). Dr. A. Kemet investigated whether or not oral glandulars were organ specific. Using radioactive isotope tracings, he found that **glandular tissues were absorbed in the blood and deposited in the corresponding organs.** He documented his findings in German medical publications of 1958 and 1972 (Balch, Presc. for Nut. Heal., p. 326). More research needs to be actively pursued in order to better understand glandular therapy.

The best source of glandular supplements are organic, freeze-dried, defatted, fresh glands because any use of heat or chemicals will destroy enzyme activity. Fat needs to be removed because fat usually contains the most toxic substances and can be oxidized and go rancid. Many different glandulars have been used in clinical practice. Although glandular therapy has been used widely in Europe since the turn of the century, further investigation needs to be done in order for it to be accepted in the United States.

One study of **Candida treatment** was conducted in mice, and was largely successful when an antifungal agent was used in combination with, "a **thymus-derived immunostimulant**". The immunostimulant from the thymus, "**promoted a recovery of normal natural killer cell activity and intracellular killing of Candida albicans**", and the researchers believed it was responsible for a **direct activation of the immunocompetence system** (Clin Exp Immunol 1994;97(3): p. 347).

Thymalin, which is another extraction from bovine thymus was **used in therapy of 44 children with relapsing stomatitis,** and it was found that the extract, "helps attain a **stable anti-relapse effect** in children at a high risk of developing stomatitis recurrences (Stomatologiia-Mosk 1994;73(1):40-4).

GLUCOSAMINE SULFATE

Glucosamine sulfate (GS) is a fairly simple structure of glucose, an amine, and sulphur. It is a **precursor substance for connective tissue, comprising part of the "cellular cement"**. It is found in high amounts in the joints, and a placebo-controlled, double-blind investigation reported that it **affords some protection against destruction of the joints,** such as in osteoarthritis (Drovanti, A. et al. Clin Ther. 1980; 3(4):260).

Cartilage that was synthesized without GS contained few, if any, normal-sized chondroitin sulphate chains and only about half of the normal serine residues. Subsequent addition of glucosamine resulted in a time-dependent recovery of sulphate incorporation after 2 hr., however the chondroitin sulphate chains were restored to normal size within 15 minutes. GS is, "required for optimal glycoconjugate synthesis" (Biochem J. 1991;273(Pt 2):283-8).

The production of the proteoglycans, which are needed to repair and build joint lining and synovial fluid, is inhibited by non-steroidal anti-inflammatory drugs (NSAIDS). Glucosamine sulfate works differently than NSAIDS; NSAIDS inhibit proteoglycan synthesis (cartilage is made from proteoglycans), whereas glucosamine prevents proteoglycan degradation, thus enhancing cartilage production.

Glucosamine sulfate was listed as one of only two substances which are "chondroprotective agents (CPA's)", out of all the agents used to treat osteoarthritis. This is because the NSAIDS and corticosteroids relieve the pain and inflammation, but inhibit prostaglandin synthesis. CPA's are used, "to stop the evolution of the disease" (Int J Tissue Reac. 1992;14(5):253-61). "In particular, GS, which naturally occurs in the human body and is almost devoid of toxicity, is suitable for long-term therapeutic use. This, with its chondrometabolic, antireactive and antiarthritic properties, represents the pharmacological rationale for the use of GS as a disease-modifying agent in osteoarthritis" (ibid, p. 253).

Glucosamine sulfate was tested on rats with several arthritis models, and compared to indomethacin. "On these models GS was found effective in oral daily doses of 50-800 mg/kg. ... Since, however, the toxicity of indomethacin in chronic toxicity experiments is 1000-4000 times larger, the therapeutic margin with regard to prolonged treatments of inflammatory disorders results (in a) 10-30 times more favourable (choice) for GS than for indomethacin. GS can therefore be considered as a drug of choice for prolonged oral treatment of rheumatic disorders" (Arzneimittelforschung. 1991 May; 41(5):542-5).

Glucosamine sulfate was tested in a multicentre, randomized, placebo-controlled, double-blind, parallel group study. It was found to be highly efficacious in 155 out-patients with knee osteoarthritis (Arzneimittelforschung. 1994 Jan; 44(1):75-80). Even though glucosamine is converted to **N-acetyl glucosamine** (NAG), the production of NAG can be blocked by antagonists such as alcohol and NSAIDS, and therefore is helpful when administered along with glucosamine sulfate. **NAG** may be considered a synergistic element, because in addition to **reducing joint pain, swelling, and restricted motion,** it plays a major role in the **secretion of the protective mucus from the intestinal mucosal cells** (it is a mucin precursor). In some cases, glucosamine sulfate may cause GI disturbances, in which case added DGL may be of some help.

GLUTAMINE

Some known properties and functions of glutamine include:

- precursor for nucleotide biosynthesis
- enhance gut immune function
- improve cell function
- increase jejunal mucosal weight and DNA content
- reduce villous atrophy and mucosal injury
- stimulate intestinal mucosal growth
- improve nitrogen balance
- reduce infection rate
- inhibit bacterial invasion from the gut
- prevent extracellular fluid expansion occuring after catabolic stress
- reduce hospital stays
- reduce severity of methotrexate-induced enterocolitis
- reduce endotoxin transmigration from the gut lumen
- increase synthesis of mucoproteins
- increase tissue healing
- acid-base regulator
- important precursor of nucleic acids
- important precursor of glutathione, a potent antioxidant and detoxifier
- increase natural killer cell activity (currently being tested in AIDS patients)
- increase normal tissue but not tumor tissue (delivers chemotherapy to breast cancer cells in animal studies)
- decrease catabolic stress and protein loss
- enhance healing of ulcers
- no toxicity shown

(Judy Schubert, MD RD & Nancy Erlich. The Ultimate Nutrient Glutamine. 1994. Avery Publ Garden City NY; Souba W. Intestinal Glutamine Metabolism and Nutrition. J Nutr Biochem1993;4:2-9; Journal of Parenteral and Enteral Nutrition. 1992; 16(6): 835-375; Ann Surg 1991; 214(4): 385-93).

L-glutamine aids in tissue healing, maintains a healthy digestive tract, and effectively treats small intestine absorption problems. It is an integral amino acid needed for the synthesis of the mucoproteins present in the intestinal mucus secretions (Texas J Med 1957; 53:840-3); the addition of glutamine can prevent small intestinal mucus atrophy (Chung Hua Wai Ko Tsa Chih 1993;31(2):94-6). Oral glutamine administration improves mucosal structure and healing (Arch Surg 1990;125(8):1040-45). Glutamine is the principle fuel used by the upper gastrointestinal tract, and provides respiratory fuel for rapidly proliferating cells (such as enterocytes and lymphocytes), regulates acid-base balance, and is an important precursor of nucleic acids. Nutrition Reviews argued in 1990 that, "Abundant evidence suggests that glutamine may become a conditionally essential amino acid" (it has since achieved this status) due to its physiological role in tissues, and that, "During stress the body's requirements for glutamine appear to exceed the individual's ability to produce sufficient amounts of this amino acid. Provision of supplemental glutamine... may enhance nutritional management..." (Nutr Rev 1990;48(8):297-309). "In this model of catabolic stress, fluid retention and expansion of the extracellular fluid compartment commonly observed after standard total parenteral nutrition, can be attenuated by administering glutamine-supplemented intravenous feedings, possibly by protecting the host from microbial invasion and associated infection" (Ann Surg 1991;214(4):385-93). Glutamine metabolism by the ileum and colon is impaired in Crohn's disease, and supplementation is indicated (Sido B et al. Langenbecks Arch Chir Suppl Kongressbd 1997;114:653-656).

Ulcers

Japanese scientists discovered glutamine as an antiulcer agent, and it is currently the most popular remedy for ulcers in Asia. Glutamine is able to prevent ulcers in rats given aspirin, because it protects the lining from mucosal damage (Okabe, S, Takeuchi K, Honda K, Takagi K. Effects of Acetylsalicyclic acid (ASA) plus L-glutamine and L-glutamine on healing of chronic gastric ulcer in the rat. Digestion 1976;14:85-88).

Food Allergies

Many foods cause immune reactions because macromolecules, or large, undigested food proteins, pass through leaks in the intestinal lining. Glutamine's ability to protect the barrier function of the gut can reduce the incidence of immune activation. This is especially important in some of the autoimmune diseases where food is suspected of being a possible trigger, i.e. rheumatoid arthritis, multiple sclerosis, dermatitis herpetiformis, etc.

Urea Cycle

Glutamine is necessary for the urea cycle, which plays an important part in elimination of toxins. Glutamine is essential for the transfer of amino groups during this process, and is also essential for amino group transfer from the tissues to the liver.

Immune System

"Arginine, glutamine, the long chain polyunsaturated omega-3 and omega-6 fatty acids, and, to a lesser extent, ribonucleic acid and the vitamins E, C, and A have pharmacological effects when given in amounts in excess of what is needed to prevent nutritional deficiency. These effects are exerted primarily via the immune system, and immunoenhancing diets that embody the recently developed principles of nutritional pharmacology have been shown to reduce infectious complications by approximately 75% in surgical patients and hospital stay by more than 20% in surgical patients and patients in the intensive care unit in three independent, prospective, randomized studies, two of which were double-blinded. These findings suggest that specialized diets can be designed that will be of benefit to patients with cancer, atherosclerosis, intestinal diseases, autoimmune diseases, infections, and trauma" (Arch Surg 1993;128(11):1242-5). "Human studies that have investigated the use of glutamine-supplemented nutrition in the host with cancer suggest that pharmacologic doses of dietary glutamine may be beneficial" (Ann Surg 1993;218(6):715-28). Glutamine also enhances chemotherapy treatment while reducing toxicity (J Parenteral and Enteral Nutrition 1992;16:835-875).

pH Balance

An oral glutamine load was given to nine subjects (2 grams dissolved in a cola drink), and 90 minutes later, plasma bicarbonate concentration and circulating growth hormone had significantly increased. "These findings demonstrate that a surprisingly small oral glutamine load is capable of elevating alkaline reserves as well as plasma growth hormone" (AJCN 1995;61:p. 1058). The increase in growth hormone is believed to be responsible for shifting fuel utilization from glucose to fatty acids in muscle (increased fat oxidation), and also for accelerating renal acid secretion. The increased fat oxidation may play an important role in weight regulation/body composition, and increased acid secretion may play, "a potentially important role during strenuous exercise when acidogenesis may limit performance" (AJCN 1995;61:p. 1061).

Contraindications/Toxicology

Glutamine is an amino acid which has been tested in AIDS patients in amounts up to 40 grams. This is a high amount, however, and is not recommended for daily ingestion. Judy Schubert, MD, takes 8 gm/day for maintenance (Judy Schubert, MD RD & Nancy Erlich. The Ultimate Nutrient Glutamine. 1994. Avery Publ Garden City NY). It should be noted that glutamine is an amino acid, and may compete with other amino acids for absorption, such as tryptophan. This is one of the reasons a stimulatory effect has been noted from larger amounts, and should probably not be taken right before bedtime. Medicinal amounts of any vitamin, mineral or specialty nutrient should only be taken with the advice of a trained licensed healthcare professional.

GLYCINE

Glycine is an amino acid which can be formed from choline in the liver or kidney. It may be helpful in **reducing gastric acidity** and is known as a **stomach soother.** Glycine is one of the three building blocks that form glutamine, which is an essential nutrient for the intestinal tract.

GOLDENSEAL (Hydrastis canadensis)

Goldenseal is a powerful herb, acting as a **detoxifier and antibiotic.** One of the most popular herbs, golden seal is known in traditional Chinese medicine as a **balancer and stimulator of internal organs**. Golden seal **reduces Candida infections, and helps hypoglycemia** (Heinerman, John. . p. 158,162).

Goldenseal contains berberine, which is **antibacterial, antipyretic antimalarial, and is used as bitters for the stomach** (Merck Index, 11th ed. Merck & Co. Inc., Rahway, N.J. 1989). The berberine accounts for the yellow color of the root, and is excellent for **treating inflammation of the cornea and iris** (Indian Journal of Opthamology March 1983, as cited in Heinerman, p. 158). Berberine **destroys microorganisms,** and has been "shown to be **effective in the treatment of E. Coli, Shigella dysenteriae, Salmonella paratyphi B, Klebsiella, Giardia lamblia and Vibrio Cholerae**." (Murray M. Enc. Nat. Med; p. 289) Berberine also **inhibits infectious organisms** and toxic formation by the organisms.

Another compound in goldenseal, **hydrastine**, has long been used as an ingredient in commercial eyewashes to **constrict tiny blood vessels and eliminate redness from tired eyes** (hydrastine can cause a rise in blood pressure when taken internally (Wild, R., ed. The Complete Book of Natural and Medicinal Cures. 1994. Rodale Press, Emmaus, Pa. p. 305).

GOTU KOLA

The varied uses of Gotu Kola range from anti-inflammatory, antibacterial, sedative, wound healing, circulation improving, and, "is also used in Ayurvedic medicine as a cure for agitation, memory loss, anxiety, insomnia, epilepsy and hyperactivity" (Wild, R., ed. The Complete Book of Natural and Medicinal Cures. 1994. Rodale Press, Emmaus, Pa. p. 306). Gotu kola should not be confused with the Kola nut, which contains more caffeine than coffee.

GUAR GUM

Guar gum is a type of **fiber** which seems to have a favorable effect on **decreasing appetite** by providing a feeling of fullness (Heinerman J. Heinerman's Encyclopedia of Fruits, Vegetables and Herbs , p. 161). It is also known to **lower cholesterol** (Indian J Nutr Diet 1980;17:297).

GYMNEMA SYLVESTRE

Gymnema sylvestre was administered to 22 type 2 diabetics (400 mg/day), for 18-20 months, and **significantly reduced blood glucose, glycosylated hemoglobin, and glycosylated proteins. This glycosylation process involves the combination of a sugar molecule with a protein (for instance, hemoglobin and glucose). When this happens, these products can disrupt blood vessels and other tissues, and can be responsible for a lot of the damage seen with high sugar levels in diabetics.** "These data suggest that the **beta cells** (produce insulin in the pancreas) may be **regenerated/repaired** in type 2 diabetic patients **on supplementation**" (J Ethnopharmacol. 1990, 30:281-94).

HAWTHORN BERRIES

Hawthorn berries have **positive actions on the cardiovascular system,** possibly through the action of flavonoids. In addition to having a tonic long term effect on the heart, hawthorn **dilates arteries, thereby reducing pressure** (Wild, R., ed. The Complete Book of Natural and Medicinal Cures. 1994. Rodale Press, Emmaus, Pa. p. 309). A phytopharmaceutical encyclopedia lists some of the areas in which hawthorn berries are utilized: cardiotonics, coronary remedies, antihypertonics, arteriosclerosis remedies, geriatric remedies, and general tonics (Grainger, NB ed., Herbal Drugs and Phytopharmaceuticals. Medpharm Scientific Publishers. CRC Press. Boca Raton, Fla. 1994).

Hawthorn berries have a favorable effect on blood pressure (Forsch Med 1993;111:352-354; Planta Medica 1981;43:313-322). This is probably due to the flavonoids having a stabilizing effect on collagen structures, such as the blood vessels and small capillaries, and by affecting vasodilation. The ability to inhibit angiotension converting enzyme (ACE) (Jpn J Pharmacol 1987;43:242-245), and to demonstrate mild diuretic activity also help reduce hypertension. The dilation of the vessels results in reduced peripheral resistance and increased coronary circulation (Hamon NW. Canad Pharm J 1988; Nov:708-724). Angiotension converting enzyme converts a relatively inactive form of angiotensin (angiotensin I) into an active, very powerful vasoconstrictor, angiotensin II. The ability of the proanthocyanidins to inhibit the converting enzyme results in relaxed blood vessels, and its action has rivaled that of the drug, Captopril (Jpn J Pharmacol 1987;43:242-245), a synthetic enzyme inhibitor used widely for hypertension.

Hawthorn berries have been traditionally used in the area of congestive heart failure, because of their ability to increase the contraction of the heart. They do this by inhibiting the enzyme cyclic AMP phosphodiesterase (Planta Medica 1981;43:183-186). Since the enzyme breaks down the energy-boosting signaller, cyclic AMP, inhibition of the enzyme results in more forceful contractions. Hawthorn berries are commonly used in conjunction with other drugs for heart failure, such as digitalis, or in combination with other herbs containing cardiac glycosides (i.e. Cereus grandifloris), as it potentiates the action of the glycosides. Since hawthorn does enhance the action of the cardiac glycosides, it allows for lower doses of adjunctive therapy to be used. A physician should be consulted when combinations are considered. Magnesium also has an enhancing action on digitalis, and can be considered a good synergistic nutrient. Double-blind studies have consistently shown that hawthorn is effective for congestive heart failure in the early stages (and also minor arrhythmias) where digitalis is not yet indicated (no adverse reactions occurred in the studies) (Forsch Med 1992;110:290-292; Forsch Med 1986;104:805-808; Forsch Med 1993;111:352-354). For moderate to severe heart failure, a health care professional can recommend a combination with other cardiac glycosides.

Persistance in supplementation is recommended, as it can take up to 2 weeks to reach a satisfactory tissue saturation level. Extended use of hawthorn berries has had a beneficial effect on cholesterol, triglycerides, and blood sugar levels in Chinese animal studies (Chung His I Choeh Ho Tsa Chih 1990;10:361).

HESPERIDIN

(See Bioflavonoids)

HONEY

Honey contains predominantly fructose and glucose, along with maltose and sucrose. Honey has a long **history as a therapeutic aid**. In a survey of most commonly used herbal remedies, honey was one of the most frequently reported (Res Nurs Health 1991. 14(5): 339-50). Honey is believed to act in a variety of ways, from **relieving sore throat to diminishing wrinkles** (Heinerman J Heinerman's Encyclopedia of Fruits, Vegetables and Herbs p. 184). Long used as a home **remedy for dyspepsia,** honey was tested by the scientific community for **antibacterial action** against helicobacter pylori, the suspected culprit in causing ulcers. Sure enough, the scientific tests bore out the reputation honey has had through the years - the helicobacter pylori growth was **completely prevented by the honey** (J R Soc Med 1994;87(1):9-12).

Honey contains flavonoids with antioxidant properties. Generally, the darker honeys have stronger antioxidant capabilities, however the light, sweet clover honey is very rich in antioxidant activity (Science News 154;170-172).

HORSETAIL (Shavegrass)

Horsetail, "is highly absorbable and is **utilized to promote bone growth and collagen formation.**..horsetail's silica content makes it useful in sitz baths, which aid in treating peripheral vascular disorders, post-thrombotic swelling, as well as treating ligaments and tendons after ankle sprains and fractures" (Weiner, M.A. Herbs that heal. 1994. Quantum Books, Mill Valley, Ca. p. 197). Its actions include those of

anti-inflammatory, diuretic, astringent, tissue healer, and as an agent to stop bleeding (Ody, Complete Medicinal Herbal).

Long-term use could be detrimental to the proper functioning of the kidneys. Larges doses of horsetail may be toxic. Large doses can cause muscle weakness, fever and abnormal pulse rate in animals, however human toxicity has not been defined. External use can cause contact dermatitis in a few sensitive individuals. Medicinal amounts of any herb should only be taken with the advice of a trained licensed healthcare professional.

HYDROCHLORIC ACID (HCL)

HCl is commonly used as a **digestive aid** alone or in combination with enzymes to support normal digestive function. Many people are deficient in HCL, and the ability to produce it decreases with age. HCl is **necessary for protein digestion.** It plays a fundamental role in **activating inactive precursor proenzymes** (such as chymotrypsinogen and trypsinogen) to their active forms (chymotrypsin and trypsin). A warm feeling in the gut when taking HCl supplements indicates that an excess has been taken, and the dosage needs to be reduced. HCl should not be given in cases of excess HCl production because it could increase irritation and create additional problems. However, many cases of gastric distress are caused by low acidity rather than excess. When HCL is lacking, the body doesn't receive the proper signals to propel the food onward, and the food ferments in the stomach, eventually causing acid to reflux into the esophagus. A vast majority of patients with gastric reflux have been helped with HCL supplementation. While hyperacidity is a general term associated with stomach distress, a more common cause of indigestion is a lack of gastric acid secretion. Hydrochloric acid is necessary for **complete digestion of nutrients, and incomplete secretion can cause nutrient deficiencies.** The acid environment of the stomach is also necessary to **prevent bacterial growth.** This is why, "Gastric **hypoacidity is associated with quantitative bacterial overgrowth and opportunistic enteric infections**" (J Infect Dis 1992 166(2):277-84). Green et al. explore the **close association between gastritis in the elderly, hypochlorhydria and gastric cancer,** and point out that, "An age-related increase in the frequency of helicobacter pylori infection in the elderly parallels the known age-related increase in the prevalence of **gastritis** (Gastroenterol Clin North Am 1990;19(2):273-92). Betaine is the carboxylic acid derived by oxidation of choline; "the hydrochloride salt is used as a **gastric acidifier**" (betaine HCL) (Dorland's Pocket Medical Dictionary, 24th ed. WB Saunders Co., Phil, Pa. 1989). (see also the self-acid test in the gastrointestinal section of this book).

INOSITOL

Inositol enhances the vitamin B complex and has lipotropic characteristics (hastens fat removal/decreases deposits in the liver); inositol niacinate is a vasodilator (Merck Index, 11th ed. Merck & Co. Inc., Rahway, N.J. 1989). It is involved in the **synthesis of phospholipids**, which are essential to the **digestion and absorption of fats.** The body can produce its own inositol from glucose, so it is really not essential. Inositol has been shown to **reduce selectins** (adhesion molecules which aggravate the inflammatory response) in vitro (cell culture), which may be why it **reduces inflammation** in vivo (in the body) (J Biol Chem 1994;269(21):15060-6). Some antiulcer medications work by increasing the turnover of mucosal phosphoinositides. Phosphotidylinositol is a mucous membrane phospholipid, which is broken down to inositol derivatives that can act as **messenger molecules. The gastric mucosal protective action** of one of these derivatives, "appears to involve the metabolism of phosphoinositide-derived messenger molecules" (Int J Biochem 1990;22(10):1179-83).

"Inositol supplementation has shown some success in the treatment of experimental animal **diabetic neuropathy** since it helps **reestablish myoinositol levels in the deficient nerve cell.** The myoinositol deficiency in nerves is believed to be due to the accumulation of sorbitol within the cell, which results in the loss of intracellular myoinositol" (Murray M and Pizzorno J Encyclopedia of Natural Medicine Prima Publ, Rocklin, Ca. 1991, p. 284).

IRISH MOSS

Irish moss is rich in **mineral content**, and has been used as a **nutritive tonic** to soothe irritated membranes. As a **natural antacid**, it is used to protect the stomach, damaged tissue, and the urinary tract.

JUNIPER BERRIES

Juniper berries, "are a **powerful diuretic** that helps the body flush away excess water...Egyptian doctors used it as a **laxative** as early as 1550 B.C." (Wild, R., ed. The Complete Book of Natural and Medicinal Cures. 1994. Rodale Press, Emmaus, Pa. p. 313).

KELP

Kelp is a sea algae with capabilities to bind heavy metals. Kelp helps to control obesity (Heinerman, John. Heinerman's Encyclopedia of Fruits, Vegetables and Herbs. p. 199), possibly through its influence on the thyroid gland. It contains iodine, which **stimulates thyroid hormones that regulate basal metabolic rate.**

L-GLUTAMINE

(See also Glutamine)

L-glutamine aids in tissue healing, maintains a healthy digestive tract, and effectively treats small intestine absorption problems. It is an integral amino acid needed for the synthesis of the mucoproteins present in the intestinal mucus secretions (Texas J Med 1957; 53:840-3); the addition of glutamine can prevent small intestinal mucus atrophy (Chung Hua Wai Ko Tsa Chih 1993;31(2):94-6). Oral glutamine administration improves mucosal structure and healing (Arch Surg 1990;125(8):1040-45). Glutamine is the principle fuel used by the upper GI tract, and provides respiratory fuel for rapidly proliferating cells (such as enterocytes and lymphocytes), regulates acid-base balance, and is an important precursor of nucleic acids. Nutrition Reviews argued in 1990 that, "Abundant evidence suggests that glutamine may become a conditionally essential amino acid" due to its physiological role in tissues, and that, "During stress the body's requirements for glutamine appear to exceed the individual's ability to produce sufficient amounts of this amino acid. Provision of supplemental glutamine... may enhance nutritional management..." (Nutr Rev 1990;48(8):297-309). "In this model of catabolic stress, fluid retention and expansion of the extracellular fluid compartment commonly observed after standard total parenteral nutrition, can be attenuated by administering glutamine-supplemented intravenous feedings, possibly by protecting the host from microbial invasion and associated infection" (Ann Surg 1991;214(4):385-93).

"Arginine**, glutamine,** the long chain polyunsaturated omega-3 and omega-6 fatty acids, and, to a lesser extent, ribonucleic acid and the vitamins E, C, and A have **pharmacological effects** when given in amounts in excess of what is needed to prevent nutritional deficiency. These **effects are exerted primarily via the immune system, and immunoenhancing diets that embody the recently developed principles of nutritional pharmacology have been shown to reduce infectious complications** by approximately 75% in surgical patients and hospital stay by more than 20% in surgical patients and patients in the intensive care unit in three independent, prospective, randomized studies, two of which were double-blinded. These findings suggest that specialized diets can be designed that will be of benefit to patients with **cancer, atherosclerosis, intestinal diseases, autoimmune diseases, infections, and trauma"** (Arch Surg 1993;128(11):1242-5). "Human studies that have investigated the use of **glutamine**-supplemented nutrition in the host with **cancer** suggest that pharmacologic doses of dietary glutamine may be beneficial" (Ann Surg 1993;218(6):715-28).

An oral glutamine load was given to nine subjects (2 grams dissolved in a cola drink), and 90 minutes later, **plasma bicarbonate concentration and circulating growth hormone had significantly increased.** "These findings demonstrate that a **surprisingly small oral glutamine load** is capable of **elevating alkaline reserves** as well as plasma **growth hormone**" (AJCN 1995;61:p. 1058). The increase in growth hormone is believed to be responsible for shifting fuel utilization from glucose to fatty acids in muscle (increased fat oxidation), and also for accelerating renal acid secretion. The increased fat oxidation may play an important role in **weight regulation/body composition,** and increased acid secretion may play, "a potentially important **role during strenuous exercise when acidogenesis may limit performance**" (AJCN 1995;61:p. 1061).

Other derivatives of glutamine: When 38 cases of senile dementia were successfully treated with acupuncture and **acupoint injection of aceglutamide (N-acetyl glutamine, a glutamine derivative**), high-density lipoprotein also significantly increased (Lancet 1993;342(8869):451-2; Acupunct Electrother Res 1992;17(2): 61-73). N_2 acetyl-L-glutamine is listed as a **bronchodilator** in the Merck Index (Merck Index, p. 23).

LACTOBACILLUS

There are many types of "friendly bacteria" that can be found in the intestinal tract. These friendly bacteria are sometimes called, "probiotics". The probiotics counteract bad bacteria and keep them in check. Several important ones include lactobacillus acidophilus, lactobacillus bifidus and lactobacillus bulgaricus. Lactobacillus provides **protection for the intestinal wall by enhancing antigen-specific immune defense. Lactobacillus varieties keep bad bacteria in check, reduce toxic load on the liver, and improve bowel motility. They also enhance digestion, especially of fiber by-products.**

LACTOBACILLUS ACIDOPHILUS

Lactobacillus acidophilus destroys disease causing bacteria including salmonella, listeria and other bacteria that causes food poisoning. Acidophilus supplementation reimplants healthy bacteria into the intestinal tract. As an ingredient in yogurt, it was tested for efficiency in digesting lactose. Because of its **microbial activity and ability to break beta-galactose bonds,** L. acidophilus **"dramatically improved digestion"** (Am J Clin Nutr 1990;54(6):1041-6). "L. acidophilus has been found to inhibit Candida albicans..." (Microbios 1990;62(250):37-46). Another research team, (Hilton, E. Isenberg, H.D. Alperstein, P et al.) reported on, "Ingestion of yogurt containing Lactobacillus acidophilus as **prophylaxis for Candidal vaginitis**", (Annals of Internal Medicine, March 1, 1992; 116(5):353-357. In a crossover trial involving 33 patients, "a **threefold decrease in infections was seen when patients consumed yogurt containing L. acidophilus.** Candidal colonization significantly decreased. "Daily ingestion of 8 oz of yogurt containing L. acidophilus **decreased both candidal colonization and infection**" (Ann Intern Med 1992;116(5):353-7).

LACTOBACILLUS BIFIDUS

"A number of pioneer bacteria, which are the first to arrive in the gut, are capable of effectively blocking growth of other bacteria introduced later in the ecosystem. In some instances, these pioneer bacteria also **inhibit production of toxins by pathogenic species**... These factors include **"bifidus factors**", which promote the growth of bifidobacterium, lactoferrin and immunoglobulins, which **prevent colonization of the gut by pathogenic enterobacteria**" (Ann Pediatr Paris 1993;40(1):13-22).

LACTOBACILLUS BULGARICUS

Lactobacillus (L) bulgaricus, as an ingredient in yogurt, was fed, along with selected products, to healthy people not able to tolerate lactose. L. bulgaricus **provided for the most complete digestion of lactose,** due to enzymes which are capable of breaking bonds in the food (Am J Clin Nutr 1990;54(6):1041-6).

LECITHIN

Lecithin is a phospholipid that is important in the **structure of all membranes.** Lecithin is an oil that is found in high concentrations in soybeans and egg yolks. Choline is combined with fatty acids, glycerol and phosphate to make lecithin. Lecithin helps in **fat emulsification** and in the **integrity of the cell membrane and nerve function.** Lecithin is high in choline and inositol.

Lecithin acts as a **surfactant to coat and protect, an emulsifier to digest fats and a lipotropic agent to metabolize fat** (Merck Index, 11th ed. Merck & Co. Inc., Rahway, N.J. 1989). Some grades of lecithin are reported to contain a potent **vasodepressor substance** (Mcquarrie & Anderson, US patent # 2,931,818 1960 to Cutter labs). Increasing doses of lecithin to human bile progressively prolonged the nucleation time and **lowered cholesterol** (Gut 1993;34(1):110-5).

LICORICE ROOT

In China, licorice is called, "the great detoxifier", and is thought to drive poisons from the body (Ody, Complete Medicinal Herbal). It has also been called, "the grandfather of herbs" because of its reputation for a wide variety of effects, including anti-inflammatory, anti-arthritic, stimulant of the adrenal cortex, blood cholesterol reducer, gastric membrane soother, and possibly anti-allergenic and expectorant (Ody P, Complete Medicinal Herbal).

Licorice is valued as a base ingredient in herbal remedies, because of its ability to help focus the purpose and direction of other herbs, as well as attenuate the harsh properties of other herbs (Landis R. Herbal Defense. 1997. Warner Books. NY, NY). Adrenal insufficiency is treated well with licorice because of the constituents that resemble the adrenal corticoid hormones, it enhances immune activity, is good for digestion, is a lung tonic and energizer, reduces spasms, decreases inflammation, and has a laxative effect (ibid).

Licorice has a strong antiviral effect; some components, including glycyrrhetinic acid (and derivatives) have been shown to both reduce healing time and pain correlated to genital herpes (Br J Ven Dis 1984;60:178-181), and glycyrrhizin has been shown to inactivate the herpes simplex virus type I, while stimulating immune parameters such as the signaller interferon (Experientia 1980;36:304-305). Recent animal studies even suggest that licorice is helpful for systemic lupus erythmatosus, but further confirmation is needed (J Ethnopharm 1996;53:1-4). The novel research that was conducted showed that licorice has a favorable effect on clearing immune complexes out of the body, a mechanism important in many diseases, especially in lupus, which is characterized by the production of immune complexes.

According to the Handbook of Medicinal Herbs, licorice root is reported to be demulcent, expectorant, estrogenic, laxative, a febrifuge (reduces fevers), and used for Addison's disease, internal inflammation, indigestion, thirst, colds, sore throats (singers chew the root to strengthen the throat), appendicitis, asthma, bladder ailments, bronchitis, cough, diabetes, diuretic, ulcer, and tuberculosis (Duke JA. Handbook of Medicinal Herbs. CRC Press. Boca Raton, Fla.1985). The estrogenic effect of licorice is due to phytoestrogens (See: Phytoestrogens). Licorice is contraindicated in large amounts with hypertensive patients; it contains glycyrrhizin, which can mimic the adrenal steroid aldosterone. The glycyrrhizin content should not exceed 400 mg/day. (See also deglycyrrhizinated licorice (DGL), which has had the glycyrrhizin removed).

MARSHMALLOW

The word "marshmallow" comes from the Greek "altho", meaning "to heal" - the root is extremely **mucilaginous and softening for the tissues** (Ody P, The Complete Medicinal Herbal). It has been used as an **expectorant, diuretic, demulcent, and wound healer** (ibid).

MICROCRYSTALLINE HYDROXYAPATITE (MCHC)

Microcrystalline hydroxyapatite is a veal bone meal that contains calcium, magnesium, phosphorus and other nutrients necessary for bone growth.

MILK THISTLE (Silybum Marianum)

Milk thistle contains silymarin, which is a very potent remedy for the liver. It works by inhibiting free radical damage and promoting synthesis of new protein to replace damaged liver cells. Milk thistle protects the liver against poisoning by chemicals, and is useful in treating liver disease (Heinerman, John. Heinerman's Encyclopedia of Fruits, Vegetables and Herbs. p. 211).

Milk thistle has its main action on kidney and liver, and has long had a reputation for being hepatoprotectant (protects the liver). Milk thistle has been employed as a cholagogue (agent to stimulate gallbladder contraction and promote bile flow) in supportive treatment of hepatic and biliary functional disorders. It has also been employed as an antimalarial, emmenagogue agent (promoting menstruation), and in disorders of the uterus and spleen (Grainger, NB ed., Herbal Drugs and Phytopharmaceuticals. Medpharm Scientific Publishers. CRC Press. Boca Raton, Fla. 1994). Milk thistle has been utilized to stimulate milk production in nursing mothers (Awang D. Can Pharm J 1993;403-404), as an antidepressant (ibid), for steroid secretory modulation (Racz K et al. J Endocrinol 1990;124:341-345), and as support for promyelocytic leukemia (Invernizzi R. et al. Haematologica 1993;78:340-341). Milk thistle components are known to stimulate protein synthesis, however they do not stimulate malignant liver tissue (Sonnenbichler J et al. Biochem Pharm 1985;34:2209-2212).

Silymarin is a lipophilic (lipid-phase) antioxidant, which, when tested against hydrophilic antioxidants, "produced significant protection" from the toxic, immunosuppressive compounds that block bile acid uptake system of hepatocytes (J Endocrinol. 1990;124(2):341-5). Silymarin is a, "known hepatoprotective agent", which brings the glutathione (GSH) level back to normal after depletion (Biochem Pharmacol. 1993;46(1):182-5). Silymarin not only prevents the depletion of GSH, it even increased the basal level of this detoxifying enzyme by 35% in one study (as cited by Murray, M.T., N.D. and Pizzorno, J.E., N.D. Enc. of Natural Medicine. 1991. Prima Publishing, Rocklin, Ca., p.82). (See also: Silymarin).

MONTMORILLINITE CLAY (Selicia)

Montmorillonite is a clay and the principal constituent of bentonite. It includes K+, Mg+ and Ca++, and is able to **carry vitamin B-12-active substances and catalysts** (Merck Index, 11th ed. Merck & Co. Inc., Rahway, N.J. 1989). Bentonite is a colloidal hydrated aluminum silicate clay native to the Midwest and Canada. It contains some magnesium, iron and calcium carbonate. It has the **property of forming highly viscous suspensions or gels with not less than 10 times its weight of water**. The property of forming gels is very much increased by the addition of small amounts of alkaline substances such as magnesium derivatives.

MOTHERWORT

Motherwort is known as a **cardiac tonic** due to its glycoside content, and has been shown to be, "**hypotensive, sedative, and antispasmodic**. It **calms palpitations and normalizes heart function** in general. Recently, Motherwort extract was shown to **inhibit myocardial cells, improve mesenteric circulation and increase coronary perfusion, in other words, to improve several aspects of coronary health**" (Mowry D. Scientific Validation, p. 138). Motherwort was commonly prescribed in Chinese medicine for menstrual disorders, for general abdominal pain, and during childbirth to aid the placenta (Weiner M. Herbs That Heal; p. 238).

MYRRH GUM

Myrrh's reputation as one of the treasures of the East is reflected in the story of how the three wise men brought it to Bethlehem. Used for **muscular pains and rheumatic plasters**, myrrh is a reported **antifungal, antiseptic, astringent, immune stimulant, bitter, expectorant, circulatory stimulant, and phlegm reducer** (Ody P, Complete Medicinal Herbal).

N-ACETYL-CYSTEINE

N-acetyl-cysteine (NAC) is a stable derivative of the amino acid cysteine, which has antioxidant properties and makes up part of the tripeptide glutathione. NAC in particular protects the liver by its antioxidant properties. Researchers at the National Academy of Scientists claim that N-acetyl-cysteine has a, "**long history of therapeutic application**", and claim to, "have discovered that N-acetyl-cysteine **protects cells**

against death induced by exposure to noxious stimuli and **against programmed cell death associated with exposure to inadequate amounts of trophic (involving nutritive processes) factors**" (Proc Nat Acad Sci 1994;91(16):7496-500). N-acetyl-cysteine is noted by Life Sciences as a "reference compound" for, "**inhibition of liver injury and lipid peroxidation**" (Life Sci 1994;55(8):PL145-50).

N-ACETYL-GLUCOSAMINE

N-Acetyl-glucosamine (NAG) is one of the **building blocks of healthy cartilage**; it is recognized in the Merck Index in an **antiarthritic therapeutic category** (p. 4353). NAG is needed for optimal synthesis of chondroitin proteoglycans; this synthesis is impossible in the absence of NAG, however, the process continues once NAG is added (Biochem J. 1991 Jan; 273(Pt 2): 283-88). One of the reasons NAG is an effective antiarthritic is because NAG can effectively inhibit the respiratory burst, and, "can inhibit the release of leukocyte elastase enzyme (elastase is an enzyme which breaks down elastin connective tissue)... and acts in a dose-related fashion" (Clin Exp Rheumatol. 1991 Jan-Feb; 9(1):17-21). When normal, white blood cells (polymorphonuclear leukocytes) were exposed to NAG, the calcium response to immune complexes was significantly reduced (calcium initiates a lot of cell signals) (J Immunol. 1993;150:4571-80). NAG inhibits the ability of the neutrophils (other white blood cells) to release the superoxide anions in response to immune complexes (J Cell Biochem 1994 Oct; 56(2):225-35). NAG doesn't interfere with the binding of the immune complex to neutrophils, rather, the authors suggest, "that these molecules interfere with a step in transmembrane signaling..." (J Cell Biochem. 1994;56(2):225-35).

N-acetyl-glucosamine was tested against lipid peroxidation in rats, and, "Administration of exogenous glucosamine resulted in its incorporation into the membranes of target organs, connective tissue and normalized the levels of endogenous NAG, which finally determined antitoxic and antioxidative properties in this amino sugar (Eksp Klin Farmakol. 1993. 56(5):53-5). NAG has been used in combination with another compound in a study where patient's liver tumors significantly regressed, up to 84% (Gan To Kagaku Ryoho. 1994 Sep; 21(13):2225-8). Applications are currently being utilized in veterinary practice, where 147 clinical cases demonstrated good healing development (J Vet Med Sci. 1993 Oct; 55(5):743-7).

NAG is known to interfere with a carbohydrate-lectin interaction, and this is believed to be one of the mechanisms in **preventing cell damage** (Int J Parasitol. 1991 Dec; 21(8):941-4). NAG even inhibits the cytopathic effect of a strain of Trichomonas vaginalis (Int J Parasitol. 1991; 21(8):941-4), and has been reported to expel worms, possibly by activating glucose metabolism in the host intestines, resulting in increased mucin synthesis and qualitative changes in mucus (J Helminthol. 1993;67(3):179-88).

Altered GAG patterns (glycosaminoglycans, of which **NAG is a component**) are described in connective tissue and/or other diseases. For instance, in Inflammatory Bowel Disease, patients cannot effectively acetylate glucosamine and make NAG. Since NAG is also a necessary component for cartilage synthesis, it should be given in conjunction with glucosamine sulfate for tissue regeneration, especially in cases of diseases where patterns to make NAG are impaired. The functions are wide-ranging, and it is expected that GAG, due to their anionic charge, "may influence some metabolic processes, such as **blood coagulation,** and they could also have a **role in urolithiasis and atherogenesis**. Moreover, they may be important in **modulating the metabolism of some lipoproteins** by affecting the rate of their catabolism" (Boll Soc Ital Biol Sper. 1992;68(12):741-7). It's possible that they could reduce the risk for atherogenesis in this way.

NETTLE

(See Stinging Nettle)

OLIVE LEAF

The olive tree is believed to be the "Tree of Life" according to the writings in the Bible. The olive branch dates back to ancient times as a symbol of rebirth and growth. Recently, an extract from the leaves of the olive branch has come to symbolize a new power of healing, due to an isolated phytochemical called, "oleuropein." In addition to the oleuropein contained in olive leaf extract, other powerful bioflavonoids are present, including rutin, hesperidin, and other flavones. Together, these ingredients work synergistically together, and are responsible for the reputation that the extract is building for purported medicinal properties, including: antibacterial, antimicrobial, antiviral, antifungal, antioxidant, antiarrhythmic, hypoglycemic, hypolipidemic, hypouricemic, hypocholesterolemic, and hypotensive (Fehri, B. et al. J Pharm Belg 1994 Mar-Apr; 49(2):101-108; Visioli, F. et al. Experientia 1995; 51:32-34; Tranter HS et al. J Applied Bacteriology 1993;74:253-259; Tassou CC et al. Biotechnology and Applied Biochemistry 1991;13:231-237; Paster N et al. Il Farmaco 1991;46(6):803-815).

OREGON GRAPE ROOT (Berberis aquafolium)

Oregon grape root, "acts as a tonic on the liver and gall bladder, and can remedy chronic and scaly skin problems such as psoriasis and eczema which are caused by systemic imbalances" (Scalzo R. Naturopathic Handbook of Herbal Formulas, 3rd ed. 1994, Kivaki Press, Durango, Co. p. 96).

OREGANO

Oregano r**educes fevers, relieves cramps, alleviates bronchitis, and helps in measles, mumps and irregular menstruation** (Heinerman, John. Heinerman's Encyclopedia of Fruits, Vegetables and Herbs. p. 207). Oil of oregano can **stop seizures** with application (ibid, p. 207). Oil of oregano is also reported to be of value in treating Candida.

OX BILE (BILE SALTS)

Bile salts are usually needed to prime the biliary system for proper bile production in any gallbladder problem. Purified bile salts act as an excellent **liver detoxifier** in certain toxic states. "**The bile acids in bile keep cholesterol from becoming too concentrated and thus forming gallstones. A bile acid given in tablet form increases the bile acid concentration within the gallbladder, which brings the solid cholesterol stone back into solution**" (Larson, D, M.D., Mayo Clinic Family Healthbook. William Morrow and Company, Inc., N.Y., 1990, p. 662.)

"Administration of crude ox-bile extract produced a dose-dependent release of **Neurotensin-like immunoreactivity"** (Endocrinology 1994;134(2):603-7). Neurotensin is released from the endocrine N cells of the ileum after meals, and studies reveal that it **stimulates bicarbonate secretion by the pancreas and duodenum** (Gastroenterol Clin Biol 1991;15(8-9):574-9). Bicarbonate secretion is necessary to raise the pH of the chyme, or pre-digested food when it reaches the small intestine. Ingestion of ox bile extract reportedly reduced steatorrhea from 134 to 9 g/24 hr, and, "supplementation reduced fat excretion markedly, but did not aggravate diarrhea (Dig Dis Sci 1992;37(6):929-33).

PARSLEY

Parsley is very high in vitamins A, B-complex, C, potassium, manganese, phosphorus, calcium and iron. Only a small amount of the juice is needed for parsley to have an effect. It is an excellent cleanser and assists in digestion.

PASSION FLOWER

Passion Flower, or Passiflora incarnata, is known for its **sedative effects**. It contains many flavonoids, which contribute to its **medicinal properties.** Chrysin, one of the flavonoids isolated in Passiflora, was found in a recent study to **prevent expression of tonic-clonic seizures** in mice, and demonstrated a, "**myorelaxant action of the flavonoid**" (Biochem Pharmacol. 1990;40:2227-31). Its beneficial effects are useful after **muscle injury** when spasms are known to occur. Passiflora is also helpful in **stimulating the uptake of amino acids into cells,** which assists in the **regeneration of tissue** (Biochem Biophys Res Comm. 1990;171:1199-204). The herb should not be confused with the common variety of garden passion flower

(Passiflora caerulea), as the garden passion flower can be toxic. It contains cyanogenic glycosides (Tyler, V. The Honest Herbal. 1993.Haworth Press, Inc. NY, NY).

PAU d' ARCO

Pau d' Arco: (lapacho, taheebo,"Tabebuia avellanedae, T. impetiginosa). This herb is produced from Brazilian tree bark. Widely used by the Indian tribes of the Amazon region for centuries as a healing herb, it has become popular as an **antibacterial, antiviral, anti-inflammatory and antifungal** agent (Mayell; Natural Health First Aid Guide p. 44). The quinone, lapachol, is a component with potential toxicity, and is one reason that the whole extract is safer and just as effective. The tea and extract are taken orally, or applied topically for stings, bites, infections, **inflammations and wound-healing properties (including snakebites)** (Mayell p.123, 133). Compounds from Pau d'arco have demonstrated **anti-candida effects** (A Textbook of Natural Medicine, John Bastyr College Publications, Seattle, Wa. 1988). Pau d'arco is contraindicated with blood-thinning drugs.

PEPPERMINT

Peppermint leaf has reported value as being an antiinflammatory, antimicrobial, and antiulcer agent. Its therapeutic properties include aiding in circulation, digestion, constipation, diarrhea, mental fatigue, viruses, and cellulitis (Mowry D. Scientific Validation, pp. 75, 192).

PHYTOCHEMICALS

Phytochemicals are natural substances found in plants that enhance the plant's immunity to disease. These phytochemicals are thought to be **protective agents** which can have many health-enhancing activities, such as being antioxidants. Phyochemicals include bioflavonoids, like rutin and hesperidin, and the proanthocyanidins, powerful bioflavonoids found in dark-colored fruits and vegetables. The proanthocyanidins are also found in concentrated form in pine bark extract and grape seed extract. (See also: Bioflavonoids and Proanthocyanidins).

PHYTOESTROGENS

Phytoestrogens is the word for a group of plant-based hormones with weak estrogenic activity. These particular "phytochemicals," or chemicals from plants, are found in some 300 foods (especially soy products, cabbage and fennel), and in some herbs, such as dong quai, red raspberry, and licorice root. Since the hormones have weak estrogenic activity, they are able to eliminate some of the symptoms of menopause and decrease the risk for osteoporosis that is associated with a lack of estrogen. Since phytoestrogens also have the power to bind to regular estrogen receptors, they can also eliminate the ill effects attributed to too much circulating estrogen, such as premenstrual tension and increased risk for breast cancer. The Japanese are commonly cited for their unique statistics of women who escape menopausal symptoms and related post-menopausal disease - this is attributed by many to their increased consumption of soy-based products which are high in the phytoestrogens. In fact, the breast cancer rates increase in Japanese women if they adopt a soy-free diet (Wash. Post, April 3, 1994).

Phytoestrogens are believed to balance estrogen dominance with the effects of an adaptogen (a substance that regulates increasing or decreasing to achieve homeostasis). In addition to the weak estrogenic activity and receptor-blocking activity that they possess, these plant estrogens bind to an enzyme called estrogen synthetase, thus inhibiting the production of too much estrogen in the body, and offering additional protection against cancer risk (Lark, S. Fibroid Tumors and Endometriosis. Celestial Arts, Berkeley, Ca. 1995; p. 125).

PLANTAGO (PLAINTAIN)

Plantago is a western herb which is excellent as a **demulcent** (soothes and moistens), therefore it is helpful in **ulcerous or pre-ulcerous conditions.** Plantain spread so quickly in the New World (brought over by European settlers), that Native Americans referred to it as, **"white man's footprint"** (Mayell M. The Natural Health First Aid Guide, p. 44).

PLEURISY ROOT

Pleurisy root reportedly helps alleviate the symptoms present in flus, colds, bronchitis, pleurisy, and respiratory ailments (Mowry, D. Scientific Validation, p. 240).

PRIMROSE OIL

(See Essential Fatty Acids – Evening primrose oil)

PROANTHOCYANIDINS

Proanthocyanidins have become the "antioxidant of the 90's" - they have potent antioxidant properties (Planta Med. 1994 Aug; 60(4):323-8), and their reputation is building for possessing many times the antioxidant potential of vitamin C and vitamin E. The potent antiradical activity is due to the ability to inhibit superoxide and xanthine oxidase, and some researchers noted that the, "remarkably high activity" was even greater than expected on the basis of quantities present in samples (Planta Med 1992; 58(4):342-4). Proanthocyanidins are prevalent in many berries, i.e. blueberries, blackberries, raspberries, hawthorn berries (very high), and cherries; they are also extremely high in grape seed extract and pine bark extract. These potent bioflavonoids have been shown to relax smooth muscle (Colombo, D., and Vescovini, R. Controlled Trial of Anthocyanosides from Vaccinium Myrtillus in Primary Dysmenorrhea. G Ital Obstet Ginecol 7:1033-1038, 1985), and, "are remarkable in their ability to **stabilize collagen** structures" (Murray M. Enc Nat Med. p. 461). The properties of these strong antioxidants offer a unique potential for therapeutic value. For instance, "Supplementation with concentrated extracts or eating plenty of berries rich in these types of flavonoids may offer significant benefit in **preventing osteoporosis**" (Murray M. Enc Nat Med. p. 461). Proanthocyanidins make up part of the green tea complex, and may be responsible for many of its touted therapeutic benefits (Prev Med. 1992 May; 21(3):334-50).

Proanthocyanidins play many roles: they are important in microcirculation (Minerva Chir 1993; 48(17):XIII); in the treatment of fibrocystic disease (Minerva Ginecol 1993; 45(12):617-21); in protecting against cytogenetic damage of DNA (Akhmadieva Akh et al, Radiobiologiia 1993;33(3):433-5; Plant Physiology 1994; 105(3):881-9); in hepatoprotection (Cell Mol Biol Noisy le grand 1993; 39(4):443-8); and in normalizing free fatty acid content (Eksp Klin Farmakol 1992; 55(6):19-21). There are even reports of a, "novel, highly sweet proanthocyanidin from the rhizomes of Selliguea feei" (J Nat Prod 1993; 56(9):1532-8).

QUASSIA

Quassia is a bitter tonic and anthelmintic (anti-worm), which is, "excellent for dyspeptic conditions, stimulates the production of saliva and digestive juices, and is also used in the expulsion of worms" (Hoffman D. The Holistic Herbal. Element, Mass. p. 226).

QUERCETIN

Quercetin, called, "the most important flavonoid" by Nutrition in Cancer, is a powerful antioxidant which has demonstrated anticarcinogenic properties (Nutr. Cancer 1993, 20:21-9). Being a potent bioflavonoid, quercetin is used in inflammatory and allergic problems. It is effective because it stabilizes cell membranes, decreases the release of inflammation mediators, and decreases the contraction of smooth muscle (Murray M. Enc of Nat Med. Prima Publ., Rocklin, Ca. 1991. p.298). Bioflavonoids also improve capillary integrity (Merck Index, 11th ed. 1989. Merck and Co. Inc. Rahway, N.J. p. 1243), and stabilize the collagen matrix by preventing free radical damage.

Quercetin regulates the permeability of the capillaries and prevents the rupture of the capillaries that causes bruising. Quercetin inhibits enzymatic breakdown of the collagen matrix, and aids in the cross linking of collagen fibers to form a more stable collagen matrix (Murray M. Enc Nat Med, Prima Publ., Rocklin, Ca. 1991. p. 330). It also decreases the amount of histamine released from cells, and reduces inflammatory leukotriene formation (a hormone-like substance that is very active in asthma). Quercetin is a powerful bioflavonoid which reduces inflammation and protects cells (Biochem. Pharmacol. 45:13-9). When bioflavonoids were tested for their ability to increase bacteria-engulfing white blood cells, the proliferation not only increased, but the stimulating activity correlated with the concentration of flavonoids (Biull. Eksp. Biol. Med. 114:520-21). Quercetin is also known as an antiviral. Bioflavonoids have demonstrated a positive, protective effect on human viruses (J. Med. Virol. 15:71-79). (See also Bioflavonoids - Quercetin)

RED BEET ROOT

Beets have been used since ancient times for medicinal purposes. The beet has been cultivated for its roots and leaves since the third or fourth century B.C. In ancient times, it was used only for medicinal purposes. Beets are a great source of minerals and have been used for liver and gallbladder disorders. They have a high content of vitamin A, which makes them a good therapeutic choice for digestive and lymphatic system problems as well as the eliminative system. (Jensen, B., Foods That Heal, Avery Publishing Group Inc., Garden City Park, NY, 1988, page114-115).

Beets aid in gall bladder function, lymphatic function, and digestion (Balch JF, Prescription for Nutritional Healing, p. 39). Red beet root has been utilized for **treating tumors**; the anti-cancer strength may be due to betaine, the natural red coloring of the beet (Australian International Clinical Nutrition review July 1986, Dr. Ferenczi, as cited in: Heinerman, John. Heinerman's Encyclopedia of Fruits, Vegetables and Herbs. Parker Publishing, West Nyack, NY pp. 29-31). The powerful ability of red beet root to **present wastes to the liver when breaking up tumors** stresses the need to detoxify the liver and colon at the same time (ibid, p. 31). The betaine in red beets has also been found to lower homocysteine levels; high homocysteine levels are believed to be an independent risk factor for heart disease.

RED RADISH

Red radish is used to **remove fat deposits, stop cough and fever, control diarrhea, prevent gallstones and kidney stones, and to treat cancer** (Heinerman, John. Heinerman's Encyclopedia of Fruits, Vegetables and Herbs. Parker Publishing, West Nyack, NY p. 295).

RUTIN

(See Bioflavonoids)

SKULLCAP

Skullcap is a **sedative** for muscle spasms and convulsions, and **reduces heart and joint inflammation** (Heinerman, John. Heinerman's Encyclopedia of Fruits, Vegetables and Herbs. Parker Publishing, West Nyack, NY p. 327). It **lowers cholesterol, increases "good" cholesterol, inhibits fat accumulation in the arteries (atherosclerosis), and ameliorates the muscle and joint swelling of arthritis** (Chemical and Pharmaceutical Bulletin 29:2308;32;2724 as cited in Heinerman, John. Heinerman's Encyclopedia of Fruits, Vegetables and Herbs. Parker Publishing, West Nyack, NY p. 327).

SLIPPERY ELM

Slippery elm **calms the inflamed mucous membranes of the stomach** (Balch JF Presc for Nutr Healing 1990, Garden City, NY). In addition to a **soothing texture that coats the stomach lining,** slippery elm contains the fiber-rich ingredient **mucilage** which **stimulates mucus secretion (protective against ulcers).**

SODIUM ALGINATE

Sodium alginate is a highly viscous polysaccharide contributing to fiber content (J Nutr 1990;120(4): 353-60).

ST. JOHN'S WORT

St. John's wort has been used as an antidepressant (and depression-related symptoms during menopause and nervous exhaustion). It appears to be effective at relieving mild to moderate depression, without the side effects of Prozac or some of the other antidepressant drugs. Although St. John's Wort is reported to be a natural, herbal alternative for some of the antidepressant drugs, it should be stressed that it is for mild to moderate depression, which should be diagnosed by a practitioner. Psychovegetative disturbances, fear, and nervous disturbances have been listed as clinical indications by the official German Commission E monograph for St. John's wort.

A dosage of 300 mg of St. John's Wort was administered to patients with mild to moderately severe depression in a double blind, placebo-controlled study, and 66% of the patients improved, compared to 26% on the placebo (Fortschr Med 1993;111:339-342). In another double-blind crossover study, 12 healthy subjects experienced improved cortical function (4th Int Congress on Phytotherapy. Munich, Germany. Sept. 10-13, 1992, abstract SL53). "Impressive" improvement was found in patients treated with St. John's Wort, in terms of depression and complaints of disturbed sleep, headache, and fatigue, in another double-blind study performed in Germany (ibid, abstract SL55).

There have been at least 27 double-blind controlled studies conducted on St. John's wort using an extract of at least 0.3% hypericin, indicating that it is as effective in relieving symptoms of depression as some of the standard antidepressants, but is better tolerated with fewer side effects. The British Medical Journal published a meta-analysis of 23 randomized trials, stating that St. John's wort was, "significantly superior to a placebo" (Linde et al.).

Since St. John's Wort is suspected of working by similar mechanisms to Prozac and other antidepressants, they should not be taken at the same time. For contraindications and drug interactions, refer to the drug-nutrient interaction chart.

References: K. Linde et al. St. John's Wort for Depression An Overview and Meta-analysis of Randomised Clinical Trials BMJ 1996;313:253-258; Morazzoni P & Bombardellie E. Hypericum perforatum. Indena, Milan, Italy, 1994; Schmidt U & Sommer H. Forschr Med 1993;111:339-342; Johnson D. 4th International Congress on Phytotherapy, Munich, Germany. Sept 10-13, 1992 [Abstract SL53]; Schlich et al. Psychol 1987;13:440-444.

STINGING NETTLE

Stinging nettle is so called because of the spiny hairs of the plant that will sting as they penetrate the skin, possibly causing skin irritation or a rash. The therapeutic qualities far outweigh the inconvenience of picking the plant. Stinging nettle is a long time favored herb for hayfever and allergies. It is a good tonic for the whole body, but especially for the lungs. Because of its high nutritional value (high in iron and vitamin C), stinging nettle is a good herb for anemia.

Stinging Nettle is reported to be a **diuretic**, and also to be useful in **arresting uterine hemorrhages.** In addition, it is used as an aid for **gout, asthma, and tuberculosis** (Weiner MA. Herbs That Heal, p. 244). Stinging Nettle is also used as a **disinfectant, to improve digestion, promote milk flow, inhibit urinary tract bleeding, and stop excessive menstrual flow** (Sharon M, MD. Complete Nutrition.; p. 142). Stinging Nettle has a reputation for helping in **weight loss** (Heinerman J. Heinerman's Encyclopedia of Fruits, Vegetables and Herbs; p. 223). Stinging nettle has also been used for asthma, diarrhea hemorrhoids and arthritic problems. In Europe, nettle extracts are being employed in the treatment of urinary retention brought on by benign prostatic hypertrophy (BPH); clinical evidence supports this, and German health authorities allow it to be used for BPH (Zeitschrift fur Phytotherapie 1989;10:175-178; Bundesanzeiger, Jan. 5, 1989; March 6, 1990).

The plant should not be eaten raw (uncooked) as it can damage the kidneys. External use can cause contact dermatitis in a few sensitive individuals. Medicinal amounts of any herb should only be taken with the advice of a trained licensed healthcare professional.

TILLANDSIA

Tillandsia usenoides (Spanish Moss), is a member of the bromeliaceous family of plants. It possesses **strong absorption properties** (Spanish moss. In: Encyclopedia Brittanica, 15th ed., Vol IX, Cambridge:400-401,1980), and when processed under low temperatures, retains its naturally occurring enzymes. A rich source of **chlorophyll,** tillandsia is also touted as a **hormone precursor and natural healer** (Profiles in Nutritional progress. Rubicon Publications, Bakersfield:40-43,1993).

THYME

Thyme is an **antiseptic, destroying viruses and infectious germs,** which accounts for its effect on colds, fevers, and flus (Heinerman, John. Heinerman's Encyclopedia of Fruits, Vegetables and Herbs. Parker Publishing, West Nyack, NY p. 338). It is also used for promoting **better blood circulation, and for treating Candida albicans** (ibid p. 339); in fact, thyme contains some of the **most powerful candida substances available** (Duke, JA. Handbook of Medicinal Herbs. CRC Press, Boca Raton, Fl. 1985). Thymol is an ingredient in thyme which is **antiviral,** and also **relieves migraines and stomach cramps by relaxing muscles and tight blood vessels** (ibid, p. 340).

UREA (carbamide)

Urea is described as an **"osmotic diuretic"** (Guyton's Textbook of Medical Physiology, 8th Edition). Urea is "not easily reabsorbed by the tubules causing increased osmotic pressure and decreased water reabsorption, so that large amounts of tubular fluid flush on into the urine" (ibid, p. 351).

Urea increases nutrient digestion (J Anim Sci 1991;69(3):1300-11), and diminishes susceptibility to infection by, "directly acting on the membranes of bacteria and fungi" (Hautarzt 1992;43(Suppl)11:9-12). It has been utilized as a treatment for troublesome urinary mucus production, especially after urinary tract reconstruction. Researchers, "report a rapidly effective, nontoxic, inexpensive method of dissolving urinary mucus by periodic instillation of a concentrated urea solution" (J Urol 1994;151(4):1036-7). In people who exhibit the syndrome of inappropriate secretion of antidiuretic hormone (water conserving hormone), "Oral urea, even during long periods, is a safe and effective therapeutic approach for patients..." (Nephron 1993;63(4):468-70). Urea's water solubility, dipolar character and electrolyte properties make urea, "a unique, physiological substance" (Acta Derm Venereol Suppl Stockh 1992;177:7-8).

UVA URSI

Uva-Ursi's purported properties include that of **anesthetic, anticarcinogenic, antibiotic, antiseptic, diuretic, and urinary disinfectant** (Mowry D. Scientific Validation pp. 67-187). It contains phenolic glycosides, which have reported **diuretic and urinary antiseptic action,** and, "is used as a tonic and specific in cases involving weakened liver, kidneys, and other glands" (Mowry D. Scientific Validation, p. 67).

VALERIAN ROOT

Called, "nature's tranquilizer", valerian has a reputation as an antispasmodic, expectorant, diuretic, and a substance that strengthens the heart and lowers blood pressure (Ody P, Complete Medicinal Herbal). It has also been used for tickling, nervous coughs. It consists of a volatile oil, which is not that pleasant to the nose. It contains valepotriates, which seem to be active ingredients in relaxing the nervous system (ibid).

In a double-blind crossover study of 128 people given 400 mg valerian, the valerian produced a significant improvement in sleep quality (Leathwood PD et al. Pharmacol Biochem Behav 1982;17:65). In another study, 450 mg produced similar results against placebo, however 900 mg did not produce any further improvement; sleep latency was reduced, sleep quality improved, and nighttime awakenings reduced (Leathwood PD & Chauffard F. Planta Med 1985;51:144). The calming effect has not been shown to be additive with alcohol in mice (Braun R et al. Dtsch Apoth-Ztg 1982;122:1109). Valerian seems to be as effective in reducing sleep latency as small doses of barbiturates or benzodiazepines, but in contrast reduces the morning sleepiness seen with those drugs (Leathwood PD & Chauffard F. Planta Med 1985;51:144). In a double-blind study of insomniacs, twenty patients received either a combination of valerian root (160 mg) and Melissa officinalis (80 mg), a benzodiazepine (triazolam 0.125 mg) or placebo. The valerian preparation was as effective as the drug, as well as increasing deep sleep stages 3 and 4. The valerian combination did not cause daytime sedation, diminished concentration, or impairment of physical performance (Dressing H. et al. Therapiewoche 1992;42:726-736). Christopher Hobbes has discussed some concern about long-term use of the valepotriates (Hobbes C. Herbal Gram 1989;21:19).

VANADYL SULFATE

A form of the mineral vanadium, vanadyl sulfate regulates blood sugar. It was tested as a glucose-lowering agent in diabetic rats, and found to be of value in lowering levels of hyperglycemia. Individual intakes of vanadyl sulfate varied depending on the severity of diabetes, with the more hyperglycemic rats consuming greater quantities of the solution (Biochem Biophys Res Commun. 1993 Dec 30; 197(3):1549-55). Because of the effect on glucose metabolism, "it is not surprising that pharmacologic levels of dietary vanadium improved oral glucose tolerance in studies on guinea pigs. Pharmacologic levels of dietary vanadium also prevented an increase in glucose, despite low insulin, in blood, and prevented the decline in cardiac performance of rats made diabetic with streptozocin" (Science. 1985; 227:1474-77). In another study, vanadyl sulfate prevented the rise in insulin and blood pressure usually seen after a fructose-enriched diet in rats. Vanadyl sulfate was found to significantly improve insulin sensitivity (Hypertension. 1994 Mar; 23(3):308-12).

Excessive vanadium can cause depressed growth, diarrhea, depressed food intake and death in some animal species. Excess vanadium has been suggested as a factor in manic-depressive illness. Large doses may interfere with the Na+ K+ ATPase pump. Medicinal amounts of any vitamin, mineral or specialty nutrient should only be taken with the advice of a trained licensed healthcare professional.

WATERCRESS

PEITC is a compound found in cruciferous vegetables, and has been found to **inhibit lung tumorigenesis in animals** (Cancer Epidemiol Biomarkers Prev 1992;1(5):383-8). To measure its uptake in humans, watercress was used, because it is rich in gluconasturtiin, a precursor of PEITC. "These results clearly showed that PEITC was released in the human body upon ingestion of watercress", and suggest that the compound found in watercress, "may be a useful marker for quantitating human exposure to this **anticarcinogen** as a tool for epidemiological investigations" (Cancer Epidemiol Biomarkers Prev 1992;1(5):p. 383).

WHITE WILLOW BARK

White Willow Bark, or Salicin, is the forerunner of aspirin, which is technically known as acetylsalicyclic acid. In ancient times, chewing on pieces of this bark were known to **alleviate pain and symptoms of inflammation**. However white willow bark does not involve the side effects of aspirin, such as stomach upset and cartilage destruction. It is suggested that aspirin can cause significant bronchoconstriction in asthma patients (Yonsei Med. J. 1989;30:339-45). Other anti-inflammatory drugs, such as ibuprofen and indomethacin, can cause headaches and dizziness.

WILD YAM

Yam is **antibacterial, antispasmodic, anti-inflammatory, muscle relaxing, and contains phytosterols** (Ody P, Complete Medicinal Herbal). Wild yam has been used to **alleviate cramps** (David B. Mowry, PhD. The Scientific Validation of Herbal Medicine. 1986. Keats Publishing, New Canaan, Conn. p. 112). Yam relieves **rheumatoid arthritis** and can be combined with celery seeds, angelica (dong quai), or willow for acute stages of rheumatoid arthritis (Ody P, Complete Medicinal Herbal). Yams have been used as a starter material for the **hydrocortisones** in non-prescription eczema creams (ibid).

"Wild yams contain diosgenin, a precursor in the synthesis of progesterone, and are the only known available source" - (Rudolf Weiss, 1985, as quoted in Ody P, Complete Medicinal Herbal). Wild yam **contains hormonal substances very similar to progesterone;** extracts of bei xie (7-lobed yam) are used in the synthesis of contraceptive pills (Ody P, Complete Medicinal Herbal). "Its main action is on the **kidneys, lungs, and stomach**, and it is included in remedies for **asthma, menopausal syndrome, urinary disorders, and weak kidney energies**" (Ody P, Complete Medicinal Herbal). Wild yam is used for general female problems. Since Wild yam contains only precursors to progesterone, the actual conversion to progesterone in the body is controversial. However, clinical results show that wild yam has beneficial effects on the female system. Natural progesterone creams are generally available which provide natural progesterone without any conversion process required, and also provide for rapid absorption into the system without being broken down in the liver. Progesterone is a hormone and should be used under supervision of a qualified, licensed health care professional.

YARROW

Yarrow is valued mostly for its ability to **tame colds and influenza,** and also for its action on the **circulatory, digestive, and urinary systems.** Among other things, it contains salicyclic acid, (which is the aspirin-component of white willow bark), and flavonoids. It supposedly works to **reduce fever and inflammation**, and is helpful in **phlegm conditions** (Ody P, Complete Medicinal Herbal).

YOGURT

Yogurt is fermented milk with healthy bacteria included. The bacteria in yogurt **breaks down the protein during the fermentation process, making the protein more digestible** than milk protein. Yogurt is an excellent source of protein, calcium, potassium, phosphorus, lactobacillus, and vitamins B-6, B-12, niacin and folic acid. Yogurt has been found to:

1) **Boost the immune system** and kill off harmful bacteria.
2) **Protect the lining of the stomach** from toxins due to its high levels of PGE2.
3) Prevent diarrhea and dysentery.
4) Have a natural **antibiotic effect** because yogurt cultures flourish in the GI tract and prevent "bad bacteria" from proliferating, and is recommended for people on antibiotic therapy.
5) Neutralize uric acid in the body.
6) Be **effective in the treatment of cancer.** The National Cancer Institute has determined that malignant tumors shrink in patients who consumed a steady diet of yogurt. Studies at the Harvard Medical School and the University of Chicago Medical School show that yogurt is especially effective against vaginal cancer (Balch PA, Pres for Cooking, p. 81). In 1970, the University of Nebraska found yogurt to have **anti-tumor** effects on bowel cancer patients.
7) Decrease cholesterol in the blood.
8) Prevent gas and bloating after meals.

Lactose is just one example of substances which have bonds that are more easily broken by the enzymes present in yogurt. "**Lactose in yogurt with live bacteria is better tolerated** than lactose in other dairy foods, partly because of the **activity of microbial beta-galactosidase (beta-gal), which digests lactose**" - In this study, where yogurt was tested for its ability to improve digestion by breaking these beta-galactose bonds, **all yogurts dramatically improved digestion** (Am J Clin Nutr 1990;54(6):1041-6).

YOHIMBE BARK

Yohimbe dilates blood vessels, thus it has been useful for treating male sexual dysfunction (Wright, J, M.D., et.al. The Natural Pharmacy, Prima Health, Rocklin, CA, 1998). Yohimbe has been used for prostatitis and low sperm count. Yocon is the brand name of a drug which is actually yohimbine hydrochloride. Even though Yocon is being used to treat male impotence, and, "is thought to be an **aphrodisiac**", its officially approved use is for **dilating pupils** (Sifton, DW, ed. The Physician's Desk Reference Family Guide to Prescription Drugs. 1994. Medical Economics Data, Montvale, New Jersey). The side effects of large doses of yohimbe are attributed to the constituent yohimbine, which is used as the drug (trade name Yocon). These effects, "have not been adequately studied or related to dosage although they appear to require high doses of the drug" (The PDR Family Guide to Prescription Drugs, ibid). Remember that this is high doses of the DRUG yohimbine hydrochloride, not the HERB yohimbe. In high doses, it can cause hypotension, abdominal distress, weakness, panic attacks, blood pressure elevation, and kidney, colon, and prostate irritation. With extremely large doses, central nervous system stimulation and paralysis can occur. Do not use yohimbe in peptic ulcers or kidney disease. Avoid when taking MAO inhibitors.

BASIC NUTRITIONAL INFORMATION: VITAMINS

A vitamin is a substance that is needed by the body to sustain life; it cannot be synthesized by the body and must be ingested. For instance, the substance ascorbic acid is not needed by animals who synthesize it, so it is not a vitamin to them. Humans, however, do not possess the enzyme to change glucose into ascorbic acid, so to humans, ascorbic acid is known as, "vitamin C". Vitamins are divided into two groups: fat-soluble and water soluble. The water soluble vitamins are readily excreted, whereas the fat-soluble vitamins are stored in the liver and fatty tissues.

GENERAL DISCLAIMER

The nutritional suggestions and research reported in this book are not offered to treat, mitigate or cure disease, and should not be used as a substitute for sound medical advice. This book is designed to be used in conjunction with the services provided by a trained, licensed healthcare practitioner.

CAUTION

Caution should be used in all conditions, especially concerning pregnancy and children, when taking herbal supplements or high potency nutrients. A physician knowledgeable in natural and preventative medicine should be consulted.

It is the reader's responsibility to be aware of certain contraindications, toxicology and drug-nutrient interactions which may occur. A concise table of drug-nutrient interactions has been provided for information, however, competent resources, such as "Shils and Young, Modern Nutrition in Health and Disease", Lea & Febiger, Phil, Pa 1988, should be consulted for the RDA's and upper limits of vitamins and minerals (Contraindications and Toxicology). As an example, vitamin C supplementation to people with iron overload disease (2% of the population) can be harmful and even fatal. Less information is available on herbs and other supplements, and several resources are recommended, such as the "Lawrence Review of Natural Products", Facts and Comparisons, St. Louis, Missouri. 1996, and the German monographs.

VITAMIN A

Sources: fish liver oils, green and yellow fruits and vegetables, liver, garlic, kelp, alfalfa, eggs.

Functions: necessary for growth and repair of body tissues, maintains epithelial and mucus surfaces, prompts secretion of gastric juices necessary for proper digestion of proteins, builds strong bones and teeth, maintains good eyesight (the vitamin A in rhodopsin, located in the rods of the cell, transmits light signals by changing its configuration), and aids in the manufacturing of red blood cells. Vitamin A assists in the healing process and is important in proper cellular reproduction.

Possible Effects of Deficiency: eye disorders (especially night blindness), frequent infections, dry, scaly skin, inhibited healing processes, nerve deterioration, acne, weak tooth enamel, sinus trouble.

Clinical Applications:

1) **Infection** - supports the mucus lining. It also appears to improve antibody response and white blood cell functions.
2) **Eye problems** - many eye problems respond favorably to vitamin A due to the many functions vitamin A has in vision.

3) **Skin problems** - has many beneficial effects on the skin and is helpful in wound healing. It may be helpful in acne.
4) **Antioxidant function** - the precursor of vitamin A, **beta carotene**, is a powerful antioxidant. It protects against pollutants, stress, smoke and chemical exposure.

<u>**Adjunctive Tips**</u>: Since vitamin A is fat-soluble, it requires fat for absorption. It also requires zinc and other minerals for complete absorption. About 90% of storable vitamin A is in the liver. Preformed vitamin A is known as retinol and is found in liver and fish liver oil. Beta-carotene, known as provitamin A, is found in yellow and green leafy vegetables. Since vitamin A is a fat-soluble vitamin that can be stored in the liver, it can become toxic in extremely large doses, either acutely (doses > 660,000 IU, adults; > 330,000, children) or chronically (14,000 IU/daily, adults; 14,000, children) (Shils ME and Young VR. Modern Nutrition in Health and Disease. (1988) Lea & Febiger, Philadelphia, p.303). Newborns have low liver reserves of vitamin A; premature infants may pose a high risk clinical situation, because their vitamin A status deteriorates within the first two months, and supplements are not well utilized (Shils & Young, p. 305). Increased intake/supplementation during pregnancy is not advised, because vitamin A is teratogenic.

<u>**Research:**</u> Supplementary treatment of vitamin A is reported by some investigators to enhance antibody and cell-mediated immune response (Levis WR & Emden RG. Proc. Am Assoc. Cancer Res. (1976); 17:112; Cohen BE & Cohen IK. J. Immunol.. (1976); 111:1376). C.F. Nockels, in, "The role of vitamins in modulating disease resistance", states that vitamin A is, "...able to protect cells and enhance humoral and cellular immune responses in disease" (Vet Clin North Am Food Anim Pract. 1988; 4(3):531-42). In one clinical trial, 300 women who had developed precancerous cells in the cervix entered a study where half of them received treatment consisting of vaginal sponges which released a synthetic relative of vitamin A. In the moderate cases, the precancerous spots disappeared in the treated women (Science News. 1994; 143(22):341). "...The addition of vitamin A to vitamin A-deficient keratinizing cells in tissue culture induces a shift to mucus-producing cells... vitamin A and its analogues, both in vivo and in vitro, markedly influence the way in which cells differentiate" (Shils and Young. p. 300).

Beta-carotene (beta-carotene is a precursor to vitamin A, but there is no RDA for beta carotene since it is not a vitamin by definition).

Beta-carotene is generally non-toxic. The only side effect reported in excessive dosages is a slight yellow-orange color in the skin. High dosages of beta-carotene should be avoided in diabetic and hypothyroid conditions (they cannot readily convert beta-carotene to vitamin A). Since beta-carotene is a precursor to vitamin A, and is made into vitamin A as needed, supplementation of beta-carotene reduces the risk of vitamin A toxicity. Beta carotene, measured in blood, has been inversely associated with lung cancer (Nomura, et al. Cancer Res. 1985; 45:2369; Willett et al. New England J Med. 1984; 310:430). It seems to have a protective antioxidant effect on DNA, and, "significantly reduces chromosome damage" (Science News. 1994; 145:126). Recent studies indicate that smokers do not decrease their risk for lung cancer by supplementing with beta-carotene. Researchers from Cornell University have determined that there may be, "some biological interaction between beta-carotene and smoking." These researchers have concluded this after reporting on data collected as part of the third National Health and Nutrition Examination survey (which includes more than 15,000 people). A recent study conducted in China by one of the Cornell researchers found that while beta-carotene is the most protective antioxidant for lung function in NONSMOKERS, SMOKERS derived more protection from selenium (Science News. 1998; 153:287).

Beta-carotene interacts with alcohol and may result in more liver damage than alcohol consumption alone. Long-term dosing of 15-60 mg/day can possibly lower vitamin E levels.

VITAMIN B COMPLEX

<u>**Sources**</u>: wheat germ, brown rice, brewer's yeast, oats and whole grains, nuts and seeds, liver.

<u>**Functions**</u>: "catalytic spark plugs" of the body; catalyze many biochemical reactions because of role as coenzymes; provide energy by converting carbohydrates into glucose, vital in the metabolism of fats and proteins, necessary for normal functioning of the nervous system, essential for maintenance of muscle tone in the GI tract and for the health of skin, hair, eyes, mouth and liver.

Possible Effects of Deficiency: beriberi, pellagra, digestive disorders, poor appetite, cardiovascular disorders, loss of hair and shine, depression, fatigue, nervous disorders, constipation, enlarged tongue that is shiny, bright red and full of grooves, cracks at the corners of the mouth, anemia (especially B-12 or folic acid deficiency).

Clinical Applications: The B vitamin complex has been shown to be useful during stress, anxiety, insomnia, hyperactivity, skin problems, PMS, menopausal symptoms and alcohol withdrawal.

Adjunctive Tips: The B vitamins are water-soluble and work together in the body. Certain B vitamins can be made in the body by bacteria, yeasts, fungi and molds in the large intestine. A refined diet high in sugar, coffee, alcohol and refined flour can deplete the B vitamins.

Research: Treatment with the B vitamins B-1, B-2, and B-6, in a 4-week randomized, placebo-controlled, double-blind study resulted in trends of, "greater improvement in scores on ratings of depression and cognitive function", and these findings, "offer preliminary support for further investigation of B complex vitamin augmentation in the treatment of geriatric depression" (Bell IR et al. J Am Coll Nutr. 1992; 11(2):159-63).

VITAMIN B-1 (Thiamine or thiamin)

Sources: wheat germ and bran, brown rice and whole grains, brewer's yeast, blackstrap molasses, nuts and seeds, peas and beans.

Functions: acts as cofactor thiamine pyrophosphate (TPP), key role in glucose metabolism, supports the nervous system and mental attitude, linked to proper growth in children, aids in HCl production, helps in motion sickness.

Possible Effects of Deficiency: Beriberi (disease caused by thiamine deficiency) which is characterized by: stunted growth in children, edema, decreased heart function, weight loss, muscle wasting and nerve degeneration. Deficiency may also result in insomnia, fatigue, confusion, memory loss, mental confusion, depression, abdominal pain and poor muscle coordination. The elderly and alcoholics are at greatest risk for deficiency. Exercise and carbohydrate intake increase the need for thiamine, and a diet high in fat/sugar, or a restricted calorie diet/fasting may cause inadequate intake of thiamine (Nutr Desk Ref p. 43).

Research: Thiamine, as part of the TPP enzyme, is essential not only for glucose metabolism, but for metabolism of the branched chain amino acids (BCAA). In maple syrup urine disease (MSUD), metabolism of the BCAA is impaired. Increasing thiamine ingestion increases TPP, and increases BCAA metabolism, "its mechanism is to stabilize the enzyme complex". Thiamine is used as adjunct therapy for MSUD, along with a diet restricting the BCAA (Shils & Young; p. 1357).

VITAMIN B-2 (Riboflavin)

Sources: Brewer's yeast, liver, eggs, millet, wild rice, sunflower seeds, beans and peas, dark, green leafy vegetables, almonds, tuna and salmon.

Functions: precursor for two important coenzymes, flavin mononucleotide (FMN) and flavin adenine dinucleotide (FAD) which act as hydrogen carriers to help make ATP through carbohydrate and fat metabolism. It is necessary for normal cell growth and is instrumental in cell respiration. It is essential for the synthesis of fatty acids and amino acids.

Possible Effects of Deficiency: inflammation of the mucus membranes of the mouth, cracks at the corners of the mouth, sore, red tongue, eye problems, nerve tissue damage and digestive problems. Alcohol abusers are at high risk for deficiency.

VITAMIN B-3 (Niacin)

Sources: liver and other organ meats, poultry, fish, peanuts, brewer's yeast, whole grains, wheat germ, avocados, dates, figs and prunes.

Functions: precursor of two important coenzymes, nicotinamide adenine dinucleotide (NAD) and nicotinamide adenine dincucleotide phosphate (NADP) that are involved in 50 different metabolic reactions in the body, including glycolysis, fatty acid synthesis, deamination (nitrogen removal) of amino acids, cholesterol metabolism, sex hormone synthesis (such as estrogen, progesterone and testosterone) and proper digestion. It is important in circulation, healthy activity of the nervous system and promotes healthy skin and nerves. Niacin taken as **nicotinic acid** lowers cholesterol, but can cause a "niacin flush", which is the result of the release of histamine by the cells, causing vasodilation. Niacin taken as niacinamide or nicotinamide does not produce the flushing reaction but these forms cannot be used to aid in lowering cholesterol levels. Niacin may stimulate extra hydrochloric acid production.

Possible Effects of Deficiency: pellagra (dermatitis, diarrhea and dementia), weakness, fatigue, anorexia, indigestion, skin eruptions, mental depression, irritability, and rough skin that is extremely sensitive to light.

Research: Nicotinic acid inhibits HMG-CoA reductase activity (the rate limiting enzyme in cholesterol synthesis), and is known for lowering cholesterol in several studies (Lipids 1993;28(7):613-19). Chronic ingestion of excessive doses of nicotinic acid can have toxic effects, such as liver damage.

VITAMIN B-5 (Pantothenic Acid)

Sources: widely available in foods including brewer's yeast, organ meats, yams, whole grains, broccoli, legumes, egg yolks, cheese, peanuts, chicken, fish.

Functions: functions as part of the molecule called coenzyme A or CoA; vital for good adrenal activity including increasing production of cortisone and other adrenal hormones; important for healthy skin and nerves, supports the synthesis of acetylcholine (a neurotransmitter), fatty acids, cholesterol, steroids, and phospholipids. It is known as the anti-stress vitamin and can be made by the bacterial flora in the intestines.

Possible Effects of Deficiency: fatigue, depression, a decrease in HCl production and other digestive problems, decreased adrenal function, problems in blood sugar metabolism (hypoglycemia), decreased immunity, vomiting, insomnia, and fatigue.

Research: Deficiency of B-5 in the rat results in a lack of cartilage growth, resulting in lesions similar to those present in osteoarthritis (Murray M. Enc Nat Med p. 451). Supplementation of pantothenic acid seems to alleviate some of the symptoms of osteoarthritis (Anand, JC. Lancet. 1963; ii, p. 1,168).

VITAMIN B-6 (Pyridoxine)

Sources: wheat germ, whole grains, organ meats (liver), fish, poultry, egg yolk, beans, bananas, prunes, potatoes, cabbage, avocados, cauliflower.

Functions: Although vitamin B-6 has three natural forms (pyridoxine, pyridoxamine, and pyridoxal), the phosphorylated form of pyridoxal, pyrioxal-5-phosphate (P-5-P), functions as the active coenzyme in a wide variety of functions. For instance, it is essential in amino acid metabolism; supports production of gamma-aminobutyric acid (GABA), which is important in central nervous system function; aids in antibody and red blood cell production, and also DNA and RNA synthesis; is important in fluid balance regulation (sodium/potassium balance); and helps maintain normal intracellular levels of magnesium. There is a high requirement during pregnancy for hormonal and fluid balance maintenance. B-6 is beneficial in fatigue, PMS, edema, carpal tunnel syndrome and amino acid metabolism.

Possible Effects of Deficiency: wide variety of symptoms including muscle weakness, nervousness, depression, irritability, dermatitis, cracks at the corner of mouth, glossitis (smoothness of tongue), visual disturbances, morning sickness, amino acid/protein abnormalities.

Research: Since it is necessary for nitrogen group transfer, B-6 is essential in protein synthesis and breakdown. The requirement for B-6 increases as dietary protein increases. This reflects the increased utilization of pyridoxal-5-phosphate, the active form, which is necessary for the breakdown of the protein to amino acids. Additionally, it is involved in glycogen breakdown, and the conversion of tryptophan to nicotinamide, a form of vitamin B-3. Since tryptophan can be converted to niacin, and vitamin B-6 is a necessary cofactor, the same pellagra-like symptoms can appear as in niacin deficiency when vitamin B-6 is marginal (Gastroenterology Clinics of North America 1990;19(2):p.482).

In diabetes, the glucose level is elevated. It then becomes "glycosolated" (forms an adduct with a protein). Often the protein it joins with is hemoglobin (Hg), and glycosolated Hg is used as an indicator of glucose control (HgA 1c) in diabetics. Glycosolated proteins then undergo free radical attack, causing vascular damage, retinopathy and cataracts. **B-6**, by forming a Schiff's base to generate **P-5-P** (a form of B6), interrupts the cycle at glycosolation, and prevents the formation of glycosolated proteins which are susceptible to free radical attack. "Solomon and coworkers have found that administration of high-dose B-6 for six weeks resulted in decreased levels of hemoglobin A 1c... these observations suggest **B-6 supplementation has a beneficial role** for persons with diabetes" (Annals NY Acad Sci., Beyond Deficiency, 1992, 669:39).

In, "A deficiency of vitamin B-6 is a plausible molecular basis of the retinopathy of patients with diabetes mellitus", the authors reported that in 18 patients, some of whom were followed up to 28 years, they, "established an association of a deficiency of vitamin B-6 with diabetes...", by monitoring enzyme activity and occurrence of carpal tunnel syndrome (they claim it has been known for a decade that carpal tunnel syndrome is caused by a B-6 deficiency). Their observation of the absence of retinopathy in the treated diabetic patients, "appears monumental" (Ellis JN et al. Biochem Biophys Res Commun 1991;179(1):615-19). Pain scores were improved in those patients following B-6 treatment, and, "vitamin B-6 has been shown to change pain thresholds in clinical and laboratory studies" (Bernstein AL. J of the Am Coll Nutr 1993; 12(1):73-6). The researchers believe that carpal tunnel, whether or not it is caused by a deficiency of B-6, responds to B-6 therapy, with some responding better than others.

Sahakian et al. report in, "Vitamin B-6 is effective **therapy for nausea** and vomiting of pregnancy: a randomized, double-blind placebo-controlled study", that there was a significant difference in mean nausea scores (severity was graded on a scale of 1-10) (Sahakian V. et al. Obstet Gynecol. 1991; 78(1):33-36). The effectiveness against nausea makes it useful for morning sickness (Wright, Jonathan V. M.D. Healing with Nutrition. 1990. Keats Publishing, Inc. New Canaan, Conn. p. 519).

In the last decade, research has shown that elevated levels of **homocysteine** (indicating faulty methionine metabolism) may be a major risk factor in the development of vascular diseases, including coronary artery disease. Although genetic factors seem to play a role, "Mild hyperhomocysteinaemia can be reduced to normal in virtually all cases by simple and safe treatment with **vitamin B-6, folic acid, and betaine**, each of which is involved in methionine metabolism. A clinically beneficial effect of such an intervention, which is currently under investigation, could make large-scale screening mandatory for this risk factor" (Boers GH. Neth J Med. 1994; 45(1):34-41). Increased **B-12** levels are also related to lower homocysteine values (Rosenberg IH. Colloquium on Homocysteine, Vitamins, and Arterial Occlusive Diseases. Experimental Biology Conference, Atlanta, Ga. 1995).

"The prognosis for patients with primary **hyperoxaluria** has been ominous, with the expectation of renal failure, poor results with transplantation, and early death.... Treatment of patients with primary hyperoxaluria with orthophosphate and pyridoxine decreases urinary calcium oxalate crystallization and appears to preserve renal function" (Milliner DS et al. New England J Med. 1994; 331(23):1553-58). Other patients, exhibiting hyperoxalemia in association with Crohn's disease- related renal failure experienced successful management with pyridoxine (Marangell M. Nephrol Dial Transplant. 1992; 7(9):960-4).

B-6 is associated with preventing hormonal water-weight gain during PMS, and the pill seems to increase the need for B-6 (Wright, Jonathan V. M.D. Healing with Nutrition. 1990. Keats Publishing, Inc. New Canaan, Conn. p. 519). B-6 also seems to help with some of the other symptoms of PMS. For instance, one of the symptoms of PMS can be a low level of brain neurotransmitters, specifically dopamine. Dopamine suppresses fluid retention hormone production, and stimulates elimination of salt and water (Murray M. Enc Nat Med p. 474). The enzyme that makes dopamine is dependent on B-6, "and high supplemental doses of vitamin B-6 result in increased hypothalamic dopaminergic activity ... in addition, pyridoxine normalizes low intracellular magnesium, lowers premenstrual oestradiol levels, and increases progesterone" (Murray M. Enc Nat Med p. 476). **B-6 should never be taken in amounts greater than 250 mg, because neurological problems have been known to result** (Murray M. Enc Nat Med p. 475).

VITAMIN B-12 (Cyanocobalamin)

Sources: meat, fish, egg yolk, milk products (especially yogurt), also manufactured by bacteria in the intestines - not found in non-animal sources, thus a concern in vegetarians (may be found in tempeh and other fermented foods and some sprouts).

Functions: essential in nervous system function, stimulates growth and appetite in children, aids in red blood cell formation, increases energy level, stimulates utilization of carbohydrates, fats and proteins, important in DNA and RNA synthesis. Vitamin B-12 contains cobalt, an essential mineral. It aids in the treatment of **pernicious anemia**, along with the intrinsic factor (a mucoprotein enzyme produced by the stomach). HCl, calcium and thyroid hormone assist in the absorption of B-12.

Possible Effects of Deficiency: Even though the B vitamins are water-soluble, the body can draw vitamin B-12 from sources such as sloughed intestinal cells, so it may take years to show a deficiency. Deficiency symptoms can include nervous symptom disorders, mood changes with mental slowness, pernicious anemia (enlarged and fewer RBC's), fatigue, weakness, menstrual problems. Vitamin B-12 works similarly to folic acid, and high folic acid levels can mask a B-12 deficiency for a period of time. Vitamin B-12 deficiency can arise due to conditions which interfere with B-12 absorption, such as inflammatory bowel disease, or gastric surgery. If people lack the ability to produce intrinsic factor, which hooks onto B-12 in the small intestine for absorption, they require B-12 shots to bypass the digestive system. There is some evidence that sublingual lozenges also have some ability to bypass the digestive system and enter directly into the bloodstream.

Research: Research has shown that elevated levels of **homocysteine** (indicating faulty methionine metabolism) may be a major risk factor in the development of vascular diseases, including coronary artery disease. Increased **B-12** levels are related to lower homocysteine values (Rosenberg IH. Colloquium on Homocysteine, Vitamins, and Arterial Occlusive Diseases. Experimental Biology Conference, Atlanta, Ga. 1995).

Vitamin B-12 supplementation has been used with some success in treating diabetic neuropathy (Murray M. Enc of Nat Med. p. 284), in shortening recovery time from hepatitis (ibid. p. 352), and in treating urticaria (vascular reaction of the upper dermis) (ibid, p. 370). B-12 injections have been helpful in treating seborrhoeic dermatitis and bursitis (ibid, pp. 68,515).

B VITAMIN - FOLIC ACID

Sources: green, leafy vegetables including spinach, kale, chard, asparagus and broccoli, bean sprouts, wheat germ, whole grains, fruits including oranges, berries, cantaloupe, pineapple and bananas.

Functions: functions as coenzyme tetrahydrofolic acid (THFA); its functions are similar to vitamin B-12. It aids in RBC production, protein utilization, RNA and DNA synthesis, and is important in pregnancy since it is needed for the division of cells in the body. It is helpful in fatigue, stress, adrenal gland support, psoriasis, folic acid deficiency anemia, depression, and cervical tissue support. Para-aminobenzoic acid (PABA) is part of the folic acid structure.

Possible Effects of Deficiency: It is essential that excess folic acid is not given when there is a B-12 deficiency. Folic acid will mask symptoms associated with a B-12-related anemia, which could potentially lead to nerve damage. Folic acid deficiency symptoms include anemia, depression, irritability, fatigue, anorexia, headache, tongue inflammation, heart palpitations, poor memory and a feeling of paranoia. Folic-acid deficiency anemia (large, irregular RBC's) is different than iron-deficiency anemia (small RBC's) and is not corrected by giving iron. Neural tube defects have been correlated to low levels of folate (The Lancet 1991; 338:131-36). Pregnant females require at least double the amount of folic acid required by non-pregnant females.

Research: Folic acid is necessary for proper immune function. It is important in the single carbon transfer reactions needed for DNA synthesis, and amino acid metabolism. In fact, deprivations of folic acid, "disrupt the tissue barriers to infection and markedly depress the cell-mediated immune system (Int J Vit Nutr Res. 49). "Any illness that increases the metabolic rate (for example, infection) or cell turnover (for example, gastrointestinal bleeding) increases folic acid requirements" (Gastroenterology Clinics of North America 1990;

19(2):482). Additionally, medications which inhibit intestinal folate absorption also increase folate requirements (ibid, p.482). Research supports the administration of folic acid to pregnant mothers to prevent neural tube defects (The Lancet Prevention of neural tube defects: Results of the Medical Research Council Vitamin Study. 1991; 338:131-36).

In the last decade, research has shown that elevated levels of **homocysteine** (indicating faulty methionine metabolism) may be a major risk factor in the development of vascular diseases, including coronary artery disease. Although genetic factors seem to play a role, "Mild hyperhomocysteinaemia can be reduced to normal in virtually all cases by simple and safe treatment with **vitamin B-6, folic acid, and betaine**, each of which is involved in methionine metabolism. A clinically beneficial effect of such an intervention, which is currently under investigation, could make large-scale screening mandatory for this risk factor" (Boers GH. Neth J Med. 1994; 45(1):34-41). Folic acid supplementation was found to be a major factor in lowering homocysteine levels in a clinical trial where the results indicated, "that folate deficiency may be an important cause of hyperhomocysteinemia in the general population" (Ubbini JB et al. J of Nutr. 1994; 124(10):1927-33).

B VITAMIN - BIOTIN

Sources: found in small amounts in egg yolks, liver, unpolished rice, brewer's yeast, milk, fish and nuts; also produced by the intestinal microflora.

Functions: essential for fat metabolism and aids in the production of DNA and RNA.

Possible Effects of Deficiency: Biotin is widely distributed in food, and a deficiency is not usually seen unless a person has consumed large amounts of raw egg white, which contains avidin (binds biotin). This is why dermatitis and depression can show up as a result of ingestion (Gastroenterology Clinics of North America 1990; 19(2):482). Deficiency symptoms include fatigue, anorexia, nausea, depression, dry, flaky skin and muscle weakness.

VITAMIN C (ASCORBIC ACID)

Sources: found only in fruits and vegetables including citrus fruits (oranges, lemons, limes, tangerines and grapefruits), berries, melons, asparagus, onions, tomatoes, spinach, greens, red and green peppers.

Functions: maintains collagen, wound healing, formation of RBC's, aids in absorption of iron, fights bacterial infections, enhances WBC production, promotes thymic hormone secretion, antioxidant, aids in the metabolism of tyrosine, folic acid and tryptophan, stimulates adrenal function, aids in thyroid hormone production and cholesterol metabolism, acts as a detoxifier of certain metals and drugs, recycles other hydrogen donors such as vitamin E, and aids in phagocytosis (digestion of damaged, dead or foreign cells).

Vitamin C is necessary for the enzyme reactions of many physiological processes, including collagen synthesis. For instance, there is an enzyme that changes the amino acid proline into a compound that is one of the main constituents of **collagen**. There is also an enzyme which changes the amino acid lysine into a compound that can be incorporated into collagen. Both of these **enzymes require iron that has been reduced by vitamin C.** Unless vitamin C is present, a bridge forms in the enzyme and inactivates it. The collagen that is synthesized can't form fibers properly, resulting in skin lesions, blood vessel fragility, and poor wound healing - in other words, the symptoms of scurvy. The **prevention of scurvy** is the function of vitamin C that is most widely recognized.

Possible Effects of Deficiency: scurvy, easily bruised, impaired digestion, poor circulation, increased infection, swollen or painful joints, slow wound healing, bleeding gums.

Clinical Applications: common cold, antioxidant function, adrenal and thyroid support, viral infections, inflammation, asthma, post-surgical support, may decrease withdrawal symptoms from addictive substances, heavy metal toxicities, diabetes, eye problems (antioxidant effect), heart disease.

Adjunctive Tips: Ascorbic acid was discovered in the 1700's when many British sailors died from scurvy. James Lind discovered that the juice of lemons and limes could prevent scurvy, and from that point on, the sailors were known as "limeys" because the ships were required to carry British West Indies limes to prevent scurvy. That is where ascorbic acid got its name, from its anti-scorbutic properties. High intake of vitamin C may be a concern in people with kidney stones because of the increased oxalic acid clearance through the kidneys due to vitamin C metabolism, and can cause diarrhea in some people. Also, in those exhibiting iron overload disease, supplementation can be harmful.

Research: (See also Antioxidants) The authors of "The CRC Handbook of Free Radicals and Antioxidants in Biomedicine" conclude that, "The presence of hypercholesterolemia, hypertension, and atherosclerosis is more frequent in humans with a low intake of vitamin C. Optimum intake of ascorbic acid to prevent these disorders ... probably exceeds tenfold the doses officially recommended and is in the range of some hundred milligrams of ascorbic acid per day" (Miquel & Quintanilha, 1989; CRC Press, Boca Raton, Fla. p. 194). The same handbook points out that prevalence of low vitamin C levels increases with age, and, "the age-related rise in serum cholesterol may result from vitamin C deficiency" (ibid, p 192). Chronic subclinical deficiency, "...may result in progressive oxidative damage which in the long run may lead to permanent degenerative diseases in the heart" (Mol Cell Biochem 1992 111:41-7). For instance, it is known that, "...regions with medium to high coronary mortality had a significantly lower vitamin C status" (Gey K et al. Am J Clin Nutr 1987;45:p.1369).

When vitamin C was given in gram amounts to hyperlipidemic subjects and to two subjects with hypertriglyceridemia, it led to a massive decrease in circulating triglycerides (Sokoloff, B, Hori, M, Saelhof, CC et al. J Am Geriatr Soc. 14:1239-60, 1966; Ginter, E, N Engl J Med. 294:559-60, 1976.; Gooly, KL, Diamond, LH. Ann Intern Med. 93:511, 1980). Vitamin C's antioxidant function prevents the oxidation of low density lipoprotein, which has been shown to be instrumental in heart disease. Chronic subclinical deficiency, "...may result in progressive oxidative damage which in the long run may lead to permanent degenerative diseases in the heart" (Mol Cell Biochem 1992 111:41-7). One puff on a cigarette depletes the plasma vitamin C content by as much as 50%. This is why increased vitamin C intake has been advised for smokers (Efstratopoulos AD & Voyaki SM J of Hypertension 1993 11(suppl 5):S112-113).

Since lipid peroxidation can cause the increase of a major blood clotter known as thromboxane, it is not a surprise that clinical trials are now showing that vitamin C can lower blood pressure. In addition, the superoxide radical can interfere with a vessel dilation factor known as nitric oxide, and may have a role in the development of hypertension. The data of Ceriello suggest that, "antioxidants might have a dilatory effect and that an imbalance of the nitric oxide-free radical interaction might facilitate the development of hypertension in humans" (Ceriello, et al. Clinical Science. 1991. 81:739-42). When Trout et al. supplemented 12 borderline hypertensives with 1 gram of vitamin C for six weeks, they demonstrated a significant reduction in blood pressure. Since the basal fasting levels of vitamin C were more than adequate, the authors postulated that even larger reductions would be seen if the hypertensives studied did not have adequate vitamin C to start (Trout, D.L. 1991. American Journal of Clinical Nutrition, 53:322S-25S).

Extra addition of vitamin C seems to **boost the immune system** by increasing cellular immune functions and stimulating neutrophils. Patients receiving 1 gram vitamin C daily had improved neutrophil activity, resulting in a dramatic reduction of infectious attacks (Anderson, R. Int J Vitam Nutr Res. Suppl. 23:23-34, 1982; Patrone, R, Dallegri, F, Bonvivi, E, et al. Acta Vitaminol Enzymol. 4:163-68, 1982). According to a recent report in Allergy and Imm. (Feb., 1993), **Vitamin C** has a "special influence" on enhancing the immune response and warding off infection. Several studies of groups taking vitamin C show that it reduces the longevity and severity of colds (Brit. J. Nutr. 67:3-16). One group, taking 600 mg. supplements, had upper respiratory tract infections reduced by 50% (Amer. J. Clin. Nutr. 57:170-74). Most importantly, vitamin C treated groups don't feel as bad while they are sick. When this means less sick days and less interference with our daily lives, vitamin C can be a great help in keeping our production levels up.

Muscle carnitine is thought to be a sensitive indicator of vitamin C status, and, "Symptoms such as fatigue and lassitude seen in vitamin C-depleted human volunteers may be the result of poor energy production due to decreased carnitine biosynthesis" (Shils & Young, p.422). Given the many varied functions of vitamin C in the body, it is no surprise that it is also essential to immunocompetence. Larger doses than the RDA, "may be useful in preventing the formation of carcinogenic nitrosamines and boosting immunity" (Gastroenterology Clinics of North America 1990;19(2):p.483). Consumption of vitamin C has been inversely related to incidences of cancer in epidemiological studies (Kromhout D. Essential micronutrients in relation to carcinogenesis. Am J Clin Nutr

1987;45:1361-7). The elderly are particularly susceptible to low plasma and tissue vitamin C and leukocyte levels (Gastroenterology Clinics of North America 1990;19(2):483).

A UCLA researcher James Enstrom says that 300 mg of vitamin C a day (half from supplements) will extend the life of men 5 or 6 years longer than those getting only 25 mg. Enstrom claims that the same amount will add two years on to a woman's life (Fort Collins Coloradoan USA Weekend, Sept 30, 1994 p. 10).

VITAMIN D

Sources: butter and milk, egg yolk, halibut, salmon, tuna, sweet potatoes, vegetable oils, cod liver oil, alfalfa, and oatmeal; manufactured in the skin when exposed to sunshine.

Functions: necessary for normal bone and cartilage mineralization, and also for maintaining normal calcium levels (essential for absorption and utilization of calcium and phosphorus from the gastro-intestinal tract), works with parathyroid hormone to control calcium metabolism, calcification of bones and teeth in children, valuable in maintaining a stable nervous system, normal blood clotting and normal heart action (all are related to the body's supply and utilization of calcium and phosphorus). If vitamin D is low, blood levels of calcium and phosphorus will decrease, causing these minerals to be pulled out of the bone, resulting in bone health problems.

Possible Effects of Deficiency: bone disease, rickets (in children) and/or osteomalacia (loss of bone minerals) in adults, calcium malabsorption, gum disease, retarded growth, osteoporosis.

Clinical Applications: maintain healthy bones and teeth, osteoporosis and other bone problems.

Adjunctive Tips: Vitamin D can be considered both a vitamin and a hormone because it is produced in one part of the body (the skin) and is released into the blood to affect other tissues (the bones).

Research: Vitamin D stimulates calcium and phosphorus transport in the intestine, and calcium reabsorption by the kidney, and may act in this capacity to prevent osteoporosis (Gastroenterology Clinics of North America 1990;19(2):p.481). Supplementation of vitamin D has been shown to reduce fracture rates (Br Med J. 1994; 308:1081-82). A recent study demonstrated that in healthy, postmenopausal women, supplementation of vitamin D up to 200 IU was enough to prevent bone loss from the femoral neck. Researchers concluded that the RDA needs to be increased in an effort to reduce bone loss from the hip, and note that 800 IU/day, "is safe and effective" (AJCN 1995; 61:1140).

VITAMIN E

Sources: wheat germ, cold-pressed oils, green, leafy vegetables, nuts, milk, eggs, brown rice, oatmeal, soybeans.

Functions: antioxidant, inhibits coagulation, strengthens capillary walls, stabilizes cell membranes, prevents proteins, lipids, hormones (such as pituitary and adrenal), and other substances from being oxidized, and promotes proper functioning of linoleic acid, an unsaturated fatty acid.

Possible Effects of Deficiency: premature aging, cardiovascular and circulatory problems, impotence, female problems, heart and nervous disorders, weakened immune system.

Clinical Applications: useful in all diseases either caused by free radical damage or resulting in free radical damage (especially diabetes and eye disorders), skin conditions, and prevention of heart disease.

Research: (See also antioxidants) In an issue of the American Journal of Clinical Nutrition (June, 1994), twenty elderly subjects were studied for glucose control. Those receiving 900 mg of vitamin E for four months has their glucose disposal "significantly potentiated", and the authors concluded that, "Plasma vitamin E concentrations seem to play an important role in the modulation of insulin action in elderly people" (AJCN, June, 1994; p. 1295). It was suggested that the beneficial effects of vitamin E on insulin action are linked to its effect in lowering lipid peroxidation, and protecting the integrity of the plasma membranes.

"Thus, one can hypothesize that daily oral vitamin E supplements might improve the physical state of plasma membranes and their related activities as insulin-mediated glucose transport" (ibid, p. 1295).

VITAMIN F (UNSATURATED FATTY ACIDS)

(See also Essential Fatty Acids in the Nutrients section)

Sources: vegetable oils, fish, seeds, butter, wheat germ.

Functions: important for respiration of vital organs, helps maintain resilience and lubrication of all cells, essential for normal glandular activity, especially thyroid and adrenal glands, essential for healthy mucous membranes and nerves, related to normal function of the reproductive system.

Possible Effects of Deficiency: heart disorders, female disorders, skin disorders, celiac disease, cystic fibrosis, intestinal disorders, high cholesterol, yeast infections, liver disorders, malformation of tissues

VITAMIN K

Sources: kelp, alfalfa, leafy green vegetables, blackstrap molasses, liver, soybeans, egg yolks, safflower oil; also synthesized by the intestinal flora.

Functions: necessary for the formation of prothrombin (needed for blood clotting), vital for normal liver function, needed for phosphorylation (glucose + phosphate = glycogen). Three other factors involved in blood clotting, besides prothrombin, depend on vitamin K: factor IX, factor VII, and factor X. Vitamin K functions in the carboxylation reactions of glutamic acid (there is a glutamic acid portion of prothrombin that it carboxylates to make active), and this action may contribute to bone mineralization by forming a calcium-binding protein called "eseocalcin" (Garrison RH and Somer E. Nutr Desk Ref. 1985. Keats Publ. New Canaan, Conn. p. 42).

Possible Effects of Deficiency: hemorrhaging, hemorrhoids and bruising, delayed blood clotting, liver disorders, intestinal disorders, hemophilia, leg ulcers, colitis and diverticulitis.

Adjunctive Tips: Some antagonists, such as the anticoagulants coumadin and heparin, can interfere with vitamin K's absorption and use. Salicylates (e.g. aspirin) can increase the need for vitamin K. Ingestion of antibiotics interfere with microbial activity, and indirectly decrease the intestinal synthesis of vitamin K. Bowel-sterilizing antibiotics, such as neomycin, can initiate a vitamin K deficiency. Some patients with liver disease are unable to utilize vitamin K, and, "should be challenged with vitamin K to determine the extent of the organic disorder preventing biosynthesis of prothrombin" (Shils and Young, p. 336). Megadoses of vitamin E can antagonize the action of vitamin K.

Research: "Vitamin K, in water- or fat- soluble forms, is effective in raising prothrombin levels and controlling hemorrhage in newborns. Newborns will show reduced plasma prothrombin concentrations because of the placenta's poor transmission of fats and the sterility of the gut the first few days. (These levels begin to rise to normal by the third or fourth day). To prevent hemorrhage, expectant mothers are given supplemental vitamin K for several days prior to delivery. The infant is given supplements during the first days of life" (Garrison and Somer, Nutr Desk Ref. p. 42).

VITAMIN P (BIOFLAVONOIDS)

(See also Bioflavonoids)

Sources: lemons, oranges, limes, grapes, grapefruit, buckwheat (high in rutin), cherries, prunes, plums, papayas, green peppers, broccoli and tomatoes.

Functions: aids in the proper absorption and use of vitamin C, assists vitamin C in maintaining collagen health, acts as an antioxidant, chelates copper from the body, maintains capillary integrity and regulates permeability, prevents rupture of the capillaries that causes bruising, decreases the amount of histamine released from cells, also known as an antiviral. Bioflavonoids are used in inflammatory and allergic problems. They are effective because they stabilize cell membranes, decrease the release of inflammation mediators, and decrease the contraction of smooth muscle (Murray M. Enc of Nat Med. p.298). Bioflavonoids also improve capillary integrity and stabilize the collagen matrix by preventing free radical damage ((Merck Index, p.1243; Murray M. Enc of Nat Med. p.330).

Possible Effects of Deficiency: varicose veins, infection, easily bruised, immune deficiency, colitis, hemorrhoids, heel and bone spurs.

Clinical Applications:

1) Colds and flus - assists in vitamin C functions.
2) Increases capillary integrity, especially for easy bruising, bleeding gums, bleeding ulcers, hemorrhoids, varicose veins and nosebleeds. Rutin is specifically beneficial for this function.
3) Spontaneous abortions.
4) Allergies, asthma, bursitis, arthritis and eye problems.

Adjunctive Tips: Bioflavonoids are otherwise known as vitamin P because of their "permeability factor" (Merck Index, p.1243). A Soviet scientist first discovered the vitamin in 1936 in the white rinds of citrus fruits. The bioflavonoids include several components that work synergistically including hesperidin, rutin, quercetin, flavones, flavonols, citrin and catechin.

Research: The bioflavonoids are closely associated with vitamin C and **enhance the effect of vitamin C** when used in treatment (Merck Index, p. 1243).. Bioflavonoids, "contribute to the maintenance of **normal blood vessel conditions** by **decreasing capillary permeability and fragility**" (Merck Index, p. 1243). Bioflavonoids have been used in the **treatment of stomach ulcers** by **strengthening the capillaries** and making them **less susceptible to HCl.** They prevent free radical damage and inhibit enzymatic breakdown of the collagen matrix, and aid in the cross linking of collagen fibers to form a more stable collagen matrix. (Murray M. Enc Nat Med, p. 330).

Bioflavonoids have a positive, **protective effect on human viruses** (J. Med. Virol. 15:71-79). They seem to **reduce inflammation**, and **protect cells** (Biochem. Pharmacol. 45:13-9). When bioflavonoids were tested for their ability to **increase bacteria-engulfing white blood cells**, the proliferation not only increased, but the stimulating activity **correlated with the concentration of flavonoids** (Biull. Eksp. Biol. Med. 114:520-21). Rutin is one of the bioflavonoids, and has been called, "the most **effective inhibitor of lymphocyte damage**". (Mutat. Research, 265:245-53). One of the most intriguing facets of rutin is a **cell-protecting ability.** (Free Rad. in Biol. and Med., 12:101-6). Interestingly, when **vitamin C** was added to rutin, a "**supra-additive effect** was noted" (Pharmacol., 42:262-72). **Rutin** is used as a treatment for **varicose veins, hemorrhoids and high blood pressure**.

Biochem. Pharmacol. (1993, 46:182-5), reports **silymarin** (a flavonoid), to be a chain-breaking antioxidant, and an effective protective agent against lipid peroxidation. "**It is generally accepted that silymarin exerts a membrane-stabilizing action preventing or inhibiting membrane peroxidation**" (Mem Inst Oswaldo Cruz 1991, 86:79-85). In a one-month double blind clinical trial of 60 patients, **silymarin** not only demonstrated protective effects, but was able to **boost the immune system** (Ital J Gastroenterol. 1990, 22:283-7).

Quercetin, called, "the most important flavonoid" (Nutr. Cancer 1993, 20:21-9) is a powerful **antioxidant** which has demonstrated **anticarcinogenic** properties. **Hesperidin**, another bioflavonoid, **inhibits histamine release** from mast cells (histamine can cause sneezing, itching, watery eyes, etc.) and has proven to have **effective anti-allergic action** (Yakugaku-Zasshi, 111:193-98).

ANTIOXIDANTS

Sources: fresh fruits and vegetables; especially cruciferous vegetables such as broccoli.

Functions: **Free radicals** carry a single electron in their outer shell, making them **highly reactive.** Unfortunately, sometimes they react with various cellular components and **destroy** them in the process. The double bond, present in the fatty acid of the cell membrane, is in a vulnerable position for the free radical to steal an electron. The **loss of the electron** converts the fatty acid into a **radical,** which in turn converts the next fatty acid into a radical, and so on, known as the "**chain reaction**" of lipid peroxidation. With the change to a radical, the composition of the fatty acid is drastically affected. Since every cell membrane is composed of a phospholipid bilayer which includes these fatty acids, the disruption eventually ends in **membrane rupture and cell death** when the chain is not interrupted.

Antioxidants, which **stabilize radicals** and **halt the chain reaction**, can **prevent** that **damage** and **maintain** the **integrity of cell membranes.** The antioxidant vitamins work in different capacities to fight against cellular damage. For instance, vitamin C is an important aqueous radical quencher, which means that it works against the beginning radical formation in the watery portion of intracellular and extracellular components. Vitamin E is known as the major lipid antioxidant, and it works mainly against the lipid peroxidation of lipid cell membranes. Vitamin E is known as the "chain-breaker", because it stops the chain reaction of damage. Beta-carotene, which is a precursor to vitamin A, is also a lipid antioxidant, however it functions mainly in areas of low oxygen concentration.

Research: The antioxidant vitamins decrease cellular damage related to many diseases, and therefore have been reported to be associated with the decreased incidence of many diseases, including gastric cancer. For instance, supplements of vitamin C, vitamin E and beta-carotene were reported in Nutrition Reviews to decrease risk of gastric cancer Rev. (Nutr Rev. 1994; 52(3):75-83).

"Vitamins A, E, C and carotenoids are able to protect cells and **enhance humoral and cellular immune responses** in disease" (Nockels, C.F. The role of vitamins in modulating disease resistance. 1988. Vet Clin North Am Food Anim Pract 4(3):531-42). In a clinical trial, 300 women who had developed precancerous cells in the cervix entered a study where half of them received treatment consisting of vaginal sponges which released a synthetic relative of **vitamin A**. In the moderate cases, the **precancerous spots disappeared** in the treated women (Science News. 1994;143(22):341). Numerous studies point to the beneficial effects of the **antioxidant vitamins** in cancer protection (Dietary carotenes, vitamin C and vitamin E as protective antioxidants in human cancers. Annu Rev Nutr 1992;12:139-59). **Beta carotene** seems to have a protective antioxidant effect on DNA, as Japanese researcher Keizo Umegaki of the National Institute of Health and Nutrition in Tokyo just reported last February that **beta-carotene, "significantly reduces chromosome damage"** (Science News. 1994; 145:126).

Antioxidants help **protect** against oxidative damage to the sensitive cells of the **digestive tract**, especially the mucosal cells, which contain the villi responsible for food breakdown and absorption. Additionally, the efficacy of natural plant medicinal products was enhanced in patients who were able to degrade them into compounds with antioxidant activity; in other words, **the ability to increase free radical scavengers dramatically increased the positive response to herbal therapy.** In patients responding the best, their gastric juice produced the most compounds with antioxidant activity, including **beta-carotene and vitamin E.** This led researchers to report that, " These findings suggest that one of the factors determining the **clinical response to natural herbal medicinal products** is the ability of the patient's digestive system to degrade the product to **liberate bioactive compounds (with antioxidant activity)"** (Planta Med 1991;57(4):299-304).

UV light can be a source of free radicals, and since the eye has a high phospholipid content, the eye is quite susceptible to free radical attack. For instance, macular degeneration was one of five retinal disorders studied in the massive **Eye Disease Case-Control Study**, which obtained data from 421 patients with macular degeneration and 615 controls. Serum levels of **carotenoids, vitamins C and E, and selenium** were evaluated, and subjects were classified by level of the micronutrient (low, medium, and high). Persons in the **medium and high carotenoid** groups had, **"markedly reduced risks"** of macular degeneration. Risk in the "high" group was reduced to one half, and risk in the "medium" group was reduced to one third, demonstrating a dose-dependent result. **"An antioxidant index which combined all four micronutrient measurements showed statistically significant reductions of risk with increasing levels of the index... these results suggest that higher blood levels of micronutrients with antioxidant potential, in particular, carotenoids, may be associated with a decreased risk of the most visually disabling form of age-related macular degeneration "** (Arch. Ophthalmol. 1993, 111:104-9).

Authors of "Antioxidant protection of the ageing macula" report epidemiological evidence that suggests **patients with macular degeneration have a lower intake of carotenoids**, and, "moreover, a preliminary therapeutic trial in patients with AMD (Age-related macular degeneration) or diabetic retinopathy showed that **supplementation with beta-carotene, vitamin C, vitamin E and selenium halted the progression of degenerative changes and in some cases even brought improvement"** (Age and ageing 1991, 20:60-69). The clinical trial they refer to involved over 500 patients who received 500 mg vitamin C, 400 IU vitamin E, 9 mg beta carotene and 250 ug selenium daily for 7 to 12 years. The authors note that even though the retina contains higher concentrations of carotenoids, vitamin E and vitamin C than many other tissues, "the fact that the development of AMD still occurs indicates that in these cases **the balance between lifelong exposure to light and antioxidant protection has been disturbed in favor of light damage.** A higher intake of these antioxidant nutrients may thus be required to counteract the influence of light" (Ibid, p. 66).

The radicals formed from UV light can alter proteins, and the accumulation of damaged proteins sometimes occludes the eye in **cataracts**. Jacque and Chylack, authors of, "Epidemiologic evidence of a role for the antioxidant vitamins and carotenoids in cataract prevention", classified their subjects into three levels of vitamin C and beta-carotene status: low, intermediate, and high. **Persons with the lowest vitamin C intake had 11 times the risk of developing cataracts** as persons with the highest intake (Am J Clin Nutr. 1991, 53:3520S-25S). In the same study, **low plasma carotenoid levels corresponded to a seven-fold risk** over those with high levels.

In a review of the research on cataracts and antioxidants, The Annals of the NY Acad Sci. notes that, "Epidemiological and laboratory studies indicate that **cataractogenesis is causally related to photooxidative stress...** It appears possible to increase eye levels of some antioxidants... **several studies noted a correlation between enhanced dietary antioxidant intake or elevated plasma antioxidant levels and diminished risk of developing cataracts.** Inasmuch as age-related degeneration of the macula may be related to nutrition in similar ways as cataracts, these observations regarding benefits of antioxidant status may have extra value" (Annals NY Acad Sci, Beyond Def, 1992; 669: p. 118).

Vitamin E comes to the rescue after free radical damage. When free radical damage has already disrupted the lipids in the cell membrane, it is up to vitamin E to "stop the chain reaction". It donates a hydrogen to the radical, and neutralizes its activity. This is why vitamin E is called the major lipid antioxidant in the body.

When the red blood cell membrane is peroxidized, it loses its ability to change shape and squeeze through the vessels, and leads to a rupturing of the membrane, or hemolysis. Vitamin E has demonstrated a protective effect against this hemolysis in blood diseases, including sickle cell anemia. "In these diseases, there is extra oxidant stress, or a decrease in other protective mechanisms, so that the effects of vitamin E are more readily seen" (Halliwell and Gutteridge, Free Radicals in Biology and Medicine, 1990. New York, Oxford University Press, p. 173).

Two MD's were prompted to recommend antioxidant supplementation in <u>The New England Journal of Medicine</u> in Nov. of 1993. They cited the studies of Rimm, et al., who examined thousands of people, and determined that vitamin E reduced the risk for heart disease (New Eng J Med, 1993; 328:1444-56). In a letter to the editor, they pointed out that, "A substantial number of physicians in the United States are sufficiently convinced of the potential benefits of vitamin E to supplement their own diets with it. If vitamin E is good enough for physicians, should it not be good enough for our patients?" (James H. O'Keefe, Jr., MD, Mid America Heart Institute, Kansas City, Mo., and Carl J. Lavie, MD, Ochsner Heart and Vascular Institute, New Orleans, La. p. 1424).

When the lipid membrane of the cell is disrupted, along with the lipid membranes of intracellular structures, it's no wonder that so many disruptions of homeostasis result. It is also no surprise that there are so many strong associations between vitamin E and related diseases. Perhaps Isadore Rosenfels, MD had this in mind when he stated that, "Vitamin E is an antioxidant whose time has come".

Due to the accumulated scientific research that points to the protective qualities of antioxidant vitamins, more and more researchers and physicians are admitting that supplementation may be necessary to achieve this protection. Russian researchers have been prompted to advise, "It is probable that an increased intake of antioxidants (**ascorbic acid, carotenes, tocopherols, bioflavonoids, selenium,** etc.) would, along with other corrective provisions, **suppress** the steep increase of **cardiovascular disease"** (Vnitr Lek 1992; 38:1096-1104).

Besides these antioxidant vitamins, there are other substance which possesses antioxidant activity (see also Bioflavonoids, or vitamin P). The minerals zinc and selenium, for instance, are reported to have this activity. Zinc is an essential element in **superoxide dismutase (SOD),** a potent radical scavenging enzyme. Research demonstrates that high levels of **SOD** , "protect mitochondria from oxidative damage that probably occurs with ageing in the retinal pigment epithelium (Invest. Ophthalmol. Vis. Sci. 1992, 33:1909-18). Selenium is an essential element in another radical scavenging enzyme, glutathione peroxidase.

Turmerin, which forms 0.1% of the weight of the spice **turmeric**, contains three residues of methionine that are partly responsible for its antioxidant activity. " **Free Radicals in Biology and Medicine** (1991, 11:277-83), found **turmeric** to be **the most effective protectant** against DNA oxidative damage in human lymphocytes, amongst the ingredients they tested.. **Turmeric used widely as a spice would probably mitigate the effects of several dietary carcinogens**" (Plant Foods Hum. Nutr 1993, 44:87-92). Other spices of nature, in the limelight for their antioxidant properties, are: **cloves, cumin, red chilies, ginger, coriander, and black pepper** (Mol Cell Biochem 1992, 111:117-24; Indian J Biochem Biophys. 1993, 30:130-4).

MINERALS

The minerals are inorganic substances which differ from the other nutrients because they are elements, not compounds. That is, they consist of molecules of atoms which are all alike. Compounds have two or more different kinds of atoms. This makes them much smaller than even the vitamins; sometimes minerals are only one atom, such as sodium (Na+). Like the vitamins, minerals do not provide any direct energy to the body, rather they assist in metabolic reactions, and give fluids necessary characteristics to function.

GENERAL DISCLAIMER

The nutritional suggestions and research reported in this book are not offered to treat, mitigate or cure disease, and should not be used as a substitute for sound medical advice. This book is designed to be used in conjunction with the services provided by a trained, licensed healthcare practitioner.

CAUTION

Caution should be used in all conditions, especially concerning pregnancy and children, when taking herbal supplements or high potency nutrients. A physician knowledgeable in natural and preventative medicine should be consulted.

It is the reader's responsibility to be aware of certain contraindications, toxicology and drug-nutrient interactions which may occur. A concise table of drug-nutrient interactions has been provided for information, however, competent resources, such as "Shils and Young, Modern Nutrition in Health and Disease", Lea & Febiger, Phil, Pa 1988, should be consulted for the RDA's and upper limits of vitamins and minerals (Contraindications and Toxicology). As an example, vitamin C supplementation to people with iron overload disease (2% of the population) can be harmful and even fatal. Less information is available on herbs and other supplements, and several resources are recommended, such as the "Lawrence Review of Natural Products", Facts and Comparisons, St. Louis, Missouri. 1996, and the German monographs.

BORON

Sources: whole grains, fruits, vegetables, nuts and seeds.

Function: decreases urinary excretion of calcium and magnesium, increases estradiol levels to aid in preventing bone loss; helps in activating vitamin D to aid in calcium absorption and utilization.

Possible Effects of Deficiency: The most consistent sign of deficiency is depressed growth. "Studies defining the signs of boron deprivation are not complete. Therefore, definitively stating deficiency signs is difficult" (Shils & Young, p. 282).

Research: Boron is a, "dynamic ultratrace element that affects major mineral metabolism in higher animals. Thus, boron nutrition might have a role in some disorders of unknown etiology that exhibit disturbed major mineral metabolism (i.e. osteoporosis)" (Shils & Young, p. 283). The essentiality of boron has been debated; "Between 1981 and 1985, however, evidence was accumulated that indicated boron might be an essential nutrient" (Shils & Young, p. 281).

Boron naturally elevates estradiol levels, and decreases urinary excretion of calcium and magnesium. Osteoarthritis patients have shown improvement when supplemented with boron (Giller, R., M.D., and Matthews, K., Natural Prescriptions, Ballantine Books, NY, p. 245). A possible mechanism is via the parathyroid gland, which contains more boron than any other tissue. Boron enhances parahormone activity, and the parathyroid gland is the primary organ controlling mineralization of bone. (Burton Goldberg Group, Alternative Medicine: The Definitive Guide, Future Medicine Publishing, Inc. WA, 533).

CALCIUM

Sources: dairy products, tofu, kelp and dulse, green, leafy vegetables, broccoli, brewers yeast, oats, sardines, salmon, prunes and figs.

Functions: builds and maintains bones and teeth (along with phosphorus), essential for healthy blood, helps regulate heartbeat, eases insomnia, assists in blood clotting, plays a part in muscle growth, muscle contraction, and nerve transmission, aids in iron utilization, activates several enzymes, regulates passage of nutrients in and out of cells.

Possible Effects of Deficiency: osteoporosis, muscle cramps, rickets, osteomalacia, insomnia, mouth and gum disease, heart disorders, colitis, colon cancer, rheumatism, hypertension, brittle nails, nervous disorders.

Research: In addition to maintaining healthy bones, calcium maintains healthy tissues also, and functions as a **natural tranquilizer,** aids certain **colon conditions, relieves cramps**, and acts as a **cofactor in many enzyme reactions** (Hendlor, Sheldon. The Doctor's Vitamin and Mineral Encyclopedia. 1990. Simon and Schuster, NY. pp. 116-123). Calcium also plays a role in the intricate balance of **ion transport, muscle contraction, heartbeat maintenance, nerve impulses, and muscle tone** (Whitney E.R. and Nunnelley, E.M. Understanding Nutrition. 4th ed. 1987. West Publishing, NY. p. 390).

Calcium is critical to normal bone function, and supplementation has been **beneficial in preventing bone loss.** In 1990, it was stated that, "The current RDA of calcium for **older adults** (800 mg) is controversial, and it has been **suggested that 1500 mg/day is required for adequate calcium balance**" (Gastroenterology Clinics of North America 1990;19(2):p.484). Since that time, the RDA has been raised closer to 1,200 mg, depending on gender and age. Pregnant and lactating mothers are advised to take at least 1600 mg of calcium a day. A National Institutes of Health panel reported that **½ of all Americans consume too little calcium** (NIH Committee, Nutrition Week 22:7, June 10, 1994).

Calcium helps **transport essential minerals t**o the site of inflammation. After periods of trauma, the system tends to be alkaline, and it is important for an acid-calcium to deliver healing nutrients to binding sites. An acid environment solubilizes and ionizes the insoluble calcium salts in the body (calcium has to be ionized in the intestines in order to be absorbed). For instance, calcium **significantly improves symptoms of pouchitis** (chronic and/or acute inflammation of the ileal reservoir (Ann Chiro 1993;47(10):1049-53).

Calcium has repeatedly shown in clinical trials that one of its effects on the cardiovascular system is to **lower blood pressure**, therefore having the potential to reduce risk for heart disease (Belizan, JM Villar J. Gonzales, L. "Calcium supplementation to prevent **hypertensive** disorders of pregnancy" NEJM 1991; 325(20): 1399-1404. Calcium supplementation on normotensive and **hypertensive** pregnant women. AJCN 1992; 55:891-95. Dietary calcium and blood pressure: modifying factors in special populations. AJCN 1991; 54:215S-21).

Calcium is a potent, but **inexpensive antacid** when chewed. Calcium combined with magnesium can provide great symptomatic relief during heartburn. "The net effect of antacid action (of calcium) is **reduction in gastric acidity and in peptic activity...**" (Postgrad Med 1993;93(6):149-50). Do not use for prolonged periods of time, because it has a **rebound effect** on the stomach by initially decreasing HCl production, which is followed by an increase in HCl secretion. It should be recognized that this is only treatment of a symptom, whereas the underlying cause is insufficient mucosal protection. Chronic abuse of **calcium containing antacids** can lead to hypercalcemia and milk-alkali syndrome, a serious condition. Kidney stone formers should not take calcium supplementation for prolonged periods of time. Eating a red meat/**high protein diet can leach calcium** from the system.

CHLORIDE

Sources: table salt, kelp, dulse, rye flour olives, fish, alfalfa, milk.

Functions: regulates correct acid/alkaline balance in the blood, stimulates production of HCl, stimulates the liver and helps clean toxic waste products out of the system.

Possible Effects of Deficiency: hair and tooth loss, poor muscular contraction and digestive problems.

CHROMIUM

Sources: whole grains, brewers yeast, liver, beef, brown rice, mushrooms, potatoes, dried beans, beets.

Functions: critical component of the glucose tolerance factor (GTF), increases effectiveness of insulin, stimulates activity of enzymes involved in glucose metabolism and fatty acid synthesis, competes with iron in the transport of protein.

Possible Effects of Deficiency: diabetes, hypoglycemia, pancreas disorders, fatigue.

Research: Chromium and insulin administration to rats increased glucose uptake in the eye, and utilization of glucose for fatty acid production and energy (Garrison & Somer, Nutr Desk Ref. p. 61). Chromium supplementation as low as 0.2 ppm has lowered cholesterol levels in sugar-fed rats (Garrison & Somer, Nutr Desk Ref. p. 61).

COPPER

Sources: liver, whole grains, shellfish, green, leafy vegetables, nuts, legumes.

Functions: Necessary for proper functioning of nerve, bone, blood and connective tissue: catalyst in the synthesis of hemoglobin and RBC's, crucial role in respiration, facilitates iron absorption, involved in protein metabolism and healing processes, required for the synthesis of phospholipids (cell membranes and myelin sheaths around nerve fibers), necessary for proper bone formation and maintenance, aids in collagen formation, needed for the production of RNA, acts as a cofactor in numerous enzyme systems, most of which are oxidases, produces energy by oxidizing cytochrome c in the electron transport system.

Possible Effects of Deficiency: arthritis, heart disorders, anemia, constipation, diarrhea, ulcers, loss of hair, Menke's syndrome, low WBC count, bone demineralization, central nervous system impairment, reduced energy metabolism. Chronic diarrhea and/or iron-deficiency anemia increase risk for deficiency.

IODINE

Sources: kelp, dulse, spinach, carrots, tomatoes, garlic, onions, pineapple, mushrooms, seafood, sea salt.

Functions: aids in the development and functioning of the thyroid gland and is an integral part of thyroxine, promotes growth and development, regulates cellular oxidation, stimulates metabolism, influences cell differentiation and protein synthesis.

Possible Effects of Deficiency: thyroid disorders (i.e. goiter, hypothyroidism), irritability, nervousness, dry hair and skin, cold feet and hands, obesity. If deficiency occurs during gestation, Cretinism can result (physical and mental retardation). Natural goitrogens (such as those found in cabbage, rutabagas, cauliflower, turnips, peanuts, mustard seeds, soybeans and turnips), can induce goiter if consumed in quantities from areas where the soil and water are deficient in iodine (Garrison & Somer, Nutr Desk Ref. p. 61).

IRON

Sources: liver, oysters, heart, whole grains, legumes, leafy, green vegetables, egg yolks.

Functions: combines with protein and copper to make hemoglobin, thus building up the quality of the blood, necessary for the formation of myoglobin, improves respiratory action.

Possible Effects of Deficiency: anemia, fatigue, dizziness, low RBC count.

Research: Iron is a necessary nutrient, and insufficient iron will cause loss of energy and anemia. However, recent epidemiological studies correlate high iron levels with higher incidence of heart disease. The theory is that high levels of iron, which is a necessary catalyst in the Fenton reaction (free radical formation of the powerful hydroxyl radical), increase free radical damage; some researchers postulate that it is a woman's lower iron status (from monthly blood loss), and not estrogen, which is the main protective factor against heart disease in that gender.

Iron poisoning in children can occur when they get into iron supplements; all iron supplement products should be kept out of the reach of children.

MAGNESIUM

Sources: fresh green vegetables, wheat germ, seafood, figs, kelp, nuts and seeds, garlic, whole grains.

Functions: important in neuromuscular contractions/relaxations (counteracts calcium), regulates acid/alkline balance, associated with regulation of body temperature, activates enzymes necessary for metabolism of carbohydrates and amino acids, stimulates the body's own production of HCl, functions in lipid and protein metabolism (essential for rebuilding after injury), cofactor for many enzymes, including those in energy metabolism.

Possible Effects of Deficiency: heart disorders, nervousness, confusion, irritability, PMS, hypertension, leg cramps, insomnia. Since pyridoxine (B-6) requires magnesium for conversion to its active form, pyridoxal-5-phosphate, a magnesium deficiency can lead to decreased activity of vitamin B-6. Excess Mg (> 1000 mg/day) can cause diarrhea and upset the mineral balance (Mindell, E. Earl Mindell's Food as Medicine. Simon & Schuster,NY, NY. 1994. p. 79).

Research: Magnesium increases the solubility and retention of calcium. Magnesium gets depleted in conditions of inflammation, and is integral to the healing process. Magnesium **decreases swelling,** and, "is effective in the treatment of inflammatory skin diseases" (Hautarzt. 1990;41:602-5). When levels of magnesium were reduced, researchers noted a profound increase of inflammatory cytokines present, along with increased levels of histamine (Am J Physiol. 1992;263:R734-7).

Very important in preventing infection after trauma, "Recent findings regarding roles for magnesium in immunocompetence confirm and extend previous knowledge of its participation in natural and adaptive immunity" (Mag Res. 1992:5:281-93). Intravenous magnesium sulfate was given to treat acid burns, and resulted in a, "reduction in burn area over time, wound depth, healing time and final scar area compared to controls...This investigation found intravenous magnesium to be an effective method for treating hydrofluoric acid burns" (J Toxicol 1994;32(2):123-36). Magnesium's function in protein metabolism and rebuilding after injury makes it useful in providing ligamental nutrient support.

Several magnesium (Mg) derivatives are used in treating gastrointestinal disorders; Mg hydroxide, Mg phosphate and Mg peroxide have antacid properties; Mg peroxide is anti-infective; Mg salicylate is used specifically as an intestinal anti-infective; Mg silicates are gastric antacids and sedatives (Merck Index, 11th ed. Merck & Co. Inc., Rahway, N.J. 1989).

Magnesium may protect against blood clots (and thus heart attack/stroke) by preventing platelets from sticking together (Mindell, E. Earl Mindell's Food as Medicine. Simon & Schuster, NY, NY. 1994). It is necessary to maintain ionic balance of calcium and sodium in the cell, and prevent the buildup of other ions intracellularly, which can increase blood pressure. Besides having a favorable effect on blood pressure, magnesium fights chronic fatigue syndrome, slows bone loss, strengthens muscles, reduces kidney stone formation, and helps in diabetes (Wright, Jonathan V. M.D. Healing with Nutrition. 1990. Keats Publishing, Inc. New Canaan, Conn. p. 205).

"Trials with magnesium have improved the well-being of patients (with chronic fatigue syndrome)"" (Nippon-Rinsho 1992 Nov; 50(11):2679-83). Older people may be able to improve their ability to metabolize glucose by taking magnesium supplements (AJCN 1992; 55:1161-1167, as ref in Mindell, E. Earl Mindell's Food as Medicine. Simon & Schuster, NY, NY. 1994, p.78). Magnesium also prevents tooth decay, by binding calcium to the enamel (Garrison & Somer, Nutr Desk Ref. p. 68).

"Magnesium deficiency is strongly implicated as a causative factor in premenstrual syndrome...The deficiency is characterized by excessive nervous sensitivity, with generalized aches and pains and a lower premenstrual pain threshold. One clinical trial of magnesium in PMS showed a reduction of nervousness in 89 per cent, of breast tenderness in 96 per cent and of weight gain in 95 per cent" (Murray M. Enc Nat Med p. 475). In a study cited in Obstetrics and Gynecology, women were given 350 mg Mg 3x/day during last two weeks of cycle, and experienced less moodiness, bloating, aches and pains (cited in Mindell, E. Earl Mindell's Food as Medicine. Simon & Schuster, NY, NY. 1994, p.78). 200 mg Mg/day reduced headaches in women, especially before/during their period (Mindell, p. 78).

Some researchers believe that, "Magnesium supplements are more important than calcium in reversing bone loss" (Lau, William. J Clin End Met. Aug 1998). In a recent study, 24 young, healthy men getting the RDA in magnesium took a 350 mg supplement for 30 days. Bone turnover was unchanged in controls, however, it slowed "dramatically" in the treated group. Magnesium was said to be, "preserving bone and fostering a net buildup" (ibid).

MANGANESE

Sources: whole grains, nuts and seeds, egg yolks, green vegetables, legumes.

Functions: activates numerous enzymes, aids in the utilization of choline, catalyst in the synthesis of fatty acids and cholesterol, necessary for normal skeletal development, important for the production of milk and formation of urea, maintains sex hormone production, nourishes the brain and nerves, essential for the formation of thyroxine.

Possible Effects of Deficiency: nerve disorders, ringing in ears, vertigo, memory loss, glucose intolerance, epilepsy.

Research: Manganese is an important component of Manganese Superoxide Dismutase (MnSOD), which battles the damaging free radicals that cause swelling. Immediately after trauma, the body starts coding for more MnSOD to be produced (J Biol Chem. 1992;267:10625-30). Repletion of manganese after inflammatory trauma is necessary to keep up the free radical defense system. Recent research has shown MnSOD to be an efficient anti-inflammatory agent in models of acute and chronic inflammation; administration has decreased swelling up to 50-70% (Free Rad Res Comm. 1991: 15:297-301). In another study, "MnSOD at 5 micrograms produced a significant suppression (44% $p<0.05$) in knee joint swelling at 24 hours... "these findings support a therapeutic potential of MnSOD in inflammatory disorders..." (Free Rad Res Comm. 1993;18:291-8).

MOLYBDENUM

Sources: whole grains, meats, legumes, dark, green leafy vegetables.

Functions: essential part of two enzymes: xanthine oxidase, which aids iron mobilization from the liver, and aldehyde oxidase, necessary for oxidation of fats, also a factor in copper metabolism.

Possible Effects of Deficiency: anemia, male impotence, mouth and gum disorders.

Research: Molybdenum works with niacin to convert irritating aldehydes produced from Candida by-products into products that can either be eliminated, or used for energy in the Kreb's cycle. It also assists in detoxifying ammonia and metabolizing sulfites into harmless sulfates. Molybdenum helps chelate the excessive copper associated with PMS and Candida infection, and also plays a role in iron metabolism. It helps to lower the toxic load on the gut duc to its intestinal adsorbent qualities, which draws numerous toxins, endotoxins and bacteria out of the body (Schmitt WH, Jr. DC. Molybdemum for Candida patients and other problems. Collective Papers, Summer, 1985)..

PHOSPHORUS

Sources: fish, poultry, meat, whole grains, nuts, seeds, legumes, eggs, garlic.

Functions: functions along with calcium and is involved in almost every chemical reaction, important in cell repair and energy production, stimulates muscle contractions, necessary for proper skeletal growth, kidney functioning, tooth development and transmission of nerve impulses, component of the phosphate groups of phospholipids, buffer for acid-base balance.

Possible Effects of Deficiency: nervous disorders, fatigue, memory loss, stunted growth, bone disorders, overweight or weight loss, appetite loss. The calcium to phosphorus ratio is important; osteoporosis can be initiated by either low calcium/phosphorus intake, or a high proportion of phosphorus to calcium (Garrison & Somer, Nutr Desk Ref. p. 72).

Research: Phosphorus is a structural component of all cells, and is an integral part of the cell membrane. It is a part of the nucleic acids which comprise the genetic code in all cells, and , "therefore, phosphorus is fundamental to the growth, maintenance and repair of all body tissues, besides being necessary for protein synthesis" (Garrison & Somer, Nutr Desk Ref. p. 72).

POTASSIUM

Sources: green, leafy vegetables, bananas, whole grains, sunflower seeds, potatoes, beans, peas, and lentils.

Functions: regulates water balance (along with sodium), necessary for normal growth, stimulates nerve impulses for muscle contraction, maintains proper alkalinity of body fluids, functions in enzyme reactions, cell metabolism and stimulates the kidneys to eliminate poisonous wastes.

Possible Effects of Deficiency: edema (kidney), heart disorders, anxiety, menstrual disorders, insomnia, irregular heartbeat, muscle damage, digestive disorders, acne.

Research: Since potassium (K+), along with sodium (Na+), maintains ionic balance through the Na+/K+ ATPase pump, it is involved in the regulation of many cell functions; supplementation of extra potassium in the diet seems to have a favorable effect on blood pressure. Many researchers believe that it may not be the amount of sodium that influences blood pressure so much, but rather a relative lack of potassium in proportion to the sodium.

In a clinical trial, supplemental dietary potassium reduced the need for **antihypertensive** drug therapy in patients (Nutrition Reviews 1992; 50(5):144). Additionally, Dr. Louis Tobain, chief of the hypertension section of the University of Minnesota Hospitals, supplemented stroke-prone rats with potassium, and only 2% of those treated with potassium died, compared to 83% of the placebo group.

SELENIUM

Sources: fish and shellfish, whole grains, chicken, turkey, garlic, onions, dairy products.

Functions: antioxidant, essential part of glutathione peroxidase enzyme, necessary for prostaglandin production, preserves elasticity of tissues by delaying oxidation of polyunsaturated fatty acids.

Possible Effects of Deficiency: premature aging, cancer, heart disorders, immune deficiency, environmental allergies, possible infertility, may be related to crib death.

Research: Selenium, as part of the glutathione peroxidase enzyme, is involved with antioxidant reactions. Additionally, however, it has reported antioxidant activity of its own, the mechanism of which is not certain (Shils & Young, p. 263). Studies on the metabolism of phenobarbitol in rats suggest that selenium is needed for normal functioning of the hepatic microsomal P-450 system, and this function is also independent of glutathione peroxidase.

Epidemiological studies suggest that many diseases, such as heart disease and cancer, are higher in areas where selenium is depleted in the soil. For instance, cultivating garlic and onion in selenium **reduced total tumor yield** up to 75%, with garlic being more powerful in cancer inhibition. This study in Carcinogenesis suggests that the high-selenium garlic/onion is an ideal food form for cancer prevention (Carcinogenesis

1994;15(9):1881-5). Qidong County in China is a high-risk area for hepatoma, and this has been correlated to low levels of selenium in the soil and in the plasma of residents (Prev Med 1993;22(5):712-22). Administration of selenium is reported to inhibit the incidence of hepatoma (Prev Med 1993;22(5):712-22).

SILICON

Sources: plant fiber, oats, barley, spinach, figs, tomatoes, seeds, kelp.

Functions: connective tissue integrity, works with calcium to make strong bones.

Possible Effects of Deficiency: soft bones and teeth, weak nails, osteoporosis, hair loss and shine.

SODIUM

Sources: celery, carrots, salt, cheese, beets, cucumbers, seafood, poultry, meat, kelp (rarely deficient in diet because found in most foods).

Functions: functions with potassium to equalize acid/alkaline factor in the blood, regulate water balance within the body, involved in muscle contraction and expansion, nerve stimulation.

Possible Effects of Deficiency: acidosis, digestive disorders, intestinal gas, vomiting, weight loss, arthritis and rheumatism.

SULFUR

Sources: eggs, onion, garlic, meat, fish, cheese and milk.

Function: keeps hair glossy and smooth and complexion clear, necessary for collagen synthesis, prevalent in keratin (protein necessary for healthy skin, hair and nails), found in insulin, found in heparin (an anticoagulant), helps liver secrete bile, plays a part in tissue respiration.

Possible Effects of Deficiency: dry, brittle hair, brittle nails, dry skin

VANADIUM

Sources: shellfish, mushrooms, parsley, dill seed, black pepper.

Functions: The functions of vanadium are still being researched. It appears that vanadium is most important for: role in glucose metabolism, role in lipid metabolism, enzyme cofactor, regulation of adenylate cyclase/cAMP, regulation of phosphoryl transfer enzymes, regulation of the Na+/K+ ATPase and the sodium pump, regulation of other ATPases, including Ca++, gastric and colon ATPases, and muscle myosin ATPases.

Possible Effects of Deficiency: The effects of vanadium are mostly attributed to its pharmacological actions, and, "no sign of vanadium deficiency can be confidently listed here" (Shils and Young, p. 290).

Research: (see also vanadyl sulfate in the nutrient section) "Since foods contain very little vanadium, ... vanadium intake may not always be optimal" (Shils and Young, p. 290). Vanadium is active in, "pharmacological reactions", and, "Because of these actions, interest in the biochemical, nutritional, and pharmacological roles of vanadium has been stimulated" (Shils and Young, p. 288).

Excessive vanadium can cause depressed growth, diarrhea, depressed food intake and death in some animal species. Excessive vanadium has been suspected as a factor in manic-depressive illness. Large doses may interfere with the Na+ K+ ATPase pump. Medicinal amounts of any vitamin, mineral or specialty nutrient should only be taken with the advice of a trained licensed healthcare professional.

ZINC

Sources: whole grains, brewers yeast, egg yolk, liver, fish, poultry, wheat bran, wheat germ, mushrooms, sunflower seeds

Functions: constituent of 25 enzymes involved in digestion and metabolism, component of insulin, plays a part in carbohydrate digestion, protein metabolism and phosphorus metabolism, essential for growth and development of reproductive organs, necessary for proper functioning of the prostate gland, important in wound healing and burns, maintains acid-base balance, and is essential to proper immune function (involved in cell growth and tissue regeneration), antioxidant properties.

Possible Effects of Deficiency: repeated infection, retarded growth, fatigue, sore throats, frequent colds/flu, delayed sexual maturity, white spots in fingernails, brittle hair and nails, menstrual problems, impotence, painful knee and hip joints. The low zinc content of many foods is due to the fact that this mineral is totally lost in processing.

Research: Zinc has antioxidant activity, stabilizes cell membranes, and provides the cofactor for many enzymes involved in visual function. Besides having antioxidant activity, zinc is an essential element in superoxide dismutase (SOD), a potent radical scavenger. Research demonstrates that high levels of SOD , "protect mitochondria from oxidative damage that probably occurs with aging in the retinal pigment epithelium (Invest. Ophthalmol. Vis. Sci. 1992, 33:1909-18).

Zinc is necessary for the proper function of WBC's and the thymic hormones. Zinc helps prevent the age-related shrinking of the thymus (involution), and is especially effective in restoring depressed cell-mediated immunity in the elderly. Zinc lozenges are especially helpful because they bathe the throat tissues where viruses multiply. In one study (Clayton Biochemical Institute, U. of Texas-Austin), people not using zinc lozenges suffered symptoms more than twice as long as those who did.

Zinc is also the important nutrient in the "zinc fingers" which are an integral part of gene expression. Zinc's important role in gene regulation has just been discovered fairly recently. In fact, as a leading scientist acknowledges, "The approaches and tools of molecular biology have been enormously valuable to all branches of biological science over the last decade. Nutrition is no exception, where studies on the influence of nutrients on gene expression and of gene products on nutrient metabolism have resulted in a much more sophisticated and detailed understanding of nutritional biochemistry. An example of this as applied to trace minerals research can be seen in the area of thyroidology... Zinc appears to be necessary for the biological functioning of not only the thyroid hormone receptor, but also many other nuclear proteins which regulate gene expression (J Am Coll Nutr 1993;12(3):p. 294). The Proceedings of the National Academy of Sciences reported as recently as December of last year that an eye-specific kinase (containing these zinc fingers) is necessary to prevent rod degeneration (Proc. Nat. Acad. Sci. 1993, 90:11157-61).

Zinc increases mucin production and prevents the release of chemical agents that weaken the stomach lining, which predisposes it to ulceration (Werbach, p. 317). A zinc compound inhibited gastric mucosal injury in rats, and study results, "suggest that the protective effect of (the zinc compound) against the aggravation of gastric mucosal injury may be due to its inhibitory effect on lipid peroxidation" (Free Radicals in Research and Communication 1991;14(4):289-96). When several mucosal protecting anti-ulcer treatments were administered to 146 peptic ulcer patients who had recently healed, the one which contained zinc was shown to be superior in preventing relapses (Rev Esp Enferm Dig1991;80(2):91-4). Zinc deficiencies have been noted in women suffering from Candidiasis (Michaud E & Feinstein A. Prevention Magazine's 30 day immune power program. Rodale Press, Emmaus, Pa. 1989 p144).

HERBAL NUTRIENTS/VITAMINS/MINERALS AND DRUG/NUTRIENT INTERACTIONS

The recommendations of a trained licensed health professional are always advised when drug-nutrient combinations are considered. The information in this area is limited and several sources have been pooled to create this table. It is possible that interactions or depletions exist that have not been recorded. Special caution is always advised for children, pregnant or lactating women, elderly, and patients with liver/kidney disease (affects drug metabolism and clearance).

Many drug-nutrient interactions are actually potentiations, in other words, an herb or vitamin might potentiate the action of a drug, in which case the two may not be prescribed together. For instance, vitamin E is able to reduce blood clotting by reducing thromboxane A2, a potent blood clotter. Warfarin (eg. trade name Coumadin) is a drug which reduces clotting by interfering with vitamin K (an integral clotting factor). The potentiated action may thin the blood too much. There are case reports where increased bleeding resulted from combining the drug and the vitamin. Note, however, that less than 400 IU of vitamin E does not seem to cause a problem. It is when the vitamin E is taken in EXCESS that this potentiation has occurred (the current RDA is 10 IU for men and 8 IU for women).

Several herbs have anti-coagulant therapy, and should be recognized for this pharmacological actions. Herbs such as ginkgo biloba and fish oil have anticoagulant effects, and although it is possible to safely combine recommended amounts of these nutrients together, or in combination with vitamin E, these nutrients should be used with extreme caution in combination with anticoagulant drugs such as warfarin.

Several other herbs (listed below in the table) have exhibited mild anti-platelet action, and they are contraindicated (in large doses) with the anticoagulant drugs not because of reported side effects, but to err on the side of caution. Likewise, the German monograph warns against consuming St. John's wort and tyramine-containing foods at the same time (all MAO inhibitors carry this warning), even though the mechanisms by which St. John's wort works are not clearly defined, and no single case of an interaction with tyramine-containing foods has ever been reported, despite the fact that over 2.7 million prescriptions for St. John's wort have been filled in Germany.

Some drugs interact with nutrients and interfere with their metabolism or deplete their concentrations in the body. Some nutrients can interfere with drug metabolism or potentiate their action. Some examples are listed in the following table. When brand names are listed (Capitalized) it is suggested to cross-check generic drug names (lower case) to include other brands.

Many drugs deplete more than the major nutrients listed, so repletion with a multi-vitamin and mineral supplement may be in order when taking the drugs that are suspected of depleting nutrients. Minerals can contribute to our well-being, and can remove toxins and metals from our body, however they can also reduce the effectiveness of some drugs and should not be taken at the same time as certain drugs. Drug-Drug interactions are not listed here and can be found in other sources.

ALL DRUGS	Nutrient Interactions
(esp. Hismanal, Sular, Procardia XL, Calan SR, Coumadin, Rythmol, Propulsid, Mevacor, Zocor, and Pravachol)	GRAPEFRUIT JUICE; DETOX NUTRIENTS CHAMOMILE

Interactions

Grapefruit juice has an interaction with several drugs, especially ones that employ the enzyme CYP 3A4 to metabolize the drugs. Grapefruit juice slows the enzyme responsible for this process, and the drugs are not metabolized as readily, hence the juice can potentiate the action of the drug. This interaction has not been seen with other juices such as orange juice. Circulating oral estrogens can be increased by a third when taken with grapefruit juice. At least one case has proved fatal (Hismanal) with one hospitalization (Procardia XL combined with Calan SR). It is possible that there may be a cumulative effect.

An intense detoxification program may decrease the effectiveness of some drugs, because some of the nutrients, such as glutathione, are effective in removing toxins (and drug metabolites) by conjugating them and preparing them for elimination.

An ingredient in chamomile, bisabolol, may delay absorption of medications taken at the same time.

ACNE MEDICINE — Nutrient Interactions

ACNE MEDICINE	Nutrient Interactions
Accutane	VITAMIN A

Interactions

Accutane is a brand name for isoretinoin, which is related to vitamin A. Taking them together could increase toxicity and/or teratogenicity (causes birth defects). Vitamin A is fat-soluble and should not be taken (even alone) in large amounts in pregnant women.

ACNE MEDICINE — Nutrient Interactions

ACNE MEDICINE	Nutrient Interactions
OTC benzoyl peroxide i.e. Acetoxyl, Acne-Aid, Benoxyl-5, Clearasil, Dermoxyl, Noxzema clear-ups, Oxy-5, Oxy-10, Topex, Xerac, etc.	CINNAMON/FOODS CONTAINING BENZOIC ACID

Interactions

Cinnamon and foods containing benzoic acid can cause a skin rash to appear.

ALCOHOL — Nutrient Interactions

ALCOHOL	Nutrient Interactions
	BETA-CAROTENE IRON

Interactions

Some animal research indicates that beta-carotene may compound the liver damage caused by chronic intake of alcohol. Additionally, alcohol may cause excess absorption of iron.

ALCOHOL — Nutrient Depletions

ALCOHOL	Nutrient Depletions
	B VITAMINS, ESP. THIAMIN (B-1), B-6, B-12, & FOLIC ACID. ALSO VITAMIN C, D, E, K AND MINERALS MAGNESIUM & ZINC

Depletions

Alcohol robs the body of many essential nutrients. The absorption and/or utilization of these nutrients can be affected with acute or chronic alcohol ingestion. When thiamin in particular is depleted, it can be involved in the development of Wernicke-Korsakoff syndrome, characterized by the brain damage usually seen in chronic alcohol abuse.

ALCOHOL-ABUSE DRUGS — Nutrient Interactions

ALCOHOL-ABUSE DRUGS	Nutrient Interactions
Disulfiram, i.e. Antabuse, Cronetal, Ro-sulfiram	VITAMIN C

Interactions

High doses of vitamin C could reduce the effectiveness of disulfiram.

ALUMINUM-BASED ANTACIDS — Nutrient Interactions

ALUMINUM-BASED ANTACIDS	Nutrient Interactions
i.e. Di-gel, Gelusil, Maalox, Mylanta, Riopan, etc.	CASCARA SAGRADA

Interactions

Cascara sagrada is a purgative herb used for constipation; in significant amounts, it may irritate the stomach or small intestine when used in combination with antacids.

ALUMINUM-BASED ANTACIDS — Nutrient Depletions

ALUMINUM-BASED ANTACIDS	Nutrient Depletions
Di-gel, Gelusil, Maalox, Mylanta, Riopan, etc.	CALCIUM, PHOSPHATE, THIAMIN

Depletions

The aluminum can form a complex with phosphate and deplete calcium. Aluminum can also interfere with thiamin utilization. Additionally, hydrochloric acid (HCL) is necessary for calcium absorption, and by lowering HCL with antacids, the amount of calcium absorbed is also lowered. Chronic use of any antacids can lead to some of the same malabsorption syndromes seen with the H2 receptor antagonists (see ulcer drugs).

ALZHEIMER'S DRUGS — Nutrient Interactions

ALZHEIMER'S DRUGS	Nutrient Interactions
selegiline, i.e. Eldepryl, Jumex, Procythol	VITAMIN E

Interactions

Selegiline, which is normally used for Parkinson's disease to delay the need for dopamine-replacement therapy, was used in a clinical trial for Alzheimer's disease which also included vitamin E, and both demonstrated positive results (New England Journal of Medicine 1997;336:1216-1222). The two together did not have an additive effect.

ANTIBIOTICS

broad spectrum, i.e. Bactrim, Mandol, Moxam, Neomycin, Septra, etc.

Nutrient Depletions

VITAMIN K, B VITAMINS

Depletions

Antibiotics kill the good bacteria in the intestines along with the bad. The intestinal bacteria are responsible for manufacturing vitamin K, along with most of the B vitamin complex. Patients on chronic antibiotic therapy may suffer symptoms of insufficient clotting due to vitamin K deficiency. Replenishment of vitamin K and/or B vitamins may be necessary. Antibiotics which are not absorbed can contribute to lactose intolerance.

ANTIBIOTICS

quinolones, i.e. Cipro, Floxin, Maxaquin, Noroxin, Penetrex

Nutrient Interactions

CALCIUM, IRON, ZINC

Interactions

Certain minerals and antacids may reduce the effectiveness of these antibiotics when taken at the same time.

ANTIBIOTICS

tetracyclines, i.e. Achromycin, Aureomycin, Minocin, Panmycin, Terramycin

Nutrient Interactions

CALCIUM, IRON, MAGNESIUM, ZINC
RIBOFLAVIN (vitamin B-1), VITAMIN C

Interactions

Some minerals can form complexes with tetracycline and reduce absorption of the antibiotics into the body. Calcium carbonate in particular can form an insoluble complex more so than other more absorbable chelated forms, such as calcium aspartate or calcium citrate. Also, chronic use of tetracycline can deplete these nutrients.

ANTIHISTAMINES

Allerdryl, Benedryl, Codehist DH, Co-Tylenol Cold, Dehist, Dimetapp DM, Efricon, Histafed, Nauseatol, Nordryl, Nyquill, P-V Tussin, Robitussin A-C, Sinusol-B, Triaminic, Vicks Formula 44, etc.

Nutrient Depletions

VITAMIN C

Depletions

Antihistamines deplete vitamin C especially.

ARTHRITIS DRUGS

acetaminophen, i.e. TylenoL

Nutrient Interactions

FASTING

Interactions

Acetaminophen has a greatly compounded effect with both alcohol and fasting, because all these substances deplete glutathione in the liver. A compounded effect can drastically reduce glutathione levels and increase acetaminophen toxicity.

ARTHRITIS DRUGS

aspirin, i.e. Anacin, Ascriptin, Bayer, Bufferin, Excedrin

Nutrient Depletions

VITAMINS A & C, FOLIC ACID, B COMPLEX, CALCIUM, POTASSIUM, IRON

Depletions

Aspirin can deplete nutrients, especially those listed. Chronic aspirin use causes small amounts of blood to be lost from the stomach, which depletes iron over time.

ARTHRITIS DRUGS

indomethacin, i.e. Indameth, Indocin

Nutrient Depletions

IRON

Depletions

Indomethacin is an NSAID (non-steroidal antiinflammatory agent) with ibuprofen as a prototype. It can irritate the stomach even more than aspirin, and the chronic low level of blood loss could lead to iron-defiency anemia.

ARTHRITIS DRUGS

methotrexate, i.e. Folex, Methotrate, Mexate, Rheumatrex

Nutrient Interactions

FOLIC ACID

Interactions

Methotrexate interferes with folic acid metabolism. Since folic acid is crucial to dividing cells, this mechanism is used for preventing cancer cells from dividing. Although methotrexate is a powerful drug which does interfere with an essential nutrient, it is being used more commonly to treat arthritis and psoriasis in addition to cancer. A physician should be consulted concerning supplementation.

ARTHRITIS DRUGS

methotrexate i.e. Folex, Methotrate, Mexate, Rheumatrex

Nutrient Depletions

VITAMIN B-12; BETA CAROTENE

Depletions

Methotrexate affects the transcellular permeability of the intestinal wall and vitamin B-12 and beta-carotene may not be absorbed as well. Vitamin B-12 gets absorbed in the distal ileum.

ARTHRITIS DRUGS

penicillamine i.e. Cuprimine, Depen etc.

Nutrient Interactions

IRON, MAGNESIUM

Interactions

Iron and magnesium can reduce the absorption and hence the effectiveness of these drugs and should not be taken at the same time.

ARTHRITIS DRUGS

penicillamine i.e. Cuprimine, Depen etc.

Nutrient Depletions

COPPPER, ZINC, VITAMIN B-6

Depletions

These drugs can deplete copper, zinc, and vitamin B-6.

ASTHMA DRUGS

theophylline, i.e. Bronkaid, Bronkodyl, Primatene, Slo-bid, Theobid, Theodur, Uniphyl, etc.

Nutrient Interactions

CHARBROILED FOODS, HOT RED PEPPERS, FAT

Interactions

Charbroiled foods increase the elimination of theophylline, possibly because the formed compounds stress the liver. Excretion of the drug can be increased up to 42% by these compounds (Clin Pharmacol Ther 1978;23:445-449). Hot red peppers can increase blood levels of theophylline. Depending on the brand, fat can either boost effectiveness (Theo-24) or decrease effectiveness (Theolair).

BIRTH CONTROL PILLS

i.e. Demulen, Norlestrin, Ortho-Novum, Ovcon, Ovral, Tri-Norinyl etc.

Nutrient Interactions

VITAMIN C

VITAMIN B-6, FOLIC ACID, VITAMIN E. Birth control pills deplete these vitamins, especially B-6.

Interactions

There is a possible interaction with vitamin C in high doses (> 1 g) increasing blood levels of estrogens from birth control pills or estrogen replacement therapy.

BLOOD PRESSURE DRUGS

(all)

Nutrient Interactions

GINSENG, GUARANA, GLYCYRRHIZIN

Interactions

The ginsengs and Siberian ginseng (not considered a true ginseng because it belongs to the same family but not the same genus) are sometimes called adaptogens. However, in large amounts, they can be contraindicated in high blood pressure, as that is one of the side effects from excess use. The Siberian ginseng is tolerated better than the other "true" ginsengs as far as the upper limits causing side effects.

Guarana is a plant which contains more caffeine by dry weight than coffee, and is not recommended by most herbalists due to its stimulatory effect. It should not be combined with blood pressure medication.

Glycyrrhizin is an ingredient in licorice root which can increase glucocorticoid activity when used in significant amounts, and is contraindicated in high blood pressure (it can also potentiate potassium loss).

BLOOD PRESSURE DRUGS

ACE inhibitors, i.e. Accupril, Altace, Capoten, Lotensin, Monopril, Prinivil, Vasotec, Zestril

Nutrient Interactions

HAWTHORN BERRIES, POTASSIUM

Interactions

Hawthorn berries demonstrate some ability to inhibit ACE (angiotensin-converting enzyme). They have been used in conjunction with other ACE inhibiting drugs, however the determination of a combination should be determined by a physician.

These medications optimize potassium levels, which is OK unless extra potassium supplementation is also being given; levels should be monitored by a physician.

BLOOD PRESSURE DRUGS

hydralizine - containing, i.e. Apresazide, Aresoline, Ser-Ap-Es etc.

Nutrient Depletions

VITAMIN B-6

Depletions

These drugs interfere with a necessary enzyme in B-6 metabolism and deplete the body of it.

BLOOD PRESSURE DRUGS

loop diuretics, such as bumetanide, i.e. Bumex, or such as furosemide, i.e. Lasix

Nutrient Depletions

POTASSIUM, MAGNESIUM, ZINC, VITAMINS B-2 & C, IODINE

Depletions

These diuretics leach minerals with the water they draw out of the body. Potassium especially can be depleted. Since all of these minerals play an important role in regulating blood pressure, special attention should be given to repletion. Cascara sagrada is a purgative herb which may increase potassium loss if given in combination with a diuretic.

BLOOD PRESSURE DRUGS

thiazide diuretics i.e. Aldoril, Diuril; and hydrochlorothiazide i.e. HydroDiuril, Ser-Ap-Es, etc.

Nutrient Depletions

POTASSIUM, MAGNESIUM PHOSPHATES, ZINC, VITAMINS B-2 & C, IODINE

Depletions

Diuretics pull nutrients out with the water they draw from the body. Thiazide diuretics can decrease calcium excretion and cause pathological changes in the parathyroid gland with hypercalcemia and hypophosphatemia during long-term therapy. Cascara sagrada is a purgative herb which may increase potassium loss if given in combination with a diuretic.

BLOOD PRESSURE DRUGS	**Nutrient Interactions**
triamterene-containing drugs i.e. Diazide, Dyrenium, Maxzide etc.	POTASSIUM

Interactions

These drugs conserve potassium levels, which is OK unless extra potassium supplementation is also being given; levels should be monitored by a physician.

BLOOD PRESSURE DRUGS	**Nutrient Depletions**
triamterene-containing drugs i.e. Diazide, Dyrenium, Maxzide etc.	FOLIC ACID

Depletions

These drugs deplete folic acid and may cause deficency unless extra folic acid is supplemented.

BLOOD PRESSURE DRUGS	**Nutrient Depletions**
alpha-adrenergic blockers such as clonidine, i.e. Catapres, Dixarit	CALCIUM, VITAMIN B COMPLEX

Depletions

These drugs can deplete these nutrients.

BLOOD PRESSURE DRUGS	**Nutrient Interactions**
beta-blockers such as nadolol, i.e. Corgard, such as propranolol, i.e. Inderal, such as metoprolol, i.e. Lopressor, and such as atenolol, i.e. Tenormin	HYDRASTINE

Interactions

Hydrastine is a concentrated extract from the plant, goldenseal, which can constrict blood vessels. Since there is little research on drug interactions, caution is advised when combining with blood pressure drugs, especially the beta-blockers.

BLOOD THINNERS

warfarin, i.e. Coumadin, Panwarfin, Warfilone etc.

Nutrient Interactions

VITAMIN E, VITAMIN C, FISH OIL, GARLIC, GINKGO BILOBA, DONG QUAI, BILBERRY, ASTRAGALUS, CAPSAICIN, FENUGREEK, VITAMIN K, COENZYME Q 10, FEVERFEW, PAU D'ARCO, GINGER, BROMELAIN

Interactions

Interactions which potentiate the drugs: Vitamin E thins the blood and should not be given (in amounts > 400 IU) at the same time as blood thinning drugs, or it could increase bleeding time. Amounts of 400 IU or less have not been reported to cause a problem. One of the reasons the eskimos have lower risk for heart disease is thought to be the blood thinning action of fish oil (the thinning may increase risk for stroke, however). Large amounts of fish oil should not be combined with anticoagulant drugs. Although the interaction is uncertain and not proven, vitamin C in large amounts (over 5 grams/day) could possibly interfere with the action of blood thinning medications. Vitamin C, like vitamin E, exhibits some effect on lowering levels of thromboxane A2, (thromboxane increases clotting).

Interaction with herbs: Several herbs also possess anticoagulant properties. It is a good idea to avoid potentiations by not combining significant amounts of these herbs with blood thinning medications. For instance, a few milligrams of garlic in a synergistic formula should not interact with blood thinning drugs. However, a standard dose of 500 mg of garlic as a single herb would definitely be contraindicated with the drugs. An interaction with the herb feverfew is suspected but has not been studied.

Some herbs possess anticoagulant properties to a lesser extent, and even though case reports have not been documented about specific interactions, it would be wise to exhibit caution with these nutrients in relation to these drugs. These include dong quai, pau d'arco, ginger, bilberry, astragalus, capsaicin, and fenugreek. Bromelain, an enzyme derived from pineapple, would be included also.

Interactions which reduce effectiveness of the drugs: Blood thinners such as Coumadin inhibit vitamin K metabolism as a mechanism of action (vitamin K is a clotting factor), so supplementation could interfere with the effectiveness of these drugs. It is recommended that people on these drugs not ingest excess amounts of vitamin K-rich foods (see vitamin K in the vitamins, minerals and nutrients section). Although vitamin K-rich foods do not have to be totally avoided, caution is advised not to go overboard. There are case reports of foods such as avocado interfering with the effectiveness of warfarin (Lancet 1991;337:914). Coenzyme Q·10 has been observed in Sweden to reduce effectiveness of Coumadin and change bleeding time in patients on Coumadin (the blood became more prone to clotting).

CANCER DRUGS

methotrexate i.e. Folex, Methotrate, Mexate, Rheumatrex

Nutrient Interactions

FOLIC ACID

Interactions

Methotrexate interferes with folic acid metabolism. Since folic acid is crucial to dividing cells, this mechanism is used for preventing cancer cells from dividing. Although methotrexate is a powerful drug which does interfere with an essential nutrient, it is being used more commonly to treat arthritis and psoriasis in addition to cancer. Supplementation of folic acid may reduce effectiveness of methotrexate since it depends on inhibition of folic acid as a mechanism to thwart cancer cells. A physician should be consulted.

CANCER DRUGS

methotrexate i.e. Folex, Methotrate, Mexate, Rheumatrex

Nutrient Depletions

VITAMIN B-12; BETA CAROTENE

Depletions

Methotrexate affects the transcellular permeability of the intestinal wall and vitamin B-12 and beta-carotene may not be absorbed as well. Vitamin B-12 gets absorbed in the distal ileum.

CHOLESTEROL DRUGS

bile acid sequesterants, such as cholestyramine (i.e. Cholybar & Questran), or such colestipol hydrochloride (prototype, cholestyramine), i.e. Cholestabyl, Colestid, Lestid

Nutrient Depletions

FAT-SOLUBLE VITAMINS, i.e. VITAMINS A, D, E, K, WATER-SOLUBLE VITAMINS, i.e. VITAMIN B-12, FOLIC ACID

Depletions

These drugs may deplete these nutrients.

CHOLESTEROL DRUGS

lovastatin, i.e. Mevacor, Mevinolin

Nutrient Interactions

NICOTINIC ACID, GARLIC

Interactions

Lovastatin works to lower cholesterol by inhibiting the major rate-limiting enzyme for cholesterol synthesis, HMG Coenzyme A reductase. Nicotinic acid is sometimes used to support normal cholesterol levels. Liver enzymes should periodically be monitored since the possibility of a potentiation exists. Garlic contains some nicotinic acid, however the small quantities may or may not cause a potentiation.

CHOLESTEROL DRUGS

lovastatin, i.e. Mevacor, Mevinolin

Nutrient Depletions

COENZYME Q10

Depletions

Lovastatin may lower levels of coenzyme Q 10.

CORTICOSTEROIDS

i.e. Aristocort, Cortef, Decadron, Delta-Cortef, Deltasone, Kenacort, Medrol, etc.

Nutrient Depletions

VITAMIN D (CALCIUM), POTASSIUM, VITAMINS A, C, B-6, B12, FOLIC ACID ZINC

Depletions

Corticosteroids can deplete these vitamins and minerals. Since vitamin D can be depleted, and vitamin D is needed for proper calcium metabolism, chronic use of these drugs could result in bone loss.

DEPRESSION DRUGS

(all)

Nutrient Interactions

HIGH-FIBER FOODS

Interactions

High-fiber foods can decrease the effectiveness of certain medications, such as digitalis glycosides and antidepressants (especially the tricyclics). Lithium, used for manic depression, reduces sodium uptake, and excess sodium reduces the effectiveness of lithium.

DEPRESSION DRUGS

MAO inhibitors i.e., Marplan, Nardil, Parnate

Nutrient Interactions

ST. JOHN'S WORT, YOHIMBINE, FENUGREEK, PARSLEY, PLEURISY ROOT, TYRAMINE-CONTAINING FOODS, PROTEIN SUPPLEMENTS

Interactions

MAO inhibitors should not be used at the same time as St. John's Wort. The mechanism of action of St. John's wort still needs to be determined; it is thought that it works more as an SSRI (selective serotonin reuptake inhibitor) than a MAO inhibitor (raises all the amine neurotransmitters). Erring on the side of caution dictates that the herb should not be used with MAO inhibitors or SSRI's in case of possible potentiation. (Prozac is an SSRI) Yohimbine, the extract from the plant, yohimbe, has MAO inhibiting activity. The activity of the whole plant as an herb is not as strong as the concentrated extract, however caution is advised with the plant for possible potentiation.

Fenugreek, parsley, and pleurisy root are herbs which are contraindicated with MAO inhibitors. Tyramine-containing foods are contraindicated because MAO inhibitors block an enzyme which breaks this substance down, potentially leading to toxic accumulation in the body. Six people on Parnate (MAO inhibitor) reached a hypertensive crisis level because they had consumed liver pate with a high content of tyramine (Am J Psychiatry. 1966;122:933-937). Anyone on MAO inhibitors should receive a list of these foods from their doctor. The action of bacteria on protein also produces tyramine, so the freshness of meats is important. Tyramine-containing foods range from avocadoes to yeast supplements, and include four types of foods: broad bean pods (fava, lima, etc.); yeast concentrates (i.e. brewer's yeast); salted, smoked, or pickled fish (especially herring); and aged cheeses. Wine has tyramine (Chianti is especially high), and one death has been reported from the interaction of a MAO inhibitor and vermouth. Fermented soybean products, such as miso and soy sauce may also cause problems, as can large amounts of chocolate. Protein supplements should not be used to excess.

DEPRESSION DRUGS

SSRI's such as fluoxetine hydrochloride, i.e. Prozac

Nutrient Interactions

ST. JOHN'S WORT

Interactions

The mechanism of action of St. John's wort still needs to be determined; it is thought that it works more as an SSRI (selective serotonin reuptake inhibitor) than a MAO inhibitor (raises all the amine neurotransmitters). Caution dictates that the herb should not be used with MAO inhibitors or SSRI's in case of possible potentiation.

DIABETIC DRUGS

Diabeta, Diabenese, Dymelor, Glucotrol, Glynase, Micronase, Orinase, Tolamide, and Tolinase

Nutrient Interactions

GLUCOMANNAN, GUAR GUM

Interactions

These dietary fibers can lower blood sugar levels and possibly change insulin requirements. Blood sugar should be closely monitored.

EPHEDRINE & PSEUDOEPHEDRINE

EPHEDRINE (i.e. Broncholate, Bronkotuss, Ephed II, Histatuss, KIE, Rynatuss, etc.), PSEUDOEPHEDRINE (i.e. Actifed, Bayhistine, DH, Contac severe cold, Dimacol, Halofed, Neofed, Pseudo, Sudafed)

Nutrient Interactions

WHITE WILLOW BARK, POPLAR, MEADOWSWEET, WINTERGREEN, GREEN TEA, BLACK TEA, UVA URSI, BLACK WALNUT, RED RASPBERRY, OAK, WITCH HAZEL

Interactions

These two drugs act like epinephrine, or adrenalin. Ephedrine dilates bronchial passages, while pseudoephedrine decreases the symptoms of allergic rhinitis. The effectiveness of these drugs is diminished if other salicylate compounds are given at the same time. Salicylate-containing herbs include white willow bark, poplar, meadowsweet and wintergreen. High-tannin herbs, such as green tea, black tea, uva ursi, black walnut, red raspberry, oak, and witch hazel can interfere with absorption of these drugs if taken at the same time.

EPILEPSY DRUGS

phenobarbital, phenytoin i.e. Dilantin, and barbiturates such as primidone, i.e. Mysoline; glutethimide

Nutrient Interactions

FOLIC ACID, VITAMIN B-6, PUDDING

Interactions

Both folic acid and vitamin B-6 can potentially reduce the effectiveness of these anticonvulsants; supplementation of these nutrients should be carefully monitored to prevent seizures. Excessive amounts of folic acid (> 2 mg) can reduce the effectiveness of Dilantin (keep in mind that folic acid is usually administered in mcg amounts). High amounts of vitamin B-6 (80 mg or greater) can reduce the effectiveness of the drug by 50%. Tests for anemia are recommended. If the reduction of B-6 is severe enough, it could affect homocysteine levels.

Pudding has been known to decrease the effectiveness of Dilantin by 50%, although exact ingredients causing the interaction have not been identified. Suspected ingredients were caseinates, corn oil starch, coconut oil, and carrageenan.

EPILEPSY DRUGS

phenobarbital, phenytoin i.e. Dilantin, and barbiturates such as primidone, i.e. Mysoline; glutethimide

Nutrient Depletions

VITAMIN D, VITAMIN K, VITAMIN C, FOLIC ACID, VITAMIN B-6

Depletions

Most epilepsy drugs interfere with folic acid, vitamin B-6, and vitamin D (and thus calcium) absorption. Supplementation may be indicated, however amounts should not exceed those listed above which may interfere with drug effectiveness. It may help to take the supplements away from the drug. Also, blood levels of vitamin K may be reduced and supplementation may be necessary. If the drugs are taken in conjunction with antibiotics that kill the bacteria that produce vitamin K, the deficiency could be compounded. Dilantin and Mysoline in particular lower vitamin K. Barbiturates deplete vitamin C. Additionally, carbamazepine (i.e. Epitol, Tegretol) dilutes blood sodium.

ETIDRONATE

Didronel, EHDP

Nutrient Interactions

MINERALS, esp. CALCIUM and MAGNESIUM, IRON

Interactions

Minerals can interfere with the absorption of etidronate. Since antacids also decrease the effect of the drug, calcium and magnesium can interfere if taken in amounts high enough to act as an antacid. Minerals should not be taken within two hours of the drug.

ETIDRONATE

Didronel, EHDP

Nutrient Depletions

VITAMIN D

Depletions

Etidronate is used as an antihypercalcemic to treat postmenopausal osteoporosis, however, it alters vitamin D metabolism, which is needed for metabolism of calcium. It is important that vitamin D and calcium intake be maintained.

GOUT DRUGS

colchicine, i.e., Novocolchine, ColBenemid

Nutrient Depletions

VITAMIN B-12, BETA- CAROTENE, MAGNESIUM, POTASSIUM

Depletions

These drugs may impair the metabolism of all these nutrients.

GOUT DRUGS

allopurinol, i.e., Alloprin, Aluline, Novopurol, Purinol, Zurinol, Zyloric, etc.

Nutrient Interactions

IRON

Interactions

The Complete Guide to Prescription and Non-prescription Drugs states that iron can accumulate in the tissues when iron supplements are given in conjunction with the drug.

HEART DRUGS

(see also blood pressure drugs) digitalis glycosides, i.e. Digoxin, Digitalis, Digitoxin, Lanoxicaps, Lanoxin, Novodigoxin

Nutrient Interactions

HIGH-FIBER FOODS; HAWTHORN BERRIES, MAGNESIUM, CEREUS GRANDIFLORIS, PLEURISY ROOT, GINSENG, CALCIUM, PRUNE JUICE, CASCARA SAGRADA, GLYCYRRHIZIN

Interactions

High-fiber foods can increase clearance of some drugs, including heart drugs, and decrease effectiveness of the drug. Caution should be exercised about taking them at the same time. Some of the flavonoids, including hawthorn berries (in significant amounts), can increase the force of contraction of the heart by inhibiting the enzyme cyclic AMP phosphodiesterase (Planta Medica 1981;43:183-186). Hawthorn is commonly used in conjunction with other drugs for heart failure, such as digitalis, or in combination with other herbs containing cardiac glycosides (i.e. Cereus grandifloris), as it potentiates the action of the glycosides. The digitalis glycosides work by different mechanisms than hawthorn berries. Since hawthorn does enhance the action of the cardiac glycosides, it allows for lower doses of adjunctive therapy to be used. Combinations of digitalis-like drugs and hawthorn berries should be prescribed with caution by a medical doctor. Double-blind studies have consistently shown that hawthorn is effective for congestive heart failure in the early stages (and also minor arrhythmias) where digitalis is not yet indicated.

Magnesium has an enhancing action on digitalis.

Pleurisy root and ginseng are contraindicated (ginseng contraindication is described under, "Blood Pressure drugs (all)").

Calcium supplements, prune juice, and high-fiber foods can all decrease the effectiveness of digitalis glycosides. Cascara sagrada is a purgative herb used for constipation; in significant amounts, it can lower potassium levels and may increase toxicity of digitalis due to the decreased potassium level. Glycyrrhizin is a component of licorice root, and in significant amounts, it will increase glucocorticoid activity. It is contraindicated with digitalis glycosides, and could cause possible irregular heart rhythms and cardiac arrest.

HEART DRUGS

(see also blood pressure drugs) digitalis glycosides, i.e. Digoxin, Digitalis, Digitoxin, Lanoxicaps, Lanoxin, Novodigoxin

Nutrient Depletions

VITAMIN B-1, B-6, ZINC

HORMONE REPLACEMENT THERAPY

Nutrient Interactions

Estrace, Estratab, Menest, Premarin, Conjugated Estrogens, C.E.S., etc.

VITAMIN C

Interactions

High amounts of vitamin C (>1 g) can possibly increase the effect of these exogenous estrogens.

HORMONE REPLACEMENT THERAPY

Nutrient Depletions

Estrace, Estratab, Menest, Premarin, Conjugated Estrogens, C.E.S., etc.

VITAMIN B-6, VITAMIN E, FOLIC ACID

LAXATIVES

Nutrient Depletions

mineral oil, i.e. Agoral, Mikinol, Neo-Cultol, etc.; phenolphthalein, i.e. Ex Lax, Feen-a-mint, Modane tablets

FAT-SOLUBLE VITAMINS, VITAMINS A,E, D, & K

Depletions

The mineral oil laxatives in particular will deplete the fat-soluble vitamins. Most all laxatives interfere with vitamin D metabolism and can result in altered calcium homeostasis and bone loss when used chronically.

PARKINSON'S DRUGS

Nutrient Interactions

levodopa i.e. Dopar, Larodopa

VITAMINS B-6, B-12, AND C

Interactions

Supplementation of vitamin B-6 should be avoided if levodopa is being taken; vitamin B-6 can reduce effectiveness of the drug.

POTASSIUM PRESCRIPTIONS

Nutrient Depletions

Kaon-Cl, Klotrix, K-tab, Micro-K, Slow K, etc.

VITAMIN B-12

Depletions

These supplements can block absorption of vitamin B-12. Chronic use of them, which is common in conjunction with diuretics, can lead to a frank deficiency. Neurological effects have been known to show up in the elderly before blood tests determine a deficiency.

SLEEPING PILLS

i.e. Doriden

Nutrient Depletions

VITAMIN D (CALCIUM)

Depletions

Doriden in particular interferes with vitamin D metabolism, which can decrease calcium metabolism because of the necessity of vitamin D for calcium metabolism.

THYROID HORMONE

levothyroxine, i.e. Synthroid, Levothroid, Levoxine, Levo-T

Nutrient Interactions

IRON

Interactions

Iron can reduce effectiveness of the thyroid hormone drugs.

TRANQUILIZERS

chlorpromazine, i.e. Thorazine; fluphenazine, i.e. Permitil, Prolixin

Nutrient Interactions

VITAMIN C, VALERIAN

Interactions

One case report showed that a high dose of vitamin C reduced blood levels of Prolixin. Interactions of valerian with tranquilizers have not been demonstrated, however valerian is an effective calming agent and potentiations should be kept in mind.

TRANQUILIZERS

chlorpromazine, i.e. Thorazine; fluphenazine, i.e. Permitil, Prolixin

Nutrient Depletions

RIBOFLAVIN (vitamin B-1), VITAMIN B-12

Depletions

Tranquilizers will deplete some of the B vitamins, most notably riboflavin and vitamin B-12.

TUBERCULOSIS DRUGS

isoniazid, i.e. INH, Isotamine, Izonid, Laniazid, Nydrazid, PMS Isoniazid, Rifamate, Rimifon, Teebaconin, Trecator-SC

Nutrient Interactions

VITAMIN B-6, ST. JOHN'S WORT, TYRAMINE-CONTAINING FOODS

Interactions

Excess vitamin B-6 can reduce effectiveness of these drugs, however, the drugs deplete vitamin B-6, and supplemented vitamin B-6 has been shown to decrease the chance of nerve damage in the extremities.

Recommended dosages of supplementation range from approximately 6-50 mg vitamin B-6. Supplements should be taken away from the drug. Since isoniazid is a MAO inhibitor, it should not be used at the same time as St. John's Wort. The mechanism of action of St. John's wort still needs to be determined; it is thought that it works more as an SSRI (selective serotonin reuptake inhibitor) than a MAO inhibitor (raises all the amine neurotransmitters). Caution still dictates that the herb, St. John's wort, should not be used with MAO inhibitors in case of possible potentiation.

Tyramine-containing foods are contraindicated in MAO inhibitors. See, "Depression drugs, MAO inhibitors" for more information.

TUBERCULOSIS DRUGS

isoniazid, i.e. INH, Isotamine, Izonid, Laniazid, Nydrazid, PMS Isoniazid, Rifamate, Rimifon, Teebaconin, Trecator-SC

Nutrient Depletions

VITAMIN B-6, VITAMIN D (CALCIUM & PHOSPHATE)

Depletions

The above tuberculosis drugs deplete niacin and vitamin B-6, and change vitamin D metabolism. The change in vitamin D metabolism can affect calcium and phosphate metabolism.

TUBERCULOSIS DRUGS

para-aminosalicylic acid, i.e. Nemasol-Sodium, P.A.S., Tubasal

Nutrient Depletions

VITAMIN B-12 & FOLIC ACID

Depletions

Para-aminosalicylic acid depletes these vitamins.

ULCER DRUGS

H2 receptor antagonists, such as ranitidine, i.e. Zantac, cimetidine, i.e.Tagamet, nizatidine, i.e. Axid, or famotidine, i.e. Pepcid AC; proton pump inhibitors such as omeprazole, i.e. Losec, Prilosec

Nutrient Interactions

CAFFEINE, SPICY FOODS, CASCARA SAGRADA

Interactions

Caffeine drinks and spicy foods can decrease the effectiveness of omeprazole. This effect has not been demonstrated in the H2 antagonists. Cascara sagrada is a purgative herb used for constipation; in significant amounts, it may irritate the stomach or small intestine when used in combination with acid suppressants.

ULCER DRUGS

H2 receptor antagonists, such as ranitidine, i.e. Zantac, cimetidine, i.e.Tagamet, nizatidine, i.e. Axid, or famotidine, i.e. Pepcid AC; proton pump inhibitors such as omeprazole, i.e. Losec, Prilosec

Nutrient Depletions

MOST NUTRIENTS

Depletions

Since hydrochloric acid (HCL) is needed for proper digestion (it starts the signals which are responsible for pancreatic/bile secretions etc.), drugs which reduce HCL could be responsible for malabsorption of some nutrients. In particular, vitamin B-12 is at high risk for deficiency. Cimetidine in particular has been reported to decrease iron. Since HCL is also responsible for maintaining a pH that discourages bacterial growth, acid suppressants could increase bacterial colonization. Some bacteria produce carcinogenic nitrosamines and are believed to increase the risk for cancer.

ULCERATIVE COLITIS

sulfasalazine, i.e. Azaline, Azulfidine, PMS Sulfasalazine, Salazopyrin, Salazosulfapyridine, Salicylazosulfapyridine, S.A.S.

Nutrient Interactions

CALCIUM, IRON, VITAMIN C

Interactions

Calcium and iron can decrease the effect of these sulfa drugs. High doses of vitamin C could cause possible kidney damage.

ULCERATIVE COLITIS

sulfasalazine, i.e. Azaline, Azulfidine, PMS Sulfasalazine, Salazopyrin, Salazosulfapyridine, Salicylazosulfapyridine, S.A.S.

Nutrient Depletions

FOLIC ACID, PABA, FRIENDLY BACTERIA

Depletions

These drugs for ulcerative colitis, which is a category of inflammatory bowel disease, will deplete folic acid. Pay special attention if combining with other drugs which interfere with folic acid metabolism, such as methotrexate. The biggest difference is that the sulfa drugs deplete folic acid, but do not rely on that as a mechanism for drug effectiveness. The mechanism of Azulfidine, for example, is unknown, but believed to be associated with its delivery of sulfapyridine and 5 aminosalicylic acid to intestinal cells. Methotrexate, on the other hand, uses reduction of folic acid to inhibit the replication of cancer cells.

URINARY TRACT INFECTION DRUGS

nitrofurantoin, i.e. Apo-nitrofurantoin, Furadantin, Furalan, Furaloid, Furan, Macrodantin, Nifuran, Ro-Antoin, Saradant, Trantoin, and Urotoin

Nutrient Depletions

FOLIC ACID

Depletions

Nitrofurantoin is an antimicrobial drug which blocks folic acid metabolism. There is usually not a problem if the drug therapy is short term. Long term application might warrant a folic acid supplement. Pay special attention if combining with other drugs which interfere with folic acid metabolism, such as sulfasalazine or methotrexate.

REFERENCES

Balch, J.F., M.D. and Balch, P.A., C.N.C. Prescription for Nutritional Healing. 1990. Avery Publishing, Garden City Park, NY.

Garrison, R.H. and Somer E. Nutrition Desk Reference. Keats Publishing, New Canaan, Conn. 1985.

Graedon, J and Graedon, T. Deadly Drug Interactions. The People's Pharmacy Guide. St. Martin's Griffin, NY. 1995.

Griffith, H.W. M.D. Complete Guide to Prescription and Non-prescription drugs. Putnam Publ. Group, NY, NY. 1992.

Hansten, PD. and Horn, JR. Drug interactions and updates. Vancouver, Wa. Applied Therapeutics, 1990.

Physician's Desk Reference. Medical Economics Co. Oradell, NJ. 1998.

PDR Family Guide to Prescription Drugs. Medical Economics Co. Montvale, NJ. 1993.

Roe, D. "Diet, Nutrition and Drug Reactions", in: Shils, M. and Young, V., (eds.) Modern Nutrition in Health and Disease., 7th ed. 1988. Lea & Febiger, Philadelphia, Pa.

Tatro, D. (ed). Drug Interaction Facts. St. Louis: Facts and Comparisons, 1992.

BIBLIOGRAPHY

Balch, P.A., C.N.C. and Balch, J.F., M.D. Prescription for Cooking. 1987. PAB Books, Tx.

Balch, J.F., M.D. and Balch, P.A., C.N.C. Prescription for Nutritional Healing. 1990. Avery Publishing, Garden City Park, NY.

Barnes, B.O., M.D. and Galton, L. Hypo-thyroidism: The Unsuspected Illness. 1976. Harper and Row Publishers, NY, NY.

Braly, J., M.D. Dr. Braly's Food Allergy and Nutrition Revolution. 1992. Keats Publishing, Inc. New Canaan, Ct.

Burton Goldberg Group. Alternative Medicine: The Definitive Guide. 1993. Future Medicine Publishing, Inc., Puyallup, Wa.

Chalmers, I. The Great Food Almanac. 1994. Collins Publishing, San Francisco, Ca.

Crook, W., M.D. The Yeast Connection. 1983. Professional Books, Jackson, Tenn.

Duke, J.A. Handbook of Medicinal Herbs. 1985. CRC Press, Boca Raton, Fl.

Dunne, L.J. Nutrition Almanac., 3rd ed. 1990. McGraw-Hill Publishing Company, NY, NY.

Giller, R.M., M.D. and Matthews, K. Natural Prescriptions. 1994. Ballantine Books, NY, NY.

Garrison, R.H. and Somer E. Nutrition Desk Reference. 1985. Keats Publishing, New Canaan, Conn.

Gittleman, A.L. Guess What Came to Dinner. 1993. Avery Publishing Group, Inc., Garden City Park, NY.

Griffith, H.W. Complete Guide to Prescription and Non-Prescription Drugs., 9th ed. 1992. Putnam Publishing Group, NY, NY.

Guyton, A.C., M.D. Textbook of Medical Physiology., 8th ed. W.B. Saunders Company, Philadelphia, Pa.

Haas, E.M., M.D. Staying Healthy with Nutrition. 1992. Celestial Arts, Berkeley, Ca.

Halliwell and Gutteridge. Free Radicals in Biology and Medicine. 1990. Oxford University Press, NY, NY.

Heinerman, John. Heinerman's Encyclopedia of Fruits, Vegetables and Herbs. 1988. Parker Publishing, West Nyack, NY.

Hendler, S.S., M.D. The Doctor's Vitamin and Mineral Encyclopedia. 1990. Simon & Schuster, NY, NY.

Hoffman, D. The New Holistic Herbal. 1992. Element, Rockport, Ma.

Krohn, J., M.D. The Whole Way to Allergy Relief and Prevention. 1991. Hartley and Marks Publishers, Point Roberts, Wa.

Larson, D.E., M.D., ed. Mayo Clinic Family Health Book. 1990. William Morrow and Company, Inc., NY, NY.

Lieberman, S. and Bruning, N. The Real Vitamin and Mineral Book. 1990. Avery Publishing Group, Inc., Garden City Park, NY.

Linder, M.C., ed. Nutritional Biochemistry and Metabolism with Clinical Applications. 1991. Appleton & Lange, Norwalk, Ct.

Mayell, M. The Natural Health First Aid Guide. 1994. Pocket Books, NY, NY.

Merck Index, 11th ed. 1989. Merck & Co. Inc., Rahway, N.J.

Michaud E & Feinstein A. Prevention Magazine's 30 day immune power program. Rodale Press, Emmaus, Pa. 1989.

Mindell, E. Earl Mindell's Food as Medicine. 1994. Simon & Schuster, NY, NY.

Mowry, David B., PhD. The Scientific Validation of Herbal Medicine. 1986. Keats Publishing, New Canaan, Conn.

Murray, M.T., N.D. Natural Alternatives to Over-the-Counter and Prescription Drugs. 1994. William Morrow and Company, Inc. NY, NY.

Murray, M.T., N.D. and Pizzorno, J.E., N.D. Encyclopedia of Natural Medicine. 1991. Prima Publishing, Rocklin, Ca.

Odds, F.C. Candida and Candidosis. 1988. Bailliere Tindall, Philadelphia, Pa.

Ody, P. The Complete Medicinal Herbal. 1993. Dorling Kindersley Ltd, London.

Prevention Magazine editors. The Complete Book of Natural & Medicinal Cures. 1994. Rodale Press, Inc., Emmaus, Pa.

Scalzo, R. Naturopathic Handbook of Herbal Formulas. 1994. Kivaki Press, Durango, Co.

Schmitt, W.H., D.C. Common Glandular Dysfunctions in the General Practice. 1981. Applied Kinesiology Study Program, Chapel Hill, NC.

Sharon, Dr. M. Complete Nutrition. 1994. Prion Publishing, London, England.

Shils, M. and Young, V., eds. Modern Nutrition in Health and Disease., 7th ed. 1988. Lea & Febiger, Philadelphia, Pa.

Tierra, L. The Herbs of Life. 1992. The Crossing Press, Freedom, Ca.

Tortora, G.J. and Anagnostakos, N.P. Principles of Anatomy and Physiology., 4th ed. 1984. Harper & Row Publishers, NY, NY.

Weiner, M.A., PhD. and Weiner, J.A. Herbs that Heal. 1994. Quantum Books, Mill Valley, Ca.

Werbach, M.R., M.D. Nutritional Influences on Illness. 1988. Keats Publishing, Inc., New Canaan, Ct.

Werbach, M., M.D. Healing Through Nutrition. 1993. Harper Collins Publishers, NY, NY.

Werbach, M., M.D. & Murray, M.T., N.D. Botanical Influences on Illness. 1994. Third Line Press, Tarzana, Ca.

Whitney, E.R. and Nunnelley, E.M. Understanding Nutrition., 4th ed. West Publishing, NY, NY.

Wild, R., ed. The Complete Book of Natural and Medicinal Cures. 1994. Rodale Press, Emmanus, Pa.

Wright, Jonathan V. M.D. Healing with Nutrition. 1990. Keats Publishing, Inc. New Canaan, Conn.

Zand, J., OMD, Walton, R., RN and Rountree, B., M.D. Smart Medicine for a Healthier Child. 1994. Avery Publishing Group, Garden City Park, NY.

INDEX

A

B

C

D

E

F

G

H

I

J

K

L

M

N

O

P

Q

R

S

T

U

V

W

Y

Z